MEDICAL WORD FINDER

Fourth Edition

test of deep
tendon reflexes

Gendrassick
maneuver

WEBSTER'S NEW WORLD

MEDICAL WORD FINDER

Fourth Edition

Compiled by
George Willeford, Jr., M.D.

Prentice Hall Press
New York

Published by New World Dictionaries/Prentice Hall Press
A Division of Simon & Schuster, Inc.
Gulf + Western Building
One Gulf + Western Plaza
New York, NY 10023

Manufactured in the United States of America

1 2 3 4 5 6 7 8 9 10

Library of Congress Cataloging-in-Publication Data

Willeford, George.
Webster's new world medical word finder.

Rev. ed. of: Medical word finder, 3rd ed. c1983.
1. Medicine—Terminology. 2. Spellers.
I. Willeford, George. Medical word finder.
II. Title. [DNLM: 1. Dictionaries, Medical.
2. Medicine—terminology. W 15 W698m]
R123.W47 1987 610'.14 87-2362
ISBN 0-13-947326-2

PREFACE

This Medical Word Finder was compiled to provide medical, dental and allied health professionals with a fast and easy way to correctly spell, syllabicate, divide and accentuate frequently used medical terms.

The list of PREFIXES and SUFFIXES will help to better understand the genesis of a medical vocabulary, thus increasing the ease of usage.

Two parts of this book are of special note:

SECTION II was prepared to save the time of medical secretaries and transcribers. The phonetic/correct spelling of often used medical words will be welcomed by those not schooled in medical terminology.

SECTION VII lists commonly used proprietary drugs and corresponding generic terms. For the busy practitioner who usually is better acquainted with proprietary names of pharmaceuticals, this will facilitate prescribing in the most cost effective way. This will also aid the interpreting of key articles in the medical literature where generic terms are nearly always used.

HOW TO USE THE WORD FINDER MOST EFFECTIVELY

SECTION I is an alphabetical list of important prefixes and suffixes found in usual medical words. This will particularly help those who are not familiar with medical vocabulary to understand and remember key words and phrases.

SECTION II is an alphabetical list of current medical and paramedical terminology. The listings are accentuated to help you with pronunciation; they are syllabicated (divided) as an aid to your transcription.

SECTION III is a list of commonly used words in several of the major medical specialities—these words are also accentuated and syllabicated. It will save time for you to use the specialized lists when the situation dictates.

SECTION IV lists the phonetic spelling of "problem words" in alphabetical order. Secretaries, transcribers and others using medical vocabulary often run across words unfamiliar to them. This section lists these "problem" words phonetically (e.g., new mo'ni a), with the corresponding correct spelling (e.g., pneumonia).

SECTION V lists alphabetically most of the arteries, veins, muscles, syndromes, diseases, laboratory tests, surgical incisions, dental surfaces, descriptive positions (i.e., anatomical). When it is necessary to spell a particular muscle or test, etc., it may be quicker to use the specialized list than to try to find it in a regular medical dictionary or in the list of alphabetical terms. This section will be particularly helpful when transcribing an operative procedure such as a limb amputation where the names of several muscles and blood vessels will need to be accurately spelled.

SECTION VI lists abbreviations frequently used in medical transcription and prescription writing.

SECTIONVII contains alphabetical lists of commonly prescribed drugs. First, the proprietary names are alphabetically listed with corresponding generic names, then the same drugs are listed with their generic names alphabetized with corresponding proprietary names. This is particularly helpful now that it is popular to buy generically. Most physicians are better informed about proprietary names, thus these lists can be time-saving.

There also is a list of commonly prescribed Class II drugs, a proprietary list and a corresponding list of generic terms.

SECTION VIII is right up to date in itemizing recognized medical specialities for handy reference and review of precise definitions.

SECTION IX contains tables of potentially important information: conversion tables of weights and measures (metric to apothecary) and an obstetrical table to determine the expected date of confinement.

SECTION X is a special section of troublesome medical words, showing how to spell them correctly and grouped here for quick reference.

SYLLABIC ACCENTUATION: The heavy or primary accent is marked by a single mark (′). The secondary accent is indicated by two accent marks (″).

George Willeford, Jr., M.D.

MEDICAL WORD FINDER

Fourth Edition

Section I

LIST OF PREFIXES AND SUFFIXES

PREFIX	*MEANING*
a-, an-	not, without, absence of, negative
ab-, ab	away from
abdomino-	relating to the abdomen
acou-	relating to hearing
acro-	relating to the extremities
acromio-	relating to the shoulder
ad-	motion toward, adherence
adeno-	relating to a gland
adipo-	relating to fat, fatty
aer-	air
alg-, algi-	pair
all-	other, different
amb-	around, on both sides
andro	relating to man or male
angio-	relating to blood vessels
ante-	before in time or position
antero-	before, in front of
anti-	against
apo-	from, opposed, detached
ara, an-	up
argento-	denoting silver
arterio-	relating to arteries
artho-	straight, normal
arthro	relating to joints
auri-	relating to the ear
aut-, auto-	self
bacillo-	related to the bacillus
bacterio-	related to bacteria
bi-	two, double
bili-	related to bile or the bile-producing system
bio-	related to life
brachio-	denoting the arm
brachy-	short
brady-	slow
bronchio-, broncho-	related to the bronchial system
cac-, caco-	bad, evil
calcaneo-	related to the heel
calori-	pertaining to heat
cardio-	related to the heart
cat-, cata-, cath-	down

PREFIX	*MEANING*
cent-	hundred
cephalo-	related to the head
cervico-	related to the neck of the body or organ
cheilo-	related to the lips
cholo-	pertaining to bile or gall
chondrio-	related to gristle, cartilage
chrom-, chromo-	color
chromato-	related to color
chrono-	pertaining to time
chylo-	related to chyle
circum-	around
cleido-	related to the collarbone
colo-	related to the colon
colpo-	pertaining to the vagina
condylo-	pertaining to a joint
contra-	against or opposite
copro-	related to feces
coraco-	pertaining to the coracoid process of the scapula
corneo-	related to the cornea
cortico-	related to the cortex
costo-	related to the rib
cranio-	related to the cranium
cryo-	pertaining to cold
cuti-	skin
cysto-	pertaining to the bladder
dacryo-	relating to tears of lacrimal glands
dactylo-	relating to fingers, toes
de-	away, not
deca-	ten
demi-	half
dent-	relating to teeth
derma-	the skin
dia-	through, apart; between
dipla-, diplo-	double
dis-	negative, apart, absence of
duodeno-	relating to the duodenum
dys-	difficult or painful
e-	out, without
ecto-	outer
ectro-	congenital absence

PREFIX	*MEANING*
endo-	within, internal
entero-	denoting the intestine
epi-	upon, over, outside
erythro-	denoting red blood cells
esophago-	pertaining to the esophagus
eu-	normal, well
ex-	beyond, from, without
extra-, exo-	outside of
galact-, galacto-	milk
gastro-	pertaining to the stomach
glosso-	pertaining to the tongue
gluco-	denoting glucose
hem, hemato-	pertaining to blood
hemi-	half
hepa-, hepar-, hepato-	pertaining to the liver
hetero-	other dissimilarity
hidro-	pertaining to sweat
holo-	all
homo-	same, similar
humero-	pertaining to the humerus
hyper-	excessive, abnormal, over
hypo-	lack, deficiency, below, less
hystero-	pertaining to the uterus
idio-	peculiar to the individual or organ
ileo-	pertaining to ileum
ilio-	pertaining to ilium
in-	into, in, within, on, not
infra-	below, beneath, within
inter-	between, among
intra-	in or within
ischio-	pertaining to ischium or hip
iso-	same, in biology, from a different organism of the same species
jejuno-	pertaining to jejunum
juxta-	near
kata-, kath-	down
kerato-	pertaining to the cornea
labio-	pertaining to the lips
lact-	milk

PREFIX	*MEANING*
laryngo-	pertaining to the larynx
latero-	side
leio-	smooth
leuko-	white
lineo-	pertaining to the spleen
lipo-	pertaining to fat
litho	pertaining to stone
lumbo-	lumbar
macro-	large, enlarged, big, long
mal-	bad
masto-, mast-	pertaining to the breast
medio-, medi-	middle
mega-, meg-	enlarged, large
melano-, melan-	relating to melanin
mento-	pertaining to the chin
mes-, meso-	middle
metro-	pertaining to the uterus
micro-, micr-	small
mio-	less, smaller
mono-, mon-	one
multi-	many, much
myo-	pertaining to muscle
myxo-, myx-	pertaining to mucus
naso-	pertaining to the nose
neo-	new
nephro-, neph-	pertaining to the kidney
neuro-	pertaining to a nerve
niter-, nitro-	nitrogen
non-	not
nucleo-	nucleus
ob-	against
occipito-	occipital
oculo-	pertaining to the eye
odonto-	pertaining to a tooth
oligo-	scant
omo-	pertaining to the shoulder
omphalo-	pertaining to the umbilicus
onco-	pertaining to tumor
oophoro-	pertaining to the ovary
ophthalmo-	pertaining to the eye
opisth-	backward

PREFIX	*MEANING*
opto-	pertaining to vision
orchio- orchi-	pertaining to the testes
oro-	pertaining to the mouth
os-	pertaining to a mouth, bone
osteo-	pertaining to bone
oto-	pertaining to the ear
ovi-	pertaining to ovum
oxy-	denoting oxygen
pachy-	thick
palato-	pertaining to the palate
pan-	all
para-	beyond, beside
path-	disease
per-	excessive, through
peri-	about, near, around
perineo-	denoting the perineum
pharyngo-	pertaining to the pharynx
phlebo-	denoting vein
phono-	sound or voice
photo-	light
pilo-, pil-	denoting hair
plano-	flat
plasmo-	pertaining to plasma
platy-	flat, broad
pleuro-	pertaining to the pleura
plur-	more
pneumo-	air, lung
poly-	many, much
post-	after
postero-	posterior
pre-	before
pro-	for, before
procto-	pertaining to the anus or rectum
proto-	first
pseudo-	false
psycho-	pertaining to the mind
psychro-	cold
pubo-	pertaining to the pubis
pulmo-	pertaining to the lung
pyelo-	pertaining to the larger collecting ducts of the kidney

PREFIX	*MEANING*
pyloro-	pertaining to the pylorus
pyo-	denoting pus
rachio-	pertaining to the spine
re-	again
recto-	rectal
retro-	behind, backward
rhino-	pertaining to the nose
sacro-	pertaining to the sacrum
salpingo-	pertaining to the auditory or uterine tube
sarco-	denoting flesh
scapulo-	pertaining to the scapula
sclero-	hard
sclero-	denoting the sclera
semi-	half
sero-	denoting serum
sialo-	denoting saliva
skeleto-	pertaining to the skeleton
spleno-	pertaining to the spleen
steato-	denoting fat
sterno-	pertaining to the sternum
sub-	beneath
super-	above, upon
supra-	above
syn-	with, together
tachy-	fast
tarso-	pertaining to the ankle or instep
tele-	distant, far
temporo-	pertaining to the temple
teno-	denoting tendon
tetra-	four
thio-	sulfur
thoraco-	pertaining to the thorax
thyro-	pertaining to the thyroid
tracheo-	pertaining to the trachea
trans-	across
tri-	three
tricho-	denoting hair
tropho-	relating to nutrition
uni-	one
uretero-	pertaining to the ureter
urino-, uro-	relating to urine or urinary system

PREFIX	*MEANING*
utero-	pertaining to the uterus
vaso-	denoting blood vessles
venter-, ventro-	the abdomen
vesico-	pertaining to the bladder
vulvo-	pertaining to the vulva
xantho-	yellow

SUFFIX	*MEANING*
-ad	in the direction of
-aemia	blood
-agra	catching
-algesis, -algia	suffering, pain
-ase	an enzyme
-blast	a formative or germ cell
-cele	a tumor, cavity or hernia
-cide	kill, cut
-cyte	a cell
-dynia	pain
-ectomy	surgical removal
-emisis	vomiting
-emia	blood
-esthesia	sensation, feeling, perceive
-form	form, shape
-fuge	to drive away, flee
-genous	kind
-gog, -gogue	to make flow
-gram	tracing, picture, record
-graphy	X-ray examination, a writing, a record, scratch
-iasis	condition, pathological state
-ism	condition, theory
-its	inflammation
-ize	to treat by special method
-kinesis	motion, move
lite, -lith	a stone, a calculus
-logia, -logy	science of, study of
-lytic	causing lysis of
-megalia, -megaly	large, great, extreme
-meter	measure
-ode	form, shape, path
-oid	like
-ology	the study or science of
-oma	tumor-like nodule or swelling
-opia, -opy	a defect of the eye
-opsia, -opsy	a condition of vision
-optosis	a falling of
-orraphy	the closure of by suturing
-orrhagia	hemorrhage
-orrhea	excessive flow or secretion

SUFFIX	*MEANING*
-osis	a state, condition
-oscopy	visual examination of, using an illuminated instrument
-otomosis	to furnish with a mouth or an outlet
-ostomy	establishment of an opening to the outside of the body or lumen of another hollow organ
-otomy	incision into
-pathy	disease of
-pexy	fixation of
-phobia	fear of
-phrenia	mental disorder
-phylaxis	protection
-plasty	plastic surgery of
-plasm	to mold, shape
-plegia	a stroke, paralysis
-poietic	producing
-rhage, rhagia	hemorrhage, flow
-raphy	a suturing or stitching
-rhea	to flow, discharge
-schisis	cleft or fissure of
-sclerosis	dryness, hardness
-scope	instrument for visual examination
-scopy	seeing or examining
-tome	instrument for cutting
-tomy	a cutting operation
-tropic	nurture
-uria	pertaining to urine

Section II

ALPHABETICAL WORD LIST

A

a ban′don ment
ab ap′i cal
ab″ap tis′ton
a bar″og no′sis
ab″ar tic′u lar
a ba′si a
a ba′sic
a bate′
a bate′ment
ab ax′i al
ab do′men
ab dom′i nal
ab dom″i no an te′ ri or
ab dom″i no cen te′sis
ab dom″i no hys″ter ec′to my
ab dom″i no hys″ter ot′o my
ab dom″i no per″i ne′al
ab dom″i no pos te′ ri or
ab dom″i nos′co py
ab dom′i nous
ab dom″i no ves′i cal
ab du′cens
ab du′cent
ab duct′
abduc′tion
ab duc′tor
ab er′rant
ab″er ra′tion
ab″er rom′e ter
a be″ta lip″o pro tein e′mi a
a bey′ance
ab′i ent
ab″i et′ic
a″bi o gen′e sis
a″bi o′sis
a bi o troph′ic
a″bi ot′ro phy
ab ir′ri tant
ab ir″ri ta′tion
ab″lac ta″tion
ab late′
ab la′ti o
ab la′tion
a bleph′a ry
a blep′si a
ab′lu ent
ab nerv′al
ab neu′ral
ab nor′mal
ab nor mal′ity
ab o′ral
a bort′
a bor′ti cide
a bor′tient
a bor″ti fa′cient
a bor′tin
a bor′tion
a bor′tion ist
a bor′tive
a bor′tus
a bra′chi a
a bra″chi o ceph′a lus
a bra′chi us
a brade′
ab ra′sion
ab ra′sive
ab ra′sor
ab″re ac′tion
a′brin
a bro′si a
ab rup′ti o
ab′scess
ab scis′sa
ab scis′sion
ab′sence
ab″sen tee′ism
ab′sinthe
ab′sinth ism
ab′so lute
ab sorb′

ab sor′bance
ab sor″be fa′cient
ab sorb′ent
ab sorp″ti om′e ter
ab sorp′tion
ab″sorp tiv′i ty
ab′sti nence
ab strac′tion
a bu′li a
a bu′lic
a bu″lo ma′ni a
a buse′
a but′
a but′ment
a ca′cia
a cal″ci co′sis
a″cal cu′li a
a camp′si a
a can″thes the′si a
a can′thi al
a can′thi on
a can″tho a mel″o blas to′ma
a can′tho cytes
a can″tho cy to′sis
a can′thoid
a can″tho ker″a to der′mi a
ac′an thol′y sis
ac″an tho′ma
a can″tho pel′vis
ac″an tho′sis
ac″an thot′ic
a can′thu lus
a cap′ni a
a cap′su lar
a car′di a
a car″di o he′mi a
a car″di o ner′vi a
a car″di o tro′phi a
a car′di us
ac″a ri′a sis
a car′i cide
ac′a rid
Ac″a ri′na
ac″a ro der″ma ti′tis
ac′a roid
ac″a ro pho′bi a
a car′pi a
a car′pous
a″cat a la′si a
a cat″a ma the′si a
ac″a tap′o sis
ac″a tas ta′si a
ac″a thex′i a
ac a thex′is
a cau′dal
ac cel′er ate
ac cel″er a′tion
ac cel′er a″tor
ac cel′er in
ac cel″er om′e ter
ac cen′tu a″tor
ac cep′tor
ac″ces so′ri us
ac ces′so ry
ac′ci dent
ac″ci den′tal ism
ac cli ma′tion
ac cli″ma ti za′tion
ac cli′ma tize
ac com″mo da′tion
ac couche′ment
ac″cou cheur′
ac″cou cheuse′
ac″cre men ti′tion
ac cre′ti o cor′dis
ac cre′tion
ac crit′i cal
ac cu′mu la″tor
a″ce nes the′si a
a cen″o cou′ma rol
a cen′tric
a ceph″a lo bra′chi a

a ceph'a lo cyst"
a ceph'a lus
a ceph'a ly
a cer" a to' sis
a cer'bi ty
a cer"bo pho'bi a
a ces'o dyne
a"ces to'ma
ac"e tab'u lar
ac"e tab"u lec'to my
ac"e tab'u lo plas"ty
ac"e tab'u lum
ac'e tal
ac"et al'de hyde
ac"et am in'o phen
ac"et an'i lid
ac"et ar'sone
ac'e tate
ace"ta zol am'ide
a'ce test
a ce'tic ac'id
ac"e tim'e ter
ac"e to a ce'tic
ac"e tom'e try
ac'e tone
ac"e to ne'mi a
ac"e to nu'ri a
a ce'tum
ac'e tyl
ac"e tyl cho'line
a cet'y lene
a cet"y li za'tion
ac"e tyl sal"i cyl'ic
ach"a la'si a
ache
a chei'li a
a chei'ri a
a chei'rus
a chieve'ment
A chil'les
a chil"lo bur si'tis
a chil"lo dyn'i a

ach"il lor'rha phy
ach"il lot'o my
a"chlor hy'dri a
ach"lu o pho'bi a
a cho'li a
ach"o lu'ri a
ach"o lu'ric
a chon"dro pla'si a
a chon"dro plas'tic
a'chor
a chre'o cy the'mi a
a chro'a cyte
a chro'ma cyte
a"chro ma'si a
a'chro mate
a"chro mat'ic
a chro'ma tin
a chro'ma tism
a chro"ma tol'y sis
a chro mat'o phil
a chro"ma top'si a
a chro"ma to'sis
a chro'ma tous
a chro"ma tu'ri a
a chro'mi a
a chro'mic
a chro"mo der'mi a
a chro"mo trich'i a
a chros'tic
Ach"ro my'cin
a chyl"a ne'mi a
a chy'li a
a cic'u lar
ac'id
ac'id al bu'min
ac"id am"in u'ri a
ac"i de'mi a
ac'id-
fast"
a cid"i fi ca'tion
a cid'i fy
ac"i dim'e ter

ac′id ism
a cid′i ty
a cid′o cyte
ac″i do cy″to pe′ni a
ac″i do cy to′sis
a cid′o phil″
ac″i doph′i lism
ac″i do re sist′ant
ac″i do′sis
ac″i dot′ic
a cid′u late
ac″i du′ri a
ac″i du′ric
ac′i ni
ac″i no tu′bu lar
ac′i nus
ac′la sis
a clas′tic
ac mas′tic
ac′me
ac′ne
ac′ne form
ac ne′mi a
ac ni′tis
a coe′li a
a co′lous
a co′mi a
a con′a tive
a con″u re′sis
ac″o re′a
a co′ri a
a cor′mus
a cou″es the′si a
ac″ou la′li on
a cou′me ter
a cou met′ ric
a cou′me try
ac″ou oph′o ny
a cou′si a
a cous′ma
a cous′tic
a cous″ti co pho′bi a
ac quired′
ac′quired im′mu no de fi ciency syn′drome
ac′ral
a cra′ni a
a cra′ni us
a cra′ti a
a crat″u re′sis
ac′rid
ac″ri fla′vine
ac″ro ag no′sis
ac″ro ar thri′tis
ac″ro as phyx′i a
ac″ro a tax′i a
ac′ro blast
ac″ro ceph al′ic
ac″ro ceph″a lo syn″dac tyl′i a
ac″ro ceph′a ly
ac″ro con trac′ture
ac″ro cy″a no′sis
ac″ro der″ma ti′tis
ac′ro dont
ac″ro dyn′i a
ac″ro e de′ma
ac″ro ger′i a
ac″rog no′sis
ac″ro hy″per hi dro′sis
ac″ro hy′po ther″my
ac″ro ker″a to′sis
ac″ro ma′ni a
ac″ro mas ti′tis
ac″ro me gal′ic
ac″ro meg′a loid ism
ac″ro meg′a ly
ac″ro mel al′gi a
a cro′mi al
a cro″mi o cla vic′u lar
a cro″mi o cor′a coid
a cro″mi o hu′mer al
a cro′mi on
a cro″mi o tho rac′ic
a crom′pha lus

ac″ro my co′sis
ac″ro my″o to′ni a
ac″ro neu rop′a thy
ac″ro neu ro′sis
ac′ro nyx
ac″ro pa ral′y sis
ac″ro par es the′sia
ac″ro pa thol′o gy
a crop′a thy
ac″ro pho′bi a
ac″ro pig men ta′tion
ac″ro pig men ta′ti o re tic″u lar′is
ac″ro pos thi′tis
ac″ro scle ro′sis
ac′rose
ac′ro some
ac″ros tel al′gi a
ac″ro ter′ic
a crot′ic
ac′ro tism
ac″ro tro″pho neu ro′sis
a cryl′ic
act
ACTH
Ac′thar
ac′tin
ac tin′ic
ac tin′i form
ac′tin ism
Ac″ti no ba cil′lus
ac″ti no der″ma ti′tis
ac tin′o gen
ac tin′o graph
ac″ti nol′o gy
ac tin′o lyte
ac″ti nom′e ter
Ac″ti no my′ces
ac″ti no my ce′tin
ac″tin o my′cin
ac″ti no my co′ma
ac″ti no my co′sis
ac″ti no my cot′ic
ac″ti no my′co tin
ac″ti no neu ri′tis
ac″ti no phy to′sis
ac″ti nos′co py
ac″ti no ther′a py
ac′tion
ac′ti vate″
ac″ti va′tion
ac′ti va″tor
ac′tive
ac tiv′i ty
ac″to my′o sin
ac′tu al
a cu″es the′si a
a cu′i ty
a cu′mi nate
ac′u pres″sure
ac′u punc″ture
a′cus
ac″u sec′tor
a cus′ti cus
a cute′
a cute′ness
a cu″ti cos′tal
a cy″a nop′si a
a cy″a not′ic
a cy′cli a
a cy′clic
a″cy e′sis
ac′yl
a cys′ti a
a dac′ry a
a dac′tyl
a dac tyl′i a
a dac′tylism
a dac′tyl ous
ad″a man′tine
ad″a man″ti no car″ci no′ma
ad″a man″ti no′ma

ad″a man′to blast
Adam′s ap′ple
ad″ap ta′tion
a dapt′er
ad″ap tom′e ter
ad′at″om
ad ax′i al
ad′der
ad′dict
ad dic′tion
Addis′ meth′od
Ad′di son ism
ad di′tion
ad du′cent
ad duct′
ad duc′tion
ad duc′tor
a de″lo mor′phous
a del′pho site
ad″en al′gi a
ad′e nase
ad″en as the′ni a
ad″en drit′ic
ad″en ec′to my
ad″en ec to′pi a
A′den fe′ver
a de′ni a
a den′i form
ad″e ni′tis
ad″e no ac″an tho′ma
ad″e no a me″lo blas to′ma
ad″e no an″gi o sar co′ma
ad″e no car″ci no′ma
ad′e no cele
ad″e no cel″lu li′tis
ad″e no chon dro′ma
ad″e no chon″dro sar co′ma
ad″e no cys to′ma
ad″e no fi bro′ma
ad″e no fi″bro sar co′ma
ad″e no gen′e sis
ad″e nog′e nous
ad″e no hy″per sthe′ni a
ad″e no hy poph′y sis
ad′e noid
ad″e noi dec′to my
ad′e noid ism
ad′e noi di′tis
ad″e no lei″o my″o fi bro′ma
ad″e no li po′ma
ad″e no li po″ma to′sis
ad″e no log″a di′tis
ad″e no lym phi′tis
ad″e no lym′pho cele
ad″e no lym pho′ma
ad″e no′ma
ad″e no ma la′ci a
ad″e no′ma toid
ad″e no′ma tome
ad″e no ma to′sis
ad″e nom′a tous
ad′e no mere
ad″e no my″o hy per pla′si a
ad″e no my o″ma to′sis
ad″e no my o′ma
ad″e no my″o me tri′tis
ad″e no my″o sar co′ma
ad″e no my o′sis
ad″e no myx″o chon″dro sar co′ma
ad″e no myx o′ma
ad″e no myx″o sar co′ma
ad″e non′cus
ad″e nop′a thy
ad″e no phar″yn gi′tis
ad″e no phleg′mon
ad″e no sal″pin gi tis
ad″e no sar co′ma
ad″e no sar″co rhab″ do my o′ma
ad″e no scle ro′sis
ad′e nose

a den′o sine
ad″en o sin″e tri phos″phate
ad″e no′sis
ad′e no tome
ad″e not′o my
ad″e no vi′rus
ad′e nyl
a der′me a
a der″mo gen′e sis
a der″mo tro′phi a
ad here′
ad her′ent
ad he′sion
ad he″si ot′o my
ad he′sive
a″di ac tin′ic
a″di ad″o cho ki ne′sis
a di″a pho ret′ic
a″di as′to le
a″di a ther′mic
Ad′ie pu′pil
ad′i ent
ad′i po cele″
ad′i po cel′lu lar
ad′i po cere″
ad″i po fi pro′ma
ad″i pol′y sis
ad″i po ne cro′sis
ad″i po pex′is
ad″i po pex′y
ad′i pose
ad″i po′sis
ad″i po si′tis
ad″i pos′i ty
ad″i po″so gen′i tal
ad″i po su′ri a
a dip′sa
a dip′si a
ad′i tus
ad just′ment
ad jus′tor
ad′ju vent
ad lib
ad me′di al
ad″mi nic′u lum
ad mix′ture
ad na′sal
ad′nate
ad nau′se am
ad ner′val
ad nex′a
ad nex′al
ad″nex i′tis
ad nex″o gen′e sis
ad″o don′ti a
ad″o les′cence
ad o′ral
ad or′bit al
ad re′nal
ad re″nal ec′to my
Ad ren′a lin
ad ren″al in e′mi a
ad ren″al in u′ri a
ad re′nal ism
ad re″na li′tis
ad′ren arch′e
ad″ren er′gic
Ad′ren ine
ad ren″o cor′ti cal
ad ren″o cor″ti co mi met′ic
ad ren″o cor″ti co tro′pic
ad ren″o cor″ti co tro′pin
Ad re′no-cor′tin
ad re″no gen′i tal
ad re′no gram
ad re″no lyt′ic
ad ren″o meg′a ly
ad ren′o pause
ad re″no tox′in
ad ren′o trope
ad ren″o tro′pic
ad ren″o tro′pin

ad″re not′ro pism
a″dri a my′cin
a dro′mi a
ad sorb′
ad sor′bate
ad sorb′ent
ad sorp′tion
ad sorp′tive
ad ster′nal
ad ter′mi nal
ad tor′sion
a dult′
dul′ter ant
a dul′ter ate
a dul″ter a′tion
ad vance′
ad vance′ment
ad″ven ti′ti a
ad″ven ti′tious
a″dy na′mi a
a″dy man′ic
A e′des Ae gyp′ti
ae′quum
a′er ate
a er a′ted
a′er at or
a″er a′tion
a er e′mi a
a″er en″do cor′di a
a″er en″ter ec ta′si a
aer′i al
a″er if′er ous
a′er i form″
a″er o an a″er o′bic
A″er o bac′ter
a′er obe
a″er o′bic
a″er o bi ol′o gy
a″er o bi′o scope
a″er o bi o′sis
a″er o bi ot′ic
a′er o cele″
a″er o col′pos
a″er o cys′to scope
a″er o cys tos′co py
a″er o″don tal′gi a
a″er o don′ti a
a″er o duc′tor
a″er o dy nam′ics
a″er o em′bo lism
a″er o em″phy se′ma
a″er o gas′tri a
a′er o gen″
a″er o gen′e sis
a″er o gen′ic
a′er o gram″
a″er og′ra phy
a″er o hy drop′a thy
a″er o i″on i za′tion
a″er o i″on o ther′a py
Aer′o lin
a″er o mam mog′ra phy
a″er o med′cine
a″er om′e ter
a″er o neu ro′sis
a″er op′a thy
a′er o pause″
a″er o per″i to ne′um
a″er o pha′gi a
aer o phil″
a″er o pho″bi a
a′er o phore″
a′er o phyte″
a″er o pi e″so ther′a py
a″er o ple thys′mo graph
a″er o pleu′ra
a′er o scope″
a″er os′co py
a″er o si la oph′a gy
a″er o si″nus i′tis
a er o′sis
a′er o sol″

a′er o spo″rin
a″er o stat′ics
a″er o tax′is
a″er o ther″a peu′tics
a″er o ther″mo ther′a py
a″er o ti′tis me′di a
a″er o to nome′e ter
a er o trop′ic
a er ot′ro pism
a″er o tym′pa nal
a″er o u re′thro scope
ae ru′go
Ae scu la′pi us
aes thet′ic
aes′tus
a fe′brile
a fe′tal
af′fect
af fect″a bil′i ty
af″fec ta′tion
af fec′tion
af fec′tive
af″fec tiv′i ty
af fec″ti mo′tor
af′fer ent
af fil″i a′tion
af fi′nal
af″fir ma′tion
af′flu ent
af′flux
af fu′sion
a fi″brin o gen e′mi a
aft′er birth″
aft′er brain
aft′er care″
aft′er cat″a ract
aft′er cur′rent
aft′er damp″
aft″er dis′charge
aft′er ef fect″
aft′er gild″ing
aft′er hear″ing
aft′er im″age
aft′er im pres″sion
aft′er pains″
aft′er per cep″tion
aft′er po ten′tial
aft′er sensa″tion
aft′er sound″
aft′er stain″
aft′er taste″
aft′er treat″ment
aft′er vi″sion
a func′tion
a″ga lac′ti a
ag″a lor rhe′a
a gam′ete
a gam′ic
a gam″ma-glob″u lin e′mi a
a gam″o cy tog′o ny
a gam″o gen′e sis
ag″a mog′o ny
a gam′o spore
a gan″gli o′nic
a′gar
a gas′tric
a gas″tro neu′ri a
a gen′e sis
ag″e ne′si a
ag″e net′ic
a gen″i o ce pha′li a
a gen′i tal ism
a gen′o so′mi a
a gen″o so′mus
a′gent
a″ge ra′si a
a geu′si a
ag′ger
ag glom′er ate
ag lu″ti na′tion
ag glu′ti nin
ag″glu tin′o gen

ag glu'ti noid
ag glu'tin o phore"
ag"glu tin"o scope
ag'gre gate
ag"gre ga'tion
ag gres"sin
ag gres"sion
ag"i tat"ed
ag"i ta'tion
a"gi ta'tor caud'ae
ag"i to graph'i a
ag"i to pha'si a
a glan'du lar
a glau cop'si a
ag'li a
a"glo mer'u lar
a glos'si a
a glos"so sto'mi a
a glos'sus
ag"lu ti'tion
a gly ce'mi a
a gly ce'mic
a gly"co su'ria
a gly"co su'ric
ag na'thi a
ag na"tho ceph'a lus
ag"na thus
ag ne'a
ag"no gen'ic
ag no'si a
ag"om phi'a sis
a gon'ad ism
ag'o nal
a go'ni a
ag'onist
ag'o ny
Ag'or al
ag"o ra pho'bi a
a gram'ma tism
a gran'u lo cyte"
a gran"u lo cy'tic
a gran"u lo cy to'sis
a gran"u lo plas'tic
a gran"u lo'sis
a graph'i a
ag'ri us
ag"ro ma'ni a
ag"ryp not'ic
a'gue
a"gyi o pho'bi a
a gy'ri a
a hyp'ni a
aich"mo pho'bi a
ail'ing
ail'ment
ain'hum
air my e log'ra phy
air'way"
A kan tha me'ba
a kar"yo cyte
ak"a thi'si a
a ker"a to'sis
ak"i ne'si a
ak"i ne'sis
a kin"es the'si a
ak"i net'ic
a'la
al'a bas"ter
a"lac ta'si a
a la'li a
a lal'ic
al'a nine
a lan'tic
a las'trim
a la'tus
al'ba
Al ba my'cin
Albers-Schönberg
dis ease'
al bes'cent
al'bi cans
al"bi du'ri a
al'bi nism
al bi'no

al″bo ci ne′re ous
Albright-McCune-Sternberg syn′drome
al″bu gin′e a
al″bu gi ni′tis
al bu′go
al bu′min
al bu′mi nate
al bu″mi nif′er ous
al bu″mi nim′e ter
al bu″mi nog′e nous
al bu′mi noid
al bu″mi nol′y sin
al bu″mi nome′e ter
al bu′mi nose
al bu″min u ret′ic
al bu″mi nu′ri a
al bu′mo scope
al″bu mo su′ri a
Al″ca lig′e nes fe cal′is
al cap″to nu′ri a
al′che my
Alcock's ca nal′
al′co hol
al′co hol ase
al′co hol ate
al″co hol′a ture
al″co hol′ic
Al″co hol′ics A non′y mous
al′co hol ism
al″co hol om′e ter
al″co hol″o phil′i a
al″co hol u′ri a
al″co hol′ysis
al″co me′ter
Al dar′sone
al′de hyde
al′dol ase
Al′do met
al dos′ter one
Aldrich's test
a lec′i thal
al″eu ke′mi a
al″eu ke′mic
a lex′i a
a lex′in
al′gae
al″ge don′ic
al ge′si a
al ge′sic
al″ge sim′e ter
al get′ic
al′gid
al″gi o mo′tor
al″gi o mus′cu lar
al″go gen′e sis
al″go gen′ic
al″go lag′ni a
al om′e ter
al″go pho′bi a
al′gor
al′go spasm
al′i ble
a′lien ist
al′i ment
al″i men′ta ry
al″i men ta′tion
al″i men″to ther′a py
al′i na′sal
al″i phat′ic
al′i quot
al″i sphe′noid
al″ka le′mi a
al″ka les′cent
al′ka li
al″ka lim′e ter
al′ka line
al″ka lin′i ty
al′ka lin ize″
al″ka li nu′ ri a
al″ka li pe′ni a
al″ka li ther′a py

al′ka lize
al″ka lo″sis
al″ka lot′ic
al″ka lo ther′a py
al kap″to nu′ri a
al′kyl
al ky′nol
al″la ches the′si a
al lan″to cho′ri on
al lan″to enter′ic
al lan″to gen′e sis
al lan toi″do an gi op′a gous
al lan′to in
al lan′tois
al lax′is
al″le gor″i za′tion
al lele′
al lel″o cat″a lyt′ic
al le′lo morph
al lel″o tax′is
al len′the sis
al′ler gen
al ler gen′ic
al ler′gic
al′ler gid
al′ler gin
al′ler gist
al″ler gi za′tion
al″ler go der′mi a
al″ler go′sis
al′ler gy
al″li ga′tion
al′li ga″tor for′ceps
Allis for′ceps
al lit″er a′tion
al″lo che′zi a
al″lo cor′tex
al″lo er′o tism
al lom′e try
al″lo mor′phism
al″lo mor′pho sis
al′lo path
al lop′a thy
al loph′ a sis
al′lo plasm
al″lo plas′tic
al′lo plas″ty
al″lo psy′che
al″lo psy′chic
al″lo ryth′mi a
al′lo some
al″lo ste″a to′des
al″lo syn ap′sis
al′lo therm
al lo to′pi a
al lot″ri o don′ti a
al lot″ri o geu′si a
al″lo tri′o lith
al lot″ri oph′a gy
al ot″ri u′ri a
al′lo trope
al″lo troph′ic
al″lo trop′ic
al lox′an
al′loy
all′spice″
al′lyl
al′mond
a lo′chi a
Al′oe ve′ra
a lo′gi a
al″o pe′ci a
al′pha
al″pha to coph′er ol
al pho′sis
al′ter ant
al″ter a′tion
al′ter a tive
al″ter e′go ism
Al″ter na′ri a
al″ter na′tion
al′ter na″tor

al′ti tude sick′ness
al′um
a lu′mi num
a lu′si a
Alvarez, Walter C.
al′ve at ed
al″ve o la′bi al
al ve′o lar
al ve′o late
al″ve o lec′to my
al ve′o li″
al″ve o lin′gual
al″ve o li′tis
al ve″o lo cla′si a
al ve″o lo con dyl′e an
al ve″o lo den′tal
al ve″o lo la′bi al
al ve′o lon
al ve ol′o plas″ty
al ve″o lo sub na′sal
al″ve o lot′o my
al ve′o lus
al vi′no lith
al′vus
a lym″pho cy to′sis
al″ys o′sis
Alz′hei mer′s dis ease′
a mal′gam
a mal′gam ate
a mal″gam a′tion
a man′i tin
a mas′ti a
am″a tho pho′bia
am′a tive ness
am″au ro′sis
am″au rot′ic
am″a xo pho′bi a
am″bi dex ter′i ty
am″bi dex′trous
am″bi lat′er al
am″bi le′vous
am″bi o′pi a
am″bi sex′u al
am biv′a lence
am biv′lent
am′bi vert
am″bly a cou′si a
am″bly chro ma′si a
am′bly ope
am″bly o′pi a
am′bly o scope″
am″bo cep″tor
Am bro′si a
am′bu lance
am′bu la to″ry
am bus′tion
a me′ba
a me′bic
am″e bi′a sis
a me′bi cide
a me′bid
a me′bo cyte
a me′boid
a me′boid ism
am e bo′ma
am″e bu′ri a
a mei o′sis
am el′e ia
a mel″i fi ca′tion
a mel′o blast
a mel″o blas to′ma
am″el o blas″to sar co′ma
am″e lo gen′e sis
a me′lus
a me′ni a
a men″o ma′ni a
a men″or rhe′a
a men′si a
a′ment
a men′ti a
am″er is′tic
a me″si al′i ty

a″me thop′ter in
a me′tri a
ame″tro he′mi a
am″e tro′pi a
am″i an′thoid
am″i an tho′sis
a″mi cro′vic
a mi′cron
a mi″cro scop′ic
a mic′u lum
am′ide
am′i din
a mi′do
a mi″do py′rine
A′mi gen
a mim′i a
a mine′
a mi′no ac′id
a mi′no a″cid u′ri a
a mi″no phyl′line
A″min op′te rin
a mi″no py′rine
a mi″no sal″i cyl′ic
a mi″no su′ri a
a″mi to′sis
am i tot′ic
ami″tryp′ty lene
am′mo nate
am mo′ni a
am″mo ni′a cal
am mon″i fi ca′tion
am mo′ni um
am mo″ni u′ri a
am″mo ther′a py
am″ne mon′ic
am ne′si a′
am′ni a
am″ni o cen te′sis
am″ni o cho′ri al
am″ni o em″bry
on′ic
am″ni o gen′e sis
am″ni og′ra phy
am′ni on
am″ni or rhe′a
am″ni ot′ic
am″ni o ti′tis
am′ni o tome
am″ni ot′o my
am″o bar′bi tal
amoe′ba
a mok′
a mo ral′i a
a mor′phic
a mor′phin ism
a morph′ism
a mor′phous
A mox′i cil″lin
amp
am per′age
am′pere
am phet′a mine
am″phi ar thro′sis
am′phi as″ter
Am phib′i a
am phib′i ous
am″phi blas′tic
am″phi blas′tu la
am″phi chro′ic
am″phi coe′lous
am″phi cra′ni a
am′phi cyte
am″phi des′mic
am″phi di″ar thro′sis
am″phi er′o tism
am″phi gas′trula
am″phi gen′e sis
am″phi ge net′ic
am phig′o ny
am″phi kar′y om
am″phi mix′is
am″phi mor′u la

Am″phi sto′ma ta
am′phi tene
am′phi the″a ter
am phit′ri chous
am″pho di plo′pi a
Am′pho jel
am′pho lyte
am phor′ic
am″pho ril′o quy
am″pho roph′o ny
am″pho ter′ic
am″pho ter′i cin
am pho ter′ism
Am′ pi cil″ lin
am″pli fi ca′tion
am′pli fi″er
am′pli tude
am′poule
am′pul
am pul′la
am pul′lar
am pul′lu la
am′pu tate
am″pu ta′tion
am″pu tee′
a mu′si a
am″y cho pho′bi a
am″y dri′a sis
a my″e len ceph′a lus
am″y e′li a
a my′el in a″ted
a my′e lus
a myg′da lase
a myg′da loid
a myg″da loid ec′to my
a myg′da lo lith
a′myl
am″y la′ceous
am′yl ase
a myl′o gen
am′y loid
am″y loi do′sis
am″y lol′y sis
am″y lo lyt′ic
am′y lon
am″y lo pec′tin
am″y lop′sin
am′yl ose
am″y lu′ri a
a my″o es the′si a
a my″o pla′si a
a my″o sta′si a
a my″o stat′ic
a my″o tax′i a
a my″o to′ni a
a my″o tro′phi a
a my″o tro′phic
A′my tal
a myx′i a
a myx″or rhe′a
an″a bio′sis
an″a bi ot′ic
an″a bol′er gy
a nab′o lin
an ab′o lism
an″a camp′tics
an″a ce″li a del′phous
an″a cid′i ty
a nac′li sis
a na clit′ic
an ac′me sis
a nac″ro a′si a
a nac′ro tism
an″a cu′si a
an″a de′ni a
an″a did′y mus
an″a dip′si a
an′aer obe
an aer o′bic
an″aer o bi′ase
an″aer o bi o′sis
an″aer o gen′ic

an″a go′ge
an″a gog′ic
an″a lep′sis
an″a lep′tic
an″al ge′si a
an″al ge′sic
an″al ge′sist
an″al ler′gic
an′a log
a nal′o gy
a nal′y sand
a nal′y ses
a nal′y sis
an′a lyst
an″a lyt′ic
an′a ly″zer
an″am ne′sis
an″am nes′tic
an am″ni ot′ic
an″a mor′pho sis
an an″a ba′si a
an an″a phy lax′is
an an″as ta′si a
an an cas′ti a
an an′dri a
an an″gi o pla′si a
an an″gi o plas′tic
an″a pau′sis
an″a pei rat′ic
an″aphal″an ti′a sis
an′a phase
an a′phi a
an″a pho re′sis
an″a pho′ri a
an aph″ro dis′i a
an aph″ro dis′i ac
an″a phy lac′tic
an″a phy lac′tin
an″a phy lac′to gen
an″a phy lac′toid
an″a phyl″a tox′in
an″a phy lax′is
an″a pla′si a
an″a plas mo′sis
an″a plas′tic
an′a plas″ty
an″a ple ro′sis
an″a poph′y sis
an″a rith′mi a
an ar′thri a
an″a sar′ca
an″a sar′cous
an″a stal′sis
a nas′ta sis
an″as tig mat′ic
a nas′to mose
a nas″to mo′sis
a nas to mot′ic
a nas″to mot′i ca
an″a tom′ic
an″a tom′i cal
a nat′o my
an″a tox′in
an″a tro′pi a
an au′di a
an″a vac′cine
an″a ven′in
an′chor age
an′chy lops
an″co ne′us
an′co noid
An″cy los′to ma
an″cy los″to mi′a sis
an″dra nat′o my
an″dri at′rics
an″dro blas to′ ma
an″dro ga lac″to se′mi a
an″dro gam′one
an′dro gen
an″dro gen′e sis
an″dro gen′ic
an drog′e nous

an′dro gyne
an drog′y nism
an drog′y ny
an′droid
an″dro ma′ni a
an″dro mor′phous
an″droph′i lous
an″dro pho′bi a
an dros′ter one
a ne′de ous
an″e lec trot′o nus
a ne′mi a
a ne′mic
an″e mom′e ter
a ne″mo pho′bi a
an en″ce pla′li a
an″en ce phal′ic
an″en ceph′a lus
an″en ceph′a ly
an en′ter ous
an ep′i a
an ep″i plo′ic
an″er ga′si a
an′er gy
an′er oid
an″e ryth″ro blep′si a
an″e ryth′ro cyte
an″e ryth″ro pla′si a
an″e ryth rop′si a
an es″the ki ne′sis
an″es the′si a
an es″the sim′e ter
an″es the″si ol′o gist
an″es the″si ol′o gy
an″es thet′ic
an es′ the tist
an es′the tize
an es′trum
an″e to der′ma
an eu′ploid
a neu′ri a
an′eu rin
an′eu rysm
an eu rys′mal
an″eu rys mec′to my
an″eu rys′mo graph
an″eu rys′mo plas″ty
an″eu rys mor′rha phy
an″eu rys mot′o my
an″eu tha na′si a
an frac″tu os′i ty
an frac′tu ous
an gei′al
an″gi ec′ta sis
an″gi ec tat′ic
an″gi ec′tid
an″gi ec′to my
an″gi ec to′pi a
an″gi i′tis
an gi′na
an gi′nal
an′gi noid
an′gi nous
an gi″no pho′bi a
an′gi o blast″
an″gi o blas to′ma
an″gi o car′di o gram″
an″gi o car″di o graph′ic
an″gi o car″di og′ra phy
an″gi o car″di op′a thy
an″gi o cav″er no′ma
an″gi o cav′ern ous
an″gi o chei′lo scope
an″gi o cho li′tis
an″gi o chon dro′ma
an″gi o der′ma pig″men to′sum
an″gi o der′ma
an″gi o der″ma ti′tis
an″gi o dys tro′phi a
an″gi o e de′ma
an″gi o el″e phan ti′a sis
an″gi o en″do the″li o′ma

an″gi o fi″bro blas to′ma
an″gi o fi bro′ma
an″gi o gen′e sis
an″gi o gli o′ma
an″gi o gli o″ma to′sis
an″gi og′ra phy
an″gi o hy″per to′ni a
an″gi o hy″po to′ni a
an′gi oid
an″gi o ker″a toi di′tis
an″gi o ker″a to′ma
an″gi o li po′ma
an′gi o lith″
an″gi ol′o gy
an″gi o lu′poid
an″gi ol′y sis
an″gi o′ma
an″gi o ma la′ci a
an″gi o ma to′sis
an″gi o meg′a ly
an″gi om′e ter
an″gi o my″o lip o′ma
an″gi o my o′ma
an″gi o my op′a thy
an″gi o my″o sar co′ma
an″gi o neu rec′to my
an″gi o neu ro′ma
an″gi o neu″ro my o′ma
an″gi o neu ro′sis
an″gi o neu ro′tic
an″gi o no′ma
an″gi o pa ral′y sis
an″gi o pa re′sis
an″gi op′a thy
an″gi o pla′ni a
an′gi o plas″ty
an″gi o pneu mog′ra phy
an″gi o poi e′sis
an″gi o poi et′ic
an′gi o pres″sure
an″gi or′rha phy
an″gi or rhex′is
an″gi o sar co′ma
an″gi o scle ro′sis
an′gi o scope″
an″gi o sco to′ma
an″gi o′sis
an′gi o spasm″
an″gi o stax′is
an″gi o ste no′sis
an″gi os″te o′sis
an″gi o stron″gy li′a sis
an″gi o tel″ec ta′si a
an″gi o ten′ic
an″gi o ten′sin
an″gi o ti′tis
an″gi ot′o my
an″gi ot′o nase
an″gi o ton′ic
an″gi ot′o nin
an′gi o tribe″
an″gi o troph′ic
an′gle
an′gor
ang′strom
an″gu la′tion
ang′u lus
an″he do′ni a
an hem″a to poi e′sis
an he″ma to′sis
an he″mo lyt′ic
an″hi dro′sis
an″hi drot′ic
an hy′drase
an″hy dra′tion
an″hy dre′mi a
an hy′dride
an hy′drous
an″hyp no′sis
a ni″a ci no′sis
an″i an′thi nop sy
an ic ter′ic

an id′e us
an′i line
a ni lin′gus
an′il ism
a nil′i ty
an′i ma
an′i mal
an″i mal′cule
an″i mas′tic
an″i ma′tion
an′i ma tism
an′i mism
an′i mus
an′i″on
an′i on″ic
an″i rid′i a
an″is ei kom′e ter
an″i sei ko′ni a
an i″so chro ma′si a
an i″so chro mat′ic
an i″so co′ri a
an i″so cy to′sis
an i″so dac′ty lous
an i′so dont
an i″so ga mete′
an″i sog′a my
an″i sog′na thous
an i″so me′li a
an i″so me′ri a
an i″so me tro′pi a
an i″so me trop′ic
a nis″o my′cin
an″i so′pi a
an″i so sphyg′mi a
an″i sos then′ic
an i″so ton′ic
an″i so tro′pic
an″i sot′ro py
an″i sur′ri a
a″ni trog′e nous
an′kle
an″ky lo bleph′a ron
an″ky lo chei′li a
an″ky lo col′pos
an″ky lo dac tyl′i a
an″ky lo don′ti a
an″ky lo glos′si a
an′ky lose
an″ky losed
an ′ky lo′sis
an′ky lo tome
an″ky lot′o my
an′la ge
an neal′
an nec′tent
An nel′i da
an′nu lar
an′nu late
an′nu lose
an″nu lo spi′ral
an′nu lus
an″o chro ma′si a
a no″ci as so″ci a′tion
a no″ci cep′tor
a no″ci the′si a
a″no coc cyg′e al
an o′dal
an′ode
an″o der′mous
an″o don′ti a
an″o don′tous
an′o dyne
an″o dyn′i a
an″o e′si a
an″o et′ic
a noi′a
a nom′a lo scope
a nom′ a lous
a nom′a ly
a no′mi a
an o′mous
an″o nych′i a

a non'y ma
an"o op'si a
a"no per"i ne'al
A noph'e les
an"o phel'i cide
an"o phel'i fuge
an"o pho'ri a
an"oph thal'mi a
an"oph thal'mos
an o'pi a
a'no plas ty
an op'si a
an or'chi a
an or'chism
an or'chus
a"no rec'tal
a"no rec'to plas"ty
a"no rec'tic
an"o rex'ia
an o rex' i a   ner vo' sa
an or gas'my
an"or thog'ra phy
an"or tho'pi a
an"or tho'sis
a'no scope
an os'mi a
an os'mic
an o"sog no'si a
a"no spi'nal
an"os to'sis
an o'ti a
an"o tro'pi a
an o'tus
a"no ves'i cal
an ov'u lar
an ov'u la to"ry
an"ox e'mi a
an ox'i a
an ox'ic
an'sa
an'sate
an'ser ine
an'si form
an'ta buse
ant ac'id
an tag'o nism
an tag'o nist
an tag"o nis'tic
ant al'ka line
ant"aph ro dis'i ac
an"te au'ral
an"te bra'chi al
an"te bra'chi um
an"te ci'bum
an"te cu'bi tal
an"te cur'va ture
an"te flex'ion
an"te hy poph'y sis
an"te-mor'tem
an"te na'ri al
an"te na'tal
An'te par
an'te par'tum
an te'ri or
an"ter o dor'sal
an"ter o ex ter'nal
an'ter o grade"
an"ter o in fe'ri or
an"ter o in te'ri or
an"ter o in ter'nal
an"ter o lat'er al
an"ter o me'di an
an"ter o pa ri'e tal
an"ter o pi tu'i tar y
an"ter o pos te'ri or
an"ter o su pe'ri or
an"te ver'sion
an'te vert ed
ant"hel min'tic
an the'ma
ant"hem or rhag'ic
an"tho pho'bi a

an'thra cene
an'thra coid
an"thra co ne cro'sis
an"thra co sil"i co'sis
an"thra co'sis
an'thrax
an"thro po gen'ic
an'thro poid
an"thro pol'o gy
an"thro pom'e ter
an"thro pom'e try
an"thro po mor'phic
an"thro poph'a gy
an"thro po phil'ic
an"thro po pho'bi a
an"thro po so"ma tol'o gy
ant"hyp not'ic
an"ti ac'id
an"ti ag glu'ti nin
an"ti ag gres'sin
an"ti al'bu mate
an"ti al bu'min
an"ti a lex'in
an"ti am"bo cep'tor
an"ti am'yl ase
an"ti an"a phy lax'is
an"ti a ne'mi a
an"ti a ne'mic
an"ti an'ti bod"y
an"ti ar"ach nol'y sin
an"ti ar thrit'ic
an"ti bac te'ri al
an"ti bi o'sis
an"ti bi ot'ic
an"ti bi'o tin
an"ti blas'tic
an'ti bod"y
an"ti bra'chi al
an"ti bra'chi um
an"ti car cin'o gen
an"ti car'di um
an"ti car'i ous
an"ti ca thex'is
an"ti cath'ode
an"ti ceph'a lin
an"ti chei rot'o nus
an"ti chol in er'gic
an"ti cho"lin es'ter ase
an"ti chro mat'ic
an"ti co ag'u lant
an"ti col la'gen ase"
an"ti com'ple ment
an"ti concep'tive
an"ti con cus'sion
an"ti con vul'sant
an"ti con vul'sive
an'ti cus
an"ti cu'tin
an"ti di"a bet'ic
an"ti dia"ar rhe'al
an"ti di"u re'sis
an"ti di"u ret'ic
an"ti do'tal
an'ti dote
an"ti drom'ic
an"ti dys"en ter'ic
an"ti e met'ic
an"ti en'zyme
an"ti fe'brile
An"ti fe'brin
an"ti fer'ment
an"ti fi"bri no ly'sin
an"ti fi bro"ma to gen'ic
an"ti fun'gal
an"ti ga lac'tic
an'ti gen
an ti gen'ic
an"ti ge nic'i ty
an"ti he'lix
an"ti he"mo lyt'ic
an"ti he"mo phil'ic
an"ti hem"or rhag'ic

an″ti hem″or rhoi′dal
an″ti hi drot′ic
an″ti his′ta mine
an″ti his′ta min ic
an″ti hor′mone
an″ti hy″a lu ron′i dase
an″ti hy drop′ic
an″ti in fec′tive
an″ti ke″to gen′e sis
an″ti li′pase
an″ti lip fa no′gen
an″ti lu et′ic
an″ti lym′pho cyte
an″ti lyt′ic
an″ti ma lar′i al
an″ti men or rhag′ic
an′ti mere
an″ti me tab′o lite
an″ti me tor′pi a
an′ti mo″ny
an″ti my cot′ic
an″ti nar cot′ic
an″ti neu ral′gic
an″ti neu rit′ic
an tin′i on
an″tin va′sin
an″ti o be′sic
an″ti o don tal′gic
an″ti op′so nin
an″ti ox′i dant
an″ti par″a lyt′ic
an″ti par″a sit′ic
an″ti pep′sin
an″ti pep′tone
an″ti per″i od′ic
an″ti per″i stal′sis
an″ti phag″o cyt′ic
an″ti phlo gis′tic
An″ti phlo gis′tine
an′ti phone
an″ti phthi′ri ac
an″ti plas′min
an″ti plas′tic
an″ti pneu″mo coc′cio
antip′o dal
an″ti pro throm′bin
an″ti pro′ton
an″ti pru rit′ic
an″ti py″o gen′ic
an″ti py re′sis
an″ti py ret′ic
an″ti py′rine
an″ti py″rin o ma′ni a
an″ti ra′bic
an″ti ra chit′ic
an″ti ren′nin
an″ti re tic′u lar
an″ti rhe′o scope
an″ti rheu mat′ic
an′ti-Rh se′rum
an″ti ri″bo fla′vin
an″ti ri′cin
an″ti sca bet′ic
an″ti scor bu′tic
an″ti sep′sis
an″ti sep′tic
an″ti sep′tol
an″ti se′rum
an″ti si al′a gogue
an″ti si al′ic
an″ti so′cial
an″ti spas mod′ic
an″ti spas′tic
an″ti spi″ro che′tic
an″ti ster′num
an″ti strep″to coc′cic
an″ti strep″to dor′nase
an″ti strep″to he″mo ly′sin
an″ti strep″to ki′nase
an″ti strep″to ly′sin
an″ti su″dor if′ic
an″ti syph″ i lit′ic

an″ti the′nar
an″ti throm′bin
an″ti throm″bo plas′tin
an″ti tox′i gen
an″ti tox′ic
an″ti tox′in
an″ti trag′i cus
an″ti tra′gus
an″ti tris′mus
an′ti trope
an″ti tryp′sin
An′ti tus′sin
an″ti tus′sive
an″ti ty′phoid
an″ti u′re ase
an″ti ve ne′re al
an″ti ven′in
an″ti vi′ral
an″ti vi rot′ic
an″ti vir′u lin
an″ti vir′us
an″ti vi′ta min
an″ti viv″i sec′tion
an″ti viv″i sec′tion ist
an″ti xen′ic
an″ti xe″roph thal′ mic
an″ti xe rot′ic
an″ti zy mot′ic
ant″lo pho′bi a
an′tral
an trec′to my
an tri′tis
an″tro at″ti cot′o my
an′tro cele
an″tro na′sal
ant′ro phose
an′tro scope″
an tros′to my
an″tro tym pan′ic
an′trum
An tu′trin-S

a nu′cle ar
an u′ri a
an u′ric
an u′rous
a′nus
a nus i′tis
an′vil
anx i′e ty
a or′ta
a″or tal′gi a
a or′tic
a or″ti co pul″mo na ry
a oe″ti co re′nal
a″or ti′tis
a″or tog′ra phy
a or″to il′i ac
a″or tot′o my
a pal″les the′si a
a pan′cre a
a pan′dri a
ap″an thro′pi a
a par″a lyt′ic
ap″ar thro′sis
a pas′ti a
ap″a thet′ic
ap′a thism
ap′a thy
ap′atite
a pei″ro pho′bi a
a pel′lous
a per′ri ent
a pe″ri od′ic
a per″i stal′sis
a per′i tive
Apert′s syn′drome
ap″er tom′e ter
ap″er tu′ra
ap′er ture
Apeu vi′rus
a′pex
a″pex car′di o gram

Apgar score
a pha′gi a
apha′ki a
a pha′kic
aph″a lan′gi a
aph″al ge′si a
a phan′i sis
a pha′si a
a pha′si ac
a phelx′i a
a phe′mi a
a phem′ic
aph″e pho′bi a
aph′e ter
a″phil an′thro py
a pho′ni a
a phon′ic
a′phose
a phra′si a
aph″ro dis′i a
aph″ro dis′i ac
aph″ro dis″i o ma′ni a
aph″ro ne′si a
aph′tha
aph thenx′i a
aph thon′gi a
aph tho′sis
aph′thous
a″pi cec′to my
ap″i ci′tis
ap″i co ec′to my
ap″i co lo′ca tor
ap″i col′y sis
a″pi o ther′a py
a″pi pho′bi a
a pis″i na′tion
a″pla cen′tal
ap″la nat′ic
a pla′si a
a plas′tic
a pleu′ri a
ap′ne a
ap neu″ma to′sis
ap neu′mi a
ap neu′sis
ap″o cam no′sis
ap″o car″te re′sis
ap″o chro mat′ic
ap″o clei′sis
ap′o crine
ap″o de″mi al′gi a
a po′di a
ap″o fer′ri tin
a pog′a mous
a pog′a my
ap″o mix′is
ap″o mor′phine
ap″o myt to′sis
a pon″eu ror′rha phy
a pon″eu ro′sis
a pon″eu ro si′tis
ap″o neu rot′ic
a pon″eu rot′o my
a pon′i a
a poph′y sate
a po phys′eal
a poph′y sis
a poph″y si′tis
ap″o plas′mi a
ap″o plec′ti form
ap′o plex″y
a pop nix′is
ap″or rhip′sis
a po′si a
ap″o sid′er in
ap″o si′ti a
ap″o sit′ic
ap′o some
a pos′po ry
a pos′ta sis
a pos′thi a
a poth′e car″ies

a poth'e car"y
ap"ox e'me na
ap"ox e'sis
ap"pa ra'tus
ap pend'age
ap"pen dec'to my
ap pen"di ce'al
ap pen'di ces"
ap pen"di ci'tis
ap pen"di clau'sis
ap pen'di co lith"
ap pen"di cos'to my
ap"pen dic'u lar
ap pen'dix
ap"per cep'tion
ap"per son"i fi ca'tion
ap'pe tite
ap'pe ti"zer
ap'pla nate
ap'pli ca"tor
ap"po si'tion
ap proach'
ap prox'i mal
ap prox'i mate
ap prox"i ma'tion
a prac"tog no'si a
a prax'i a
A pres'o line
a proc'ti a
a proc'tous
a"pro sex'i a
a"pro so'pi a
ap sel"a phe'si a
ap"si thy'ri a
ap sych'i a
ap ty'a lism
a'pus
a py'e tous
a py'rene
a"py ret'ic
a"py rex'i a
a"py rex'i al
aq'ua
a quat'ic
Aq'ua phor
aq'ue duct
a'que ous
Ar'a bic
a rach"i don'ic
ac'id
A rach'ni da
A rach'nid ism
a"rach ni don'ic
ar"ach ni'tis
a rach"no dac'ty ly
a rach'noid
a rach noid'al
a rach'noid ism
a rach"noi di'tis
a rach'noid-u re"ter os'to my
A'ra len
Ar'a mine
ar bo're al
ar"bo res'cent
ar"bor i za'tion
ar'bor vi'tae
ar"bo vi'rus
arc
ar cade'
ar ca'num
ar'cate
arch
ar cha'ic
ar"che go'ni um
ar chen'ter on
ar"che o ki net'ic
ar che py'on
ar'che type
ar"chi a'ter
ar'chi coele
ar"chi gas'tru la
ar"chi neph'ron
ar"chi pal'li um
ar"chi tec ton'ic

ar′cho plasm
ar chu′si a
ar″ci form
arc ta′tion
ar′cu ate
ar″cu a′tion
ar′cus
a′re a
ar″e a′tus
a″re flex′i a
a″re gen″er a′tion
ar″e na′ceous
ar″e na′tion
ar′ene
a″re no vi′rus
a re′o la
a re′o lar
ar gam″bly o′pi a
ar′ge ma
ar gen′taf fin
ar″gen taf fi no′ma
ar gen′tic
ar gen′to phile
ar gen′tous
ar″gil la′ceous
ar′gi nase
ar′gi nine
ar′gon
Argyll Robertson
ar gyr′i a
ar gyr′ic
Ar′gy rol
ar gy′ro len tis
ar gy′ro phile
ar″gy ro′sis
a rhin″en ce pha li′a
Arias-Stella phe″nom′e non
ari″bo fla″vi no′sis
a ris″to gen′ic
Aristotle
a rith″mo ma′ni a
ar′ky o chrome″
arm ar″ma men tar′i um
ar mil′la
arm′pit″
Arnold-Chiari syn′drome
ar″o mat′ic
ar rec′tor
ar rest′
ar″rhe no blas to′ma
ar″rhe no′ma
ar″rhe not′o ky
ar rhin″en ce pha′li a
ar rhin′i a
ar rhyth′mi a
ars a man′di
ar′se nate
ar′se nic
ar sen′i cal
ar sen″i co der′ma
ar se′ni ous
ar′se nite
ar″se no ther′a phy
ars phen′a mine
ar′te fact
ar ter′en ol
ar ter′i al
ar te″ri al i za′tion
ar te″ri arc′ti a
ar″te ri′a sis
ar te″ri ec′ta sis
ar te″ri ec′to my
ar te″ri ec to′pi a
ar te″ri o cap′il lar″y
ar te″ri o fi bro′sis
ar te′ri o gram″
ar te′ri o graph″
ar te″ri og′ra phy
ar te″ri o′la
ar te′ri ole
ar te′ri olith″
ar ter″i o li′tis

ar ter″ri o″lo ne cro′sis
ar te″ri o″lo scle ro′sis
ar te″ri o lo scle rot′ic
ar te″ri o ma la′ci a
ar te″ri o ne cros′sis
ar te″ri op′a thy
ar te″ri o pla′ni a
ar te″ri o plas′tic
ar te″ri o plas′ty
ar te″ri o pres′sor
ar te″ri o punc′ture
ar te″ri o re′nal
ar te″ri or′rha phy
ar te″ri or rhex′is
ar te″ri o scle ro′sis
ar te″ri o scle rot′ic
ar te′ri o spasm″
ar te″ri o ste no′sis
ar te″ri os to′sis
ar te″ri o strep′sis
ar te′ri o tome″
ar te″ri ot′o my
ar te″ri o ve′nous
ar te″ri o ver′sion
ar″te ri′tis
ar′ter y
ar thral′gi a
ar thral′gic
ar threc′to my
ar″thre de′ma
ar″thres the′si a
ar thri′tes
ar thrit′ic
ar thrit′i des
ar thri′tis
ar′thro cele
ar″thro cen te′sis
ar″thro chon dri′tis
ar″thro cla′si a
ar thro de′sis
ar thro′di a
ar″thro dyn′i a
ar″thro dyn′ic
ar″thro dys pla′si a
ar″thro em py e′sis
ar″thro en dos′co py
ar″thro er ei′sis
ar throg′ra phy
ar″thro gry po′sis
ar″thro ka tad′y sis
ar′thro lith″
ar″thro li thi′a sis
ar throl′o gy
ar throl′y sis
ar throm′e ter
ar thron′cus
ar throp′a thy
ar′thro phyte
ar″thro plas′tic
ar′thro plas″ty
ar′thro pod
ar″thror rha′gi a
ar′thro scope
ar thros′co py
ar thro′sis
ar′thro spore
ar thros′to my
ar″thro tro′pi a
ar′throus
Arthus re ac′tion
ar tic′u lar
ar″tic u lar′is ge′nus
ar tic′u late
ar tic″u la′ti o
ar tic″u la′tion
ar tic′u la″tor
ar tic′u lus
ar′ti fact
ar″ti fi′cial
ar″y ep″i glot′tic
ar′yl ene
ar″y te″no ep″i glot′i cus

a ryt'e noid
ar"y te"noi dec'to my
ar"y te"noi di'tis
ar"y te noi'do pex"y
ar"y vo cal'is
as"a fet'i da
as"a phi'a
a sar'ci a
as bes'tos
as"bes to'sis
as"ca ri'a sis
as car'i cide
As'ca ris
as cend'ing
Aschheim-Zondek test
Aschoff nod'ule
as ci'tes
as cit'ic
As"co my ce'tes
a scor'bate
a scor'bic ac'id
a se'mi a
a sep'sis
a sep'tic
a sex'u al
ash
Asherman's
dis ease'
a"si a'li a
A si ne'to bac ter
a so'cial
a so'ma
a so'ni a
asp
as"pal a so'ma
as par'a gin
as par'a gin ase
as par'tic
a spas'tic
a"spe cif'ic
as"per gil'ic
as"per gil'lin
as"per gil lo'ma
as per"gil lo'sis
As" per gil'lus
a sper mat'ic
a sper'ma tism
a sper"ma to gen'e sis
a sper'mi a
asper'mous
as phyx'i a
as phyx'i ant
as phyx'i ate
as pid'i um
as'pi rate
as"pi ra'tion
as'pi ra"tor
as'pi rin
a spo"ro gen'ic
a spo'rous
a spor'u late
as sault'
as say'
as sim'il ate
as sim"i la'tion
as so"ci a'tion
as'so nance
as'sue tude
a sta'si a
as tat'ic
a ste"a to'sis
as'ter
a ster"e og no'sis
as te'ri on
as"ter ix'is
a ster'nal
a ster'ni a
as'ter oid
as the'ni a
as then'ic
as"the no bi o'sis
as"the no co'ri a
as"the no ge'ni a
as"the nol'o gy

as″the nom′e ter
as″the no pho′bi a
as″the no′pi a
as″the no sper′mi a
as″the nox′i a
asth′ma
asth mat′ic
as′ti ban
At′ i van
a stig′ma graph
as″tig mat′ic
a stig′ma tism
as″tig mom′e ter
a stig′mo scope
a stom′a tous
a sto′mi a
as trag′a lar
as trag″a lec′to my
as trag′a lus
as′tral
as″tra pho′bi a
as trin′gent
as′tro blast
as″tro blas″to-as″tro cy to′ma
as″tro blas to′ma
as′tro cytes
as″tro cy to′ma
as trog″li o′ma
as′troid
as″tro pho′bi a
as′tro sphere
a styph′i a
a stys′i a
a″syl la′bi a
a sy′lum
a″sym bo′li a
a″sym met′ric
a″sym met′ri cal
a sym′me try
a sym′phy tous
a″symp to mat′ic
as″ymp tot′ic
a syn′chro nism
a syn′cli tism
a syn′de sis
a″syn ech′i a
as″y ner′gi a
as″y ner′ gic
a syn′er gy
a″syn e′si a
as″y no′di a
a″syn tax′i a dor sa′lis
a sys″tem at′ic
a sys′to le
a″sys to′li a
a″sys tol′ic
A′ta brine
at″a bri no der′ma
a tac′tic
a tac′ti form
a″tac til′i a
at ar ac′tic
At′ar ax
at″a rax′ic
a tav′i cus
at′a vism
a tax″a pha′si a
a tax′i a
a tax′i a graph″
a tax′ic
a tax″i o pho′bi a
at″e lec′ta sis
at″e lec tat′ic
a tel″en ce pha′li a
a te″li o′sis
at″e lo car′di a
at″e lo ceph′a lous
at″e lo chei′li a
at″e lo chei′ri a
at″e lo en″ce pha′li a
at″e lo glos′si a
at″e log nath′i a

at″e lo mit′ic
at″e lo my e′li a
at″e lo po″di a
at″e lo pro so′pi a
at″e lo ra chid′i a
at″e lo sto′mi a
at″e pho′bi a
a the′li a
ath″er o gen′e sis
ath″er o′ma
ath″er o″ma to′sis
ath″er om′a tous
ath″er o″scle ro′sis
ath′e toid″
ath″e to′sis
ath″e tot′ic
a thi″a min o′sis
a threp′si a
a thy′mi a
a thy′mic
a thy re o′sis
at lan″to ax′i al
at lan″to bas i lar′is in ter′nus
at lan″to ep″i stroph′ic
at lan″to-oc cip′i tal
at′las
at lod′y mus
at mom′e ter
at′mos phere
at″mos pher′ic
a to′ci a
at′om
a tom′ic
at″o mic′i ty
at″om i za′tion
a to′ni a
a ton′ic
at′o ny
at′o pen
a top′ic
a top″og no′si a
at′o py
a tox′ic
a tre′mi a
a tre′si a
a tre′sic
a tre″to ceph′a lus
a tre″to cor′mus
a tre″to cys′ti a
a tre″to gas′tri a
a tre″to le′mi a
a tre″to me′tri a
at″re top′si a
a tret″or rhi′ni a
a tre″to sto′mi a
a tret″u re′thri a
a′tri a
a′tri al
at″ri cho′sis
at′ri chous
a″tri o sep″to pex′y
a″tri o ven tric′u lar
a″tri o ven tric″u lar′is
a′tri um
A′ tro mid
at″ro pho der′ma
at″ropho der″ma to′sis
at′ro phy
at′ro pine
at′ro pin ism
at ro″pin i za′tion
at′ro pin ize
at′tar
at ten′tion
at ten′u ate
at ten′u at ed
at ten″u a′tion
at′tic
at″ti co an trot′o my
at″ti co mas′toid
at″ti cot′o my
at′ti tude

at ton′i ty
at trac′tion
at tri′tion
a typ′i cal
au″di mu′tism
au″di o ep″i lep′tic
au″di o gen′ic
au′di o gram″
au″di ol′o gist
au″di ol′o gy
au″di om′e ter
au″di o met′ric
au″di om′e try
au″di o vis′u al
au di′tion
au′di tive
au″di tog no′sis
au″di to psy′chic
au′di to″ry
au″di to sen′so ry
Auerbach plex′us
aug′ment
aug″men ta′tion
aug na′thus
au″lo pho′bi a
au′lo phyte
au′ra
au′rae
au′ral
Au″re o my′cin
au′ric
au′ri cle
au ric′u lar
au ric″u la′re
au″ric u lar′is
au ric″u lo fron tal′is
au ric″u lo tem′po ral
au ric″u lo ven tric′u lar
au′ris
au′rist
au ro″ra pho′bi a
au″ro ther′a py
au′rous
aus′cu late
aus cult′
aus″cul ta′tion
aus″cul′ta to ry
au′ta coid
au te′cious
au te mi′si a
au′tism
au tis′tic
au″to ac″ti va′tion
au″to ag glu″ti na′tion
au″to ag glu′ti nin
au″to al″go lag′ni a
au″to a nal′y sis
au″to an″am ne′sis
au″to an″ti bi o′sis
au″to an′ ti bod″y
au″to an′ti gen
au″to au′di ble
au′to blast
au″to ca tal′y sis
auto cat′al yst
au″to ca thar′sis
au toch′tho nous
au toc′la sis
au′to clave
au″to con″den sa′tion
au″to con duc′tion
au″to cy″to tox′in
au″to di ges′tion
au″to ech″o la′li a
au″to ech″o prax′i a
au″to ec″ze ma ti za′tion
au″to e mas″cu la′tion
au″to e rot ic
au″to er ot′i cism
au″to er′o tism
au″to fel la′ti o
au tog′a mous

au tog′a my
au″to gen′ic
au tog′e nous
au′to graft″
au′to graph″
au″to he mol′y sis
au″to he″mo ther′a py
au″to hy drol′y sis
au″to hyp no′sis
au″to hyp not′ic
au″to hyp′no tism
au″to im mune′
au″to im mun″i za′tion
au″to in fec′tion
au″to in fu′sion
au″to in oc″u la′tion
au″to in tox′i cant
au″to in tox″i ca′tion
au″to i″so ly′sin
au″to kin e′sis
au tol′o gous
au tol′y sate
au tol′y sin
au tol′y sis
au″to lyt′ic
au′to lyze
au″to mat′ic
au tom′a tin
au tom″a tin′o gen
au tom′a tism
au tom″a ti za′tion
au″to mat′o gen
au tom′a ton
au″to my″so pho′bi a
au″to ne phrec′to my
au″to no ma′si a
au″to nom′ic
au ton′o mous
au″to-oph thal′mo scope
au′to-ox″i da′tion
au top′a thy
au″to pha′gi a
au″to phil′i a
au″to pho′bi a
au″to pho″no ma′ni a
au toph′o ny
au′to plast
au′to plas′tic
au′to plas″ty
au″to pneu″mo nec′to my
au″to pro tol′y sis
au′top sy
au″to psy′che
au″to psy′chic
au″to psy cho′sis
au″to ra′di o gram
au″to ra′di o graph
au″to ra″di og′ra phy
au″to re in fu′sion
au″to sen″si ti za′tion
au′to site
au″to som′al
au′to some
au″to sug ges′tion
au″to syn′de sis
au″to syn noi′a
au tot′o my
au″to top ag no′si a
au″to trans form′er
au″to trans fu′sion
au″to trans″plan ta′tion
au′to troph
au″to vac″ci na′tion
au″to vac′cine
aux an′o gram
aux″a nog′ra phy
aux e′sis
aux et′ic
aux″o bar′ic
aux″o car′di a
aux′o chrome
aux′o cyte

aux′o drome
aux om′e ter
av′a lanche
a val′vu lar
a vas′cu lar
a vas″cu lar i za′tion
a ve′nin
A ven′tyl
av′er age
A′ver tin
a′vi an
a vid′i ty
a vir′u lent
a vi″ta min o′sis
a vo ca′li a
Avogadro′s law
av″oir du pois′
a vul′sion
ax″an thop′si a
ax″i a′tion
ax if′u gal
ax il′la
ax′ill ary
ax′is
ax″o den drit′ic
ax″o fu′gal
ax′oid
ax″o lem′ma
ax om′e ter
a za cy′ti dine
ax′on
ax′o neme″
ax″o nom′e ter
ax″on ot me′sis
ax op′e tal
ax′ o plasm″
Ayerza′s
dis ease′
a yp′ ni a
a ze′ o trope
az′ide
az′ine
az″o ben′zene
az″o car′mine
az′o dyes
a zo″o sper′mi a
az″o pro′te in
az o ru′bin
az″o te′mi a
Az″o to bac′ter
az″o tom′e ter
az″o tor rhe′a
az″o tu′ri a
az′ure
a zu′ro phile″
az″y go ag′na thus
a″zyg og′raphy
az′y gos
a zy′mi a
a zym′ic

B

Babinski sign
Ba be′sia
ba be′si o sis
ba′by
bac′ci form
bac′il lar″y
bac″il le′mi a
ba cil′li
ba cil′li form
ba cil″lo my′cin
ba cil″lo pho′bi a
bac″il lu′ri a
ba cil′lus
ba″ci tra′cin
back′ache″
back′bone″
back′ward ness
bac′lo fen
bac″te re′mi a
bac te′ri a

Bac te″ri a′ce ae
bac te ri cid′al
bac te′ri cide
bac″te ri ci′din
bac′te rid
bac ter″i o chlor′o phyll
bac te″ri o ci′din
bac te″ri oc′la sis
bac te″ri o er′y thrin
bac te″ri o flu″o res′cin
bac te″ri o gen′ic
bac te″ri o he″mo ly′sin
bac te′ri oid
bac te″ri o log′ic
bac te″ri ol′o gist
bac te″ri ol′o gy
bac te″ri o ly′sin
bac te″ri ol′y sis
bac te′ri o phage
bac te″ri o phag′ic
bac te″ri o pha gol′o gy
bac te″ri o pho′bi a
bac te″ri o pro′te in
bac te″ri op′so nin
bac te″ri os′co py
bac te″ri os′ta sis
bac te′ri o stat″
bac te″ri o stat′ic
bac te″ri o ther a peu′tic
bac te″ri o ther′a py
bac te″ri o tox′ic
bac te″ri o tox′in
bac te″ri o trop′ic
bac te″ri ot′ro pin
Bac te′ri um
bac te″ri u′ri a
bac′ter oid
Bac″ter o′i des
baf′ fle
ba″gas so′sis
Ba hi′a ul′cer
Baker′s cyst

BAL
bal′ance
ba lan′ic
bal′a nism
bal″a ni′tis
bal″a no chlam″y di′tis
bal′a no plas″ty
bal″a no pos thi′tis
bal″a no pre pu′tial
bal″a nor rha′gi a
bal″an or rhe′a
bal″an ti di′a sis
Bal″an tid′i um
bal′a nus
bald′ness
Bal′four
bal′lism
bal lis″to car′di o gram
bal lis″to car′di o graph
bal lis″to pho′bi a
bal lonne ment′
bal loon′ing
bal lotte ment′
balm
bal″ne ol′o gy
bal″ne o ther′a py
bal′sam
band′age
Bandl′s ring
Bang′s dis ease′
ban′minth
ban′thine
Banti′s dis ease′
Banting
bar″ag no′sis
barb
bar′ba
bar″bar a la′li a
bar′bi tal
bar′bi tone
bar bit′u rate
bar″bi tu ric

bar′bi tu rism
bar bo tage′
bar″es the′si a
bar″es the″si om′e ter
bar″i to′sis
ba′ri um
bar′ley
barn
bar″o cep′tor
bar″o don tal′gi a
bar″og no′sis
bar′o graph
bar″o ma crom′e ter
bar o met′ric
bar″o pho′bi a
bar″ o re cep″ tor
bar′o scope
ba ros′min
bar″o tal′gi a
bar″o ti′tis
bar″o trau′ma
bar′ren ness
bar′ri er
Bartholin's gland
bar″tho lin i′tis
bar″to nel lo′sis
bar″y la′li a
bar″y pho′ni a
ba′sal
bas″ cu la′tion
bas′cule
base
base′ment
bas-fond
ba″si al ve′o lar
ba″si bran′chi al
ba″si chro′ma tin
ba sic′i ty
ba″si cra′ni al
ba sid′i o phore″
ba sid′i o spore″
ba sid′i um
ba″si fa′cial
ba″si hy′al
ba′si lar
ba″si lat′er al
ba sil′ic
ba sil″o breg mat′ic
ba sil″o men′tal
ba sil″o pha ryn′ge al
ba″si na′sal
ba″si o al ve′o lar
ba″si oc cip′i tal
ba′si on
ba′si o tribe″
ba′si o trip″sy
ba″si pho′bi a
ba″si pre sphen′oid
ba″si rhi′nal
ba′sis
ba″si sphe′noid
ba″si syl′vi an
ba″si tem′po ral
ba″si ver′te bral
bas′ket
ba′so phil
ba″so phil′i a
ba″so phil′ic
ba soph′i lism
ba″so pho′bi a
ba″so pho′bic
ba′so plasm
bas″si net′
bath
bath″es the′si a
bath″o pho′bi a
bath″y car′di a
bath″y chro′mic
bat″o pho′bi a
bat′ta rism
bat′ter ed
bat′ter y
baux′ite

BCG
bead'ed
beam
beat
bed'bug"
bed'fast"
Bednar's
aph'thae
bed'pan"
bed'rid"den
bed'sore"
be ha'vi or"ism
bel
bel'che
bel'la don'na
bel len'gol
bel lones'
bel'ly
bel'ly ache"
bel"o ne pho'bi a
Ben'a dryl
Bence-Jones's pro'te in
Bender-Gestalt
bends
Benedict's re a'gent
be'nign
Ben'tyl
benz'a thine
ben'ze drine
ben'zene
ben'zi dine
ben'zo ate
ben'zo di az"e pine
ben zo'ic
ben'zo ic ac'id
ben'zo in
ben'zyl
Ber'i-Ber'i
be ryl"li o'sis
be ryl'li um
bes"ti al'i ty
be'ta
be'ta cism
be'ta ine
be"ta to'pic
be'ta tron
be'tel
be'va tron
bev'el
be'zoar
bi ax'i al
bib'li o clast"
bib"li o klep"to ma'ni a
bib"li o ma'ni a
bib"li o pho'bi a
bib"li o ther'a py
bi cap'i tate
bi car'bon ate
bi car'di o gram
bi'ceps
bi chlo'ride
bi chro'mate
bi cil'lin
bi cor'nate
bi cus'pid
bi dac'ty ly
bi"e lec trol'y sis
bi fa scic'u lar block
bi'fid
bi fo'cal
bi for'min
bi'fur cate
bi"fur ca'tion
bi gem'i nal
bi gem'i ny
bi'labe
bi lat'er al
bile
bil"har zi'a sis
bil'i ar"y
bi lig'u late
bil"i hu'min
bil"i neu'rine
bil'ious

bil'ious ness
bil"i pha'in
bil"i ru'bin
bil"i ru"bi ne'mi a
bil'i ru"bin-glo'bin
bil"i ru"bi nu'ri a
bil"i ther a'py
bil"i u'ri a
bil"i ver'din
Billroth op"e ra'tion
bi lo'bate
bi loc'u lar
bil'ron
bi man'u al
bi'na ry
bi na'sal
bin au'ral
bind'er
Binet's test
bin oc'u lar
bi'o as say"
bi"o aut og'ra phy
bi'o blast
bi"o chem'i cal
bi"o chem'is try
bi'o chrome
bi"o dy nam'ic
bi"o-e lec"tric'i ty
bi'o feed' back
bi"o flav'o noids
bi"o gen'e sis
bi og'en ous
bi"o ki net'ics
bi'o lac
bi o log'ic
bi"o log'i cal
bi ol'o gist
bi ol'o gy
bi"o lu"mi nes'cense
bi"o math"e mat'ics
bi"o me chan'ics
bi om'e ter
bi om'e try
bi"o mi cros'co py
bi'o phore
bi"o pho tom'e ter
bi"o phys'ics
bi op'la sis
bi'op sy
bi'ose
bi"o sta tis'tics
bi"o syn'the sis
Biot's breath'ing
bi ot'ic
bi'o tin
bi'o type
bi"o ty pol'o gy
bip'a ra
bi par"a sit'ic
bi"pa ri'e tal
bip'a rous
bi'ped
bi ped'al
bi pen'ni form
bi po'lar
bi"po lar'i ty
bi"po ten"ti al'i ty
bi"re frac'tive
bi"re frin'gence
bi rhin'i a
bi ri'mose
birth
birth'mark"
birth rate
bi sex'u al
bis fe'ri ous
bis il'i ac
bis is'chi al
bis'muth
bis mu'thi a
bis"muth o'sis
bis'sa

bis″sy no′sis
bis′tou ry
bi sul′fide
bi sul′fite
bite′wing
bi thi′o nal
Bitot's spots
bit′ters
bi tu′men
bi″u ret′re ac′tion
biv′a lence
bi va′lent
bi′valve″
bi ven′ter
black′damp″
black′head″
black′leg″
black′out″
black′tongue″
blad′der
Blalock,
Alfred
blas te′ma
blas′tin
blas′to chyle
blas′to coele
blas′to cyst
blas′to derm
blas′to disk
blas″to gen′e sis
blas tog′e ny
blas″to ki ne′sis
blas tok′o lin
blas tol′y sis
blas to′ma
blas tom″a to gen′ic
blas′to mere
Blas″to my′ces
Blas″to my ce′tes
blas″to my co′sis
blas″to neu′ro pore
blas′to pore
blas′to sphere
blas′to spore
blas tot′o my
blas′tu la
bleb
bleed′er
blen″noph thal′mi a
blen″nor rha′gi a
blen″nor rhe′a
Ble o my′cin
bleph″ar ad″e ni′tis
bleph′a ral
bleph″a rec′to my
bleph″ar e de′ma
bleph″ar e lo′sis
bleph′a rism
bleph″ar it′is
bleph″a ro ad″e ni′tis
bleph″a ro ad″e no′ma
bleph″a ro ath″er o′ma
bleph″a ro blen″nor rhe′a
bleph″a ro chal′a sis
bleph″a ro chrom″hi dro′sis
bleph″a ro clei′sis
bleph″a roc′lo nus
bleph″a ro col″o bo′ma
bleph″a ro con junc″ti vi′tis
bleph″a ro di as′ta sis
bleph″a ro dys chroi′a
bleph″a ro me las′ma
bleph′a ron
bleph″a ron′cus
bleph″a ro pa chyn′sis
bleph″a ro phi mo′sis
bleph″a roph ry plas′ric
bleph″a roph′ry plas′ty
bleph″a ro phy′ma
bleph′a ro plast″
bleph′a ro plas″ty
bleph″a ro ple′gi a
bleph″a rop to′sis
bleph″a ro py″or rhe′a

bleph″a ror′rha phy
bleph′a ro spasm″
bleph″a ro sphinc″ter ec′to my
bleph′a ro stat″
bleph″a ro ste no′sis
bleph″a ro sym′phy sis
bleph″a ro syn ech′i a
bleph″a rot′o my
bleph″so path′i a
blight
blind′ness
blink′ing
blis′ter
bloat
blood
blow′fly″
Bodansky's meth′od
bod′y
Boeck's sar′coid
boil
bo lom′e ter
bo′lus
Bon′a mine
bo′rate
bo′rax
bor″bo ryg′mus
bor′der
bo′ric ac′id
bo′ron
Bor re′li a
bot′a ny
bot′fly″
both′ri oid
both′ri um
bot′ry oid
bot″ry o my co′sis
bot′u li form
bot u li′nus
bot′u lism
bou″gie′
bouil″lon′
bour′bo nac
bour donne ment′
bo′vine
bow′el
bow′leg″
brace
bra′chi a
bra′chi al
bra″chi al′gi a
bra″chi a′lis
bra′chi form
bra″chi o cyl lo′sis
brach″i o ra″di al′sis
bra″chi ot′o my
bra′chi um
brach″y car′di a
brach″y ce pha′li a
brach″y ce phal′ic
brach″y chei′li a
brach″y chei′rous
brach″y dac tyl′i a
brach″y glos′sal
brach″y glos′si a
brach″yg nath′ous
brach″y ker′kic
brach″y me tap′o dy
brach″y mei o′sis
brach″y morph′ic
brach″y mor′phy
brach″y pel′lic
brach″y pha lan′gi a
brach″y po′dous
brach″y pro sop′ic
brach″y rhin′i a
brach″y rhyn′chus
brach″y skel′ic
brach″y staph′y line
brach″y sta′sis
brach″y u ran′ic
brad″y ar′thri a
brad″y aux e′sis
brad″y car′di a

brad″y crot′ic
brad″y di as′to le
brad″y glos′si a
brad″y ki ne′si a
brad″y ki net′ic
bra″dy ki′nin
brad″y la′li a
brad′y lex′i a
brad″y pha′si a
brad″y phre′ni a
brad″y pne′a
brad″y pra′gi a
brad″y prax′i a
brad″y rhyth′mi a
brad″y tel″e o ki ne′sis
Braille, Louis
brain
bran′chi al
branch′ing
bran″chi o gen′ic
bran″chi og′e nous
bran″chi o′ma
bran′chi o mere″
bran″chi om′er ism
bran′dy
brawn′y
Braxton Hicks's con trac′tion
break′bone″ fe′ver
breast
breast′bone
breath
breath′ing
breech
breg′ma
breg mat′ic
breg mat″o dym′i a
Bre′thine
Bre tyl′i um
brev″i col′lis
brev″i lin′e al
bridge
bridge′work″
bri′dle
bright′ness
bril′liance
broach
Broadbent's sign
Broca, Pierre
Brodie's ab′scess
bro′mate
bro″ma tom′e try
bro″ma to ther′a py
bro″ma to tox′in
brom″hi dro′sis
bro′mide
bro′mine
bro′min ism
bro′mism
bro″mo cre′sol green
Bro mo crip′tine
bro″mo der′ma
bro″mo hy″per hi dro′sis
bro″mo ma′ni a
bro″mo men″ or rhe′a
bro″mo phe′nol blue
Bro″mo Selt′zer
bro″mo thy′mol blue
Brom phen ir′a mine
brom″sul′pha lein
bronch ad″e ni′tis
bron′chi
bron′chi al
bron″chi ec′ta sis
bron″cho i o al ve′o lar
bron″chi o gen′ic
bron chi′o lar
bron′chi ole
bron″chi o lec′ta sis
bron″chi o li′tis
bron chit′ic
bron chi′tis
bron′cho cele″
bron″cho con stric′tor
bron″cho dil″a ta′tion

bron″cho di la′tor
bron″ cho e de′ma
bron″cho e soph″a ge′al
bron″cho e soph″a gol′o gy
bron″cho e soph″a gos′co py
bron″cho gen′ic
bron′cho gram
bron chog′ra phy
bron′cho lith
bron″cho li thi′a sis
bron chol′o gy
bron″cho mo ni li′a sis
bron″cho mo′tor
bron″cho my co′sis
bron chop′a thy
bron choph′o ny
bron′cho plas″ty
bron″cho pleu′ral
bron″cho pneu mo′ni a
bron″cho pneu″mo ni′tis
bron″cho pul′mo na ry
bron chor′rha phy
bron″chor rhe′a
bron′cho scope
bron chos′copy
bron′cho spasm
bron″cho spi″ro che to′sis
bron″cho spi rog′ra phy
bron″cho spi rom′e ter
bron″cho spi rom′e try
bron″cho ste no′sis
bron chos′to my
bron chot′o my
bron″cho ve sic′u lar
bron′chus
bron″to pho′bi a
Brown-Séquard,
Charles E.
Bru cel′la
bru″cel ler′gen
bru cel′lin
bru″cel lo′sis
bruc′ine
Brudzinski's re′flex
bruise
bruisse ment′
bruit
brux′ism
brux″o ma′ni a
bryg′mus
bu′bo
bu″bon ad″e ni′tis
bu″bon al′gi a
bu bon′ic plague
bu bon′o cele
bu bon′u lus
bu car′di a
buc′ca
buc′cal
buc′ci na″tor
buc″co ax′i al
buc″coc clu′sal
buc″co cer′vi cal
buc″co dis′tal
buc″co fa′cial ob′tu ra″tor
buc″co gin′gi val
buc″co la′bi al
buc″co lin′gual
buc″co me′si al
buc″co na′sal
buc″co na″so pha ryn′ge al
buc″co pha ryn′ge al
buc″co phar yn′ge us
buc″co pulp′al
buc″co ver′sion
buc′cu la
Buerger's
dis ease′
bu′fa gins
buff′er
bug′gery
bulb
bul″bo cav″er no′sus
bul″bo nu′cle ar

bul″bo spon″gi o′sus
bul″bo u re′thral
bulb′ous
bul″bo ven tric′u lar
bul′bus
bul′bus ar te″ri o′sus
bul′bus cor′dis
bu le′sis
bu li″ma rex′i a
bu lim′i a
bu lim′ic
bul′la
bull′ae (pl.)
bul la′tion
bul′lous
bun′dle
bun′ion
bun″ion ec′to my
bu′no dont
buph thal′mi a
buph thal′mus
bur
bu ret′
burn
bur′nish er
bur′row
bur′sa
bur sat′tee
bursec′to my
bur si′tis
bur′so lith
bursop′a thy
bur sot′o my
bu spi′rone
bu″ta bar′bi tal
bu′ta caine″
bu″ta di ene
bu′tane
bu ti no phe′none
Bu′ti sol
but′ter
but′tock
but′tress
bu′tyl
bu tyr′ic
bu′tyr oid
bys″si no′sis
bys′soid

C

ca ca′o
ca chec′tic
ca chet′
ca chex′i a
cach″in na′tion
ca″chou′
cac″o de mo′ni a
cac′o dyl
cac′o dyl ate
cac o phon′ic
ca coph′o ny
ca cos′mi a
ca dav′er
ca dav′er ic
ca dav′erine
ca dav′er ous
cad′mi um
ca du′ce us
cae″ru lo plas′min
cafe′ au lait
caf′er gone
Caf′er got
caf′fe ine
caf′fe in ism
cai″no pho′bi a
cais′son
Cajal, Ramón
Cal′a bar swel′lings
ca lage′
cal′a mine
ca′la mus scrip to′ri us
cal ca′ne al

cal ca″ne o ca′vus
cal ca″ne o cu′boid
cal ca″ ne o dyn′i a
cal ca″ne o na vic′u lar
cal ca″ne o val′gus
cal ca′ne us
cal′car
cal car′e ous
cal car″i u′ri a
cal ce′mi a
cal′cic
cal″ci co′sis
cal cif′er ol
cal cif′ic
cal″ci fi ca′tion
cal′ci fied
cal′ci fy
cal cig′er ous
cal′ci grade
cal cim′e ter
cal″ci na′tion
cal″ci no′sis
cal″ci pe′ni a
cal″ci to′nin
cal′ ci um
cal″ci u′ri a
cal″co glob′u lin
cal″co sphe′rite
cal″cu lo gen′e sis
cal″cu lo′sis
cal′cu lous
cal′cu lus
cal″e fa′cient
calf
calf′-bone
cal′i brate
cal″i bra′tion
cal′i bra″tor
cal′i pers
cal″is then′ics
cal″li ec′ta sis
cal″li pe′di a
cal″lo ma′ni a
cal lo′ sal,
cal los′i tas
cal los′i ty
cal lo″so mar′gin al
cal lo′sum
cal′lous
cal′lus
cal′o mel
cal′or
cal″o ra′di ance
cal″o res′ cence
ca lor′ic
cal′o rie
cal″ o rif′ic
ca lor″i gen′ic
cal″o rim′e ter
ca lor″i met′ric
cal″o rim′e try
cal va′ri a
Calve,
Jacques
cal vi′ti es
cal′vous
calx
ca′lyx
cam′bi um
cam′er a
cam′i sole
cam′phene
cam′phor
cam″pho ra′ceous
cam′phor ate
cam′phor ism
cam″phor o ma′ni a
cam pim′e ter
camp″to cor′mi a
camp″to dac′ty ly
camp′to spasm
ca nal′
can″a lic′u lar
can″a lic′u li

can al ic″u lo plas′ty
can″a lic′u lus
ca nal″i za′tion
can″al og′ra phy
can′cel lous
can′cer
can″cer o′gen
can″cer ol′o gist
can″cer ol′o gy
can″cer o pho′bi a
can′croid
can′crum o′ris
can″di ci′din
Can′di da al′bi cans
can″di di′as is
can″di did′
can′dle
ca nel′la
ca′nine
ca ni′nus
ca ni′ti es
can′ker
can″na bid′i ol
can′na bine
can nab′in oc
can nab′i nol
can′na bis
Can′na bis sa ti′via
can′na bism
can″ni bal is′tic
can′nu la
can′nu lar
can″tha ri′a sis
can thar′i des
can thec′to my
can thi′tis
can thol′y sis
can′tho plas″ty
can thor′rha phy
can thot′ o my
can′thus
can′ nu la″ tion
ca pac′i tance
ca pac′i tate
ca pac′i tor
ca pac′i ty
cap″il lar″ec ta′si a
cap″il la rim′e ter
cap″il lar′i ty
cap″il la ros′co py
cap′il lar″y
cap″il li′ti um
cap″il lo ve′nous
ca pil′lus
cap′i tate
cap″i ta″tum
cap″i tel′lum
ca pit′u lar
ca pit′u lum
cap′ra col
ca″pre o my′cin
cap′ric
ca pro′ic
ca pryl′ic
cap′su lar
cap′sule
cap″su lec′to my
cap″su li′tis
cap′su lo plas″ty
cap″su lor′rha phy
cap′su lo tome″
cap″su lot′o my
cap ta′tion
cap″ture
ca′put
car′a pace
car ba maz′e pine
car″ba mi no he″mo glo′bin
Car′bar sone
car′ba sus
carb he″me glo′bin
car′bi nol
car″bo cy′clic
car″bo hy′drase

car″bo hy′drate
car″bo hy″dra tu′ri a
car′bo late
car bol′ic
car′bo lism
car″bo lu′ri a
car bo my′cin
car′bon
car′bon ate
car′bon a″ted
car bo′nic
car bo′ni um
car″bon i za′tion
car′bon ize
car″ bon om′e ter
car″bon u′ri a
car″bo run′dum
carbo′wax
car box″y he″mo glo′bin
car box′yl
car box′yl ase
car′bun cle
car bun′cu lar
car′bun″cu lo′sis
car″ ci no em bry on′ ic
car cin′o gen
car″ci no gen′e sis
car″ci no gen′ic
car′ci noid
car″ci no′ma
car″ci nom′a toid
car″ci no″ma to′sis
car″ci no′ma tous
car″ci no sar co′ma
car′ci nous
car′di a
car′di ac
car″di al′gi a
car″di am′e ter
car″di a neu′ri a
car″di asth′ma
car″di ec′ta sis
car″di ec′to my
car″di o ac cel′er a″tor
car″di o ac′tive
car″di o an″gi ol′o gy
car″di o-a or′tic
car″di o ar te′ri al
car′di o cele
car″di o cen te′sis
car″di o cir rho′sis
car″di oc′la sis
car″di o di la′tor
car″di o di o′sis
car″di o dy nam′ics
car″di o dy″na mom′et ry
car″di o dyn′i a
car″di o e soph″a ge′al
car″di o gen′e sis
car″di o gen′ic
car′di o gram″
car′di o graph″
car″di o graph′ic
car″di og′ra phy
car″di o he pat′ic
car′di oid
car″di o in hib′i to″ry
car″di o ki net′ic
car″di o ky mog′ra phy
car″di o lip′in
car′di o lith
car″di ol′o gist
car″di ol′o gy
car″di ol′y sis
car″di o ma la′ci a
car″di o meg′a ly
car″di o mel″a no′sis
car″di o men′su ra tor
car″di o men′to pex″y
car″di om′e ter
car″di om′e try
car″di o my′o pex″y

car″di o my ot′o my
car″di o nec′tor
car″di o neph′ric
car″di o neu′ral
car″di o pal′u dism
car′di o path
car di o path′ic
car″di o pa thol′o gy
car″di op′a thy
car″di o per″i car′di o pex″y
car″di o per″i car di′tis
car″di o pho′bi a
car′di o phone
car′di o plas″ty
car″di o ple′gi a
car″di o pneu mat′ic
car″di o pneu′mo graph
car″di op to′sis
car″di o pul′mo nar y
car″di o punc′ture
car″di o py lor′ic
car″di o re′nal
car″di o re spir′a to″ry
car″di o roent′gen o gram″
car″di roent″gen og′ra phy
car″di or′rha phy
car″di or rhex′is
car″di os′chi sis
car′di o scope″
car′di o spasm″
car″di o spec′tro gram
car″di o spec′tro graph
car″di o ste no′sis
car″di o ta chom′e ter
car″di o ther′a py
car″di ot′o my
car″di o ton′ic
car″di o tox′ic
car″di o vas′cu lar
car″di o vas′cu lar-re′nal
car″di o vec tog′ra phy
car di o ver′sion
car di′tis
car″di val″vu li′tis
car″e bar′i a
ca′ri es
ca ri′na
car″i o gen′ic
car min′a tive
car′mine
car″ni fi ca′tion
car″no si ne′mi a
car′ob
car′o tene
car″o te ne′mi a
car″o te″no der′ma
ca rot′e noid
car″o te no′sis
ca rot′ic
ca rot″i co cli′noid
ca rot″i co tym pan′ic
ca rot′id
ca rot′is
car″ot o dyn′i a
car′pal
car pec′to my
car phol′o gy
car pi′tis
car″po met″a car′pal
car″po pe′dal
car″po pha lan′ge al
car′pus
car′ri er
car sick′ness
car′ti lage
car″ti la gin″i fi
ca′tion
car″ti lag′in ous
car′un cle
car un′cu lar
car″y o clas′tic
car″y o phyl′lin
cas car′a
case

ca′se ase
ca′se ate
ca″se a′tion
ca′sec
ca′se in
ca″se in′o gen
ca′se ose
ca′se ous
cas″sette′
cast
cast′ing
cas′tor
cas′trate
cas tra′tion
cas″tro phre′ni a
cas′u al ty
cas″u is′tics
cat″a ba′si al
ca tab′a sis
cat a bol′ic
ca tab′o lin
ca tab′o lism
ca tab′o lite
cat″a clo′nic
cat″ a clo′nus
cat″a cous′tics
cat″a crot′ic
cat ac′ro tism
cat″a gel″o pho′bi a
cat′a lase
cat′a lep″sy
cat a lep′tic
cat″a lep″to le thar′gic
ca tal′y sis
cat′a lyst
cat″a lyt′ic
cat′a ly″zer
cat″a me′ni a
cat″am ne′sis
cat″am nes′tic
cat″a mor′pho sis
cat′a pasm
cat″a pha′si a
ca taph′o ra
cat″a pho re′sis
cat″a pho′ri a
cat″a phor′ic
cat″a phy lax′is
cat″a pla′si a
cat′a plasm
cat″a plec′tic
cat′a plex″y
cat′a ract
ca tarrh′
ca tarrh′al
cat″a stal′sis
cat′a state
cat″a thy′mi a
cat″a to′ni a
cat″a ton′ic
cat″a tro′pi a
cat′e chol″am′ines
cat″e lec″trot′o nus
cat′er pil″lar
cat′gut″
ca thar′sis
ca thar′tic
ca thect′
ca thep′sin
ca ther′e sis
cath″e ret′ic
cath′e ter
cath′e ter ism
cath″e ter i za′tion
cath′e ter ize
cath′e ter o stat″
ca thex′is
cath′od al
cath′ode
ca thod′ic
cat′i″on
cat ion′ic

cat′lin
cat′a dont
ca top′trics
ca top′tro scope
cau′da
cau′dad
cau′dal
cau da′tum
cau″do ceph′al ad
caul
cau′line
cau″lo ple′gi a
cau″mes the′si a
cau sal′gi a
cause
caus′tic
cau′ter ant
cau″ter i za′tion
cau′ter ize
cau′ter y
ca′va
cav′al ry bone
cav′ern
car″ern i′tis
cav″er no′ma
cav″er no si′tis
cav er nos′to my
cav″er no′sum
cav′er nous
cav′i tas
cav″i ta′tion
cav′i ty
ca′vus
ce″bo ce pha′li a
ce″bo ceph′ a lus
ce″bo ceph′a ly
ce cec′to my
ce ci′tis
ce′ci ty
ce′co cele
ce″co co los′to my
ce″co il″e os′to my
ce′co pex″y
ce″co pli ca′tion
ce″cop to′sis
ce cor′rha phy
ce″co sig″moid os′to my
ce cos′to my
ce cot′o my
ce′cum
ce′dar
Ce″di lan′id
ce′li ac
ce″li a del′phus
ce″li ec ta′si a
ce″li o col pot′o my
ce″li o en″ter ot′o my
ce″li o gas trot′o my
ce″li o hys″ter ec′to my
ce″li o hys″ter ot′o my
ce″li o my″o mec′to my
ce″li o par″a cen te′sis
ce″li or′rha phy
ce″li os′co py
ce″li ot′o my
ce li′tis
cell
cel′la
cel loi′din
Cel′lo phane
cell′u lar
cel′lu lase
cel′lule
cel″lu lif′ u gal
cel″lu li′tis
cel′lu lo′sa
cel′lu lose
ce′lo scope
ce″lo so′ma
ce″lo so′mus
ce″lo the″li o′ma
ce ment′

ce men′ti cle
ce men″ti fi ca′tion
ce men′to blast
ce men″to blas to′ma
ce men″to den′ti nal
ce men″to gen′e sis
ce″men to′ma
ce men″to per″i os ti′tis
ce″men to′sis
ce men′tum
ce″nes the′si a
ce″nes thet′ic
ce″nes thop′a thy
ce″no gen′e sis
cen′sor ship
cen′ter
cen′ter ing
cen te′sis
cen′ti bar
cen′ti grade
cen′ti gram
cen′ti li″ter
cen′ti me″ter
cen″ti nor′mal
cen′ti pede
cen′ti poise
cen′trad
cen′trage
cen′tra phose
cen″trax o′ni al
cen″tren ce phal′ic
cen tric′i put
cen trif′u gal
cen′tri fuge
cen′tri ole
cen trip′e tal
cen′tro cyte
cen″tro des′mose
cen″tro lec′i thal
cen′tro mere
cen′tro phose
cen′tro some
cen′tro sphere″
cen′trum
ceph′al
ceph′al ad
ceph″a lal′gi a
ceph′a lal″gic
ceph″a le′a
ceph″ al he″ ma to′ ma
ceph a lex′in
ceph″al′gi a
ceph″al he″ma to′ma
ceph″al hy′dro cele
ce phal′ic
ceph′a lin
ceph″a li za′tion
ceph″a lo cau′dal
ceph′a lo cele″
ceph″a lo cen te′sis
ceph′a lo chord″
ceph″a lo di pro′so pus
ceph″a lo gen′e sis
ceph″a lo gly′cin
ceph′a lo graph″
ceph″a log′ra phy
ceph″a lo gy′ric
ceph″a lo he mat′o cele″
ceph″a lo he mom′e ter
ceph′a loid
ceph a lo′ma
ceph″a lom′e lus
ceph″a lo me′ni a
ceph″a lo men″in gi′tis
ceph″a lom′e ter
ceph″a lom′e try
ceph″a lo′ni a
ceph″a lo-or′bi tal
ceph″a lop′a gus
ceph″a lop′a thy
ceph″a lo pel′vic
ceph″a lo pha ryn′ge us

ceph″a lo ple′gi a
ceph″a los′co py
ceph″a lo spo′rin
ceph″a lo spo″ri o′sis
Ceph″a lo spo′ri um
ceph″a lo tho rac′ic
ceph″a lo tho″ra cop′a gus
ceph′a lo tome
ceph″a lot′o my
ceph″a lo trac′tor
ceph′a lo tribe
ceph″a lo trid′y mus
ceph′a lo trip″sy
ceph″a lo trip′tor
ceph″a lo try pe′sis
ceph″a lox′i a
cer″a to cri′coid
cer″a to phar yn′ geus
cer ca′ri a
cer ca′ri al
cer clage′
ce′re a flex″i bil′i tas
cer″e bel′lar
cer″e bel lif′u gal
cer″e bel lip′e tal
cer″e bel li′tis
cer″e bel lo pon′tine
car″e bel lo ret′i nal he″man gi
o blas″to ma to′sis
cer″e bel″lo ru′bral
cer″e bel″lo ru″bro spi′nal
cer″e bel″lo spi′nal
cer″e bel′lum
cer′e bral
cer″e bra′tion
cer′e bric
cer″e brif′u gal
cer′e brin
cer″e brip′e tal
cer″e bri′tis
cer″e bro ma la′ci a
cer″e bro med′ul lar″y
cer″e bro phys″i ol′o gy
cer″e bro pon′tine
cer″e bro scle ro′sis
cer′e brose
cer′e bro side
cer″e bro spi′nal
cer″e bro to′ni a
cer″e bro to′nin
cer″e bro vas′cu lar
cer′e brum
ce′re ous
ce′ri um
ce′roid
ce ro′sis
cer′ti fi″a ble
cer tif′i cate
ce′ru lo″plas min
ce ru′men
ce ru″ mi no′ ma
ce ru″mi no′sis
ce ru′min ous
cer′vi cal
cer″vi cec′to my
cer″vi ci′tis
cer″vi co ax′i al
cer″vi co brach′i al″gi a
cer″vi co buc′cal
cer″vi co buc″co ax′i al
cer″vi co dyn′i a
cer″vi co fa′cial
cer″vi co la′bi al
cer″vi co lin′gual
cer″vi co pu′bic
cer″vi co rec′tal
cer″vi co u′ter ine
cer″vi co vag′i nal
cer″vi co vag″i ni′tis
cer″vi co ves′i cal
cer′vix
Ce sar′e an sec′tion

Ces to′da
ces′tode
ce″vi tam′ic ac′id
Chadwick′s sign
chae to′min
cha′fing
Chagas′ dis ease′
cha la′si a
cha la′za
cha la′zi a
cha la′zi on
chal co′sis
chal″i co′sis
chalk
chal′one
cha lyb′e ate
cham′ber
cham″e ceph′a lus
cham″e ceph′a ly
cham′e conch″
cham″e cra′ni al
cham″e pro sop′ic
chan′cre
chan′croid
chan croi′dal
chan′nel
chap
char′ac ter
char′coal″
Charcot′s joint
Charcot-Marie-Tooth dis ease′
charge
char′la tan
char′la tan ism
char′ley horse
char′tu la
chaul moo′gra oil
cheek
cheek′bone″
chees′y
chei lal′gi a
chei lec′to my
chei″lec tro′pi on
chei li′tis
chei″lo an′gi o scope″
chei log′na tho pal″a tos′chi sis
chei log″na tho pros″o pos′chi
sis
chei log′na tho u″ra nos′chi sis
chei′lo plas″ty
chei lor′rha phy
chei los′chi sis
chei lo′sis
chei los″to mat′o plas″ty
chei lot′o my
chei″ma pho′bi a
che′late
che′lat ing
che la′tion
chem′i cal
chem″i co cau′ter y
chem″i lu″mi nes′cence
chem″i o tax′is
chem′ist
chem′is try
che″mo bi ot′ic
chem′o cep″tor
chem″o co ag″u la′tion
chem″o dec to′ma
chem″o pro″phy lax′sis
chem′o re cep″tor
chem″o re′flex
che mo′sis
chem′o stat
chem″o sur′ger y
chem″o tax′is
chem″o ther′a py
che″mo troph′
che″mo troph′ic
che mot′ro pism
chem′ur gy
Che″no po′di um

che′o plas ty
cher″o ma′ni a
cher″o pho′bi a
cher′ry
cher′u bism
chest
Cheyne-Stokes res″pi ra′tion
Chiari's net′work
chi′asm
chi as′ma
chi as′mal
chi as′ma ta
chick′en pox″
chig′ger
chil′blain″
child
child′bed″
child′birth″
child′crow″ing
chill
chi′mer ism
chin′i o fon
chi″o na blep′si a
chi″o no pho′bi a
chi rag′ra
chi ral′gi a
chi rap′si a
chi′rap sy
chi″rar thri′tis
chi ris′mus
chi″ro kin″es thet′ic
chi rol′o gy
chi″ro meg′a ly
chi′ro plas″ty
chi rop′o dist
chi rop′o dy
chi″ro pom′pho lyx
chi″ro prac′tic
chi′ro prac tor
chi′ro scope
chi′ro spasm
chi′tin
chi′tin ous
chlam′ y di al
chlam′y do spore″
chlo as′ma
chlor ac′ne
chlor bu′ta nol
chlo′ral
chlor″am phen′i col
chlo″ra ne′mi a
chlo′rate
chlor′dane
chlor′ di az″ e pos′ ide
chlor hy′dri a
chlo′ric
chlo′ride
chlo″ri du′ri a
chlo′ri nat″ed
chlo″rin a′tion
chlo′rine
chlo′rite
chlo″ ro cy′ cli zine
chlo′ro form
chlo′ro form ism
chlo″ro form″i za′tion
chlo ro′ma
Chlo″ro my cet′in
chlo″ro per′cha
chlo′ro phyll
chlo′ro plast
chlo″ro plas′tin
chlo rop′si a
Chlo′ro quin
chlo ro′sis
chlo rot′ic
chlor pro′ma zine
chlor″tet ra cy′cline
Chlor-tri′me ton
cho′a na
cho′a nal
choke

chol′a gogue
chol″an gi ec′ta sis
chol″an″gi o car″ci no′ma
chol″an″gi o gas tros′to my
chol″an gi og′ra phy
chol an″gi o li′tis
cho lan″gi o′ma
chol″an gi os′to my
chol″an gi ot′o my
chol″an gi′tis
chol″e bil″i ru′bin
chole″e cal cif′er ol
chol″e chrom e re′sis
chol″e chro″mo poi e′sis
chol″e chry″o cy to′sis
chol″e cy′a nin
chol′e cyst
chol″e cyst′a gogue
chol″e cyst al′gi a
chol″e cyst ec ta′si a
chol″e cyst ec′to my
chol″e cyst en″ter or′rha phy
chol″e cyst en″ter os′to my
chol e cys′tic
chol″e cys ti′tis
chol″e cys″to co los′to my
chol″e cys″to du″o de′nal
chol″e cys″to e lec″tro co ag″u
lec′to my
chol″e cys″to gas tros′to my
chol″e cys′to gram
chol″e cystog′ra phy
chol″e cys″to il e os′to my
chol″e cys″to jej″u nos′to my
chol″e cys″to ki net′ic
chol″e cys″to ki′nin
chol″e cys″to li thi′a sis
chol″e cys″to lith ot′o my
chol″e cys′to pex″y
chol″e cys tor′rha phy
chol″e cys tos′to my
chol″e cys tot′o my
cho led′o chal
cho led″o chec ta′si a
cho led″o chec′to my
cho led″o chi′tis
cho led″o cho do chor′rha phy
cho led″o cho du″o de nos′to
my
cho led″o cho en″ter os′to my
cho led″o cho gas tros′to my
cho led″o cho lith i′a sis
cho led″o cho li thot′o my
cho led″o cho lith′o trip″sy
cho led″o cho plas′ty
cho led″o chor′rha phy
cho led″o chos′to my
cho led″o chot′o my
cho led′o chus
cho′ le dyl
chol″e glo′bin
chol″e he′ma tin
cho le′ic
chol′e lith
chol″e li thi′a sis
chol″e li thot′o my
chol″e lith′o trip″sy
cho lem′e sis
cho le′mi a
cho le′mic
chol″e poi e′sis
chol″e poi et′ic
chol″e pra′sin
chol″e pyr′thin
chol′era
chol er a′ic
chol er e′sis
chol′er ic
chol′er i form″
chol″er i za′tion
chol′er oid
chol″er o pho′bi a

chol″er rha′gi a
cho″les cin′ti gram
cho le sta′sis
cho les″te a to′ma
cho les″te a to′ma tous
cho les″te a to′sis
cho les′ter ase
cho les″ter i nu′ri a
cho les′ter ol
cho les′ter ol ase″
cho les″ter ol er′e sis
cho les″ter ol o poi e′sis
cho les″ter o′sis
cho′lic
cho′line
cho″lin er′gic
cho″lin es′ter ase
chol′o chrome
chol′o gogue
chol′o lith
chol or rhe′a
cho lu′ri a
chon′dral
chon drec′to my
chon′dri fy
chon′dri gen
chon′drin
chon′dri o cont″
chon′dri o gene″
chon″dri o kin e′sis
chon′dri ome
chon dri′tis
chon″dro al bu′mi noid
chon′dro blast
chon″dro blas to′ma
chon″dro cal ci no′sis
chon″dro car″ci no′ma
chon dro cla′sis
chon′dro clast
chon″dro cos′tal
chon″dro cra′ni um
chon′dro cyte
chon″dro der″ma ti′tis
chon″dro dys pla′si a
chon″dro dys tro′phi a
chon″dro dys′tro phy
chon″dro ec″to der′mal
chon″dro ep″i tro chle′a ris
chon″dro fi bro′ma
chon″dro fi″bro sar co′ma
chon′dro gen
chon″dro gen′e sis
chon drog′e nous
chon″dro glos′sus
chon″dro hu mer al′is
chon′droid
chon dro′i tin
chon″dro lip″o sar co′ma
chon dro′ma
chon″dro ma la′ci a
chon″dro ma to′sis
chon dro′ma tous
chon′dro mere
chon″dro mu′coid
chon″dro myx o hem an″gi o end″o the″li o sar co′ma
chon″dro myx o′ma
chon″dro myx″o sar co′ma
chon″dro os″te o dys′tro phy
chon″dro-os″te o′ma
chon″dro-os″te o sar co′ma
chon drop′a thy
chon″dro pha ryn′ge us
chon′dro plast
chon′dro plas″ty
chon″dro po ro′sis
chon″dro pro′te in
chon″dro sar co′ma
chon′dro sin
chon dro′sis
chon″dro ster′nal
chon′dro tome

chon drot′o my
chor′da
chor″da blas′to pore
chor′dae ten dine′ a e
chor′dal
chor″da mes′o blast
chor″da mes′o derm
Chor da′ta
chor′date
chor dee′
chord″en ceph′a lon
chor di′tis
chor do′ma
chor dot′o my
cho re′a
cho′re al
cho re′i form
cho″re o ath′e toid
cho″re o ath″e to′sis
cho″ri o ad″e no′ma
cho″ri o al″lan to′ic
cho″ri o al lan′to sis
cho″ri o an″gi op′a gus
chor″i o blas to′sis
cho″ri o cap″il la′ris
cho″ri o car″ci no′ma
cho′ri o cele
cho″ri o ep″i the″li o′ma
cho″ri o gen′e sis
cho′ri oid
cho″ri o′ma
cho″ri o men″in gi′tis
cho′ri on
cho″ri on ep″i the″li o′ma
cho″ri o ni′tis
cho″ri o ret′i nal
cho″ri o ret″i ni′tis
cho″ri o ret″in op′a thy
chor′i sis
cho ris″to blas to′ma
cho″ri sto′ma
cho′roid
cho roi′dal
cho″roid e re′mi a
cho″roid i′tis
cho roi″do cy cli′tis
cho roi″do i ri′tis
cho roi″do ret″i ni′tis
chre″ma to pho′bi a
chro maf′fin
chro″maf fi no′ma
chro maf″fi nop′a thy
chro′ma phil
chro′ma phobe
chro ma′si a
chro′mate
chro″ma te lop′si a
chro mat′ic
chro mat′ic ness
chro′ma tid
chro′ma tin
chro″ma to der″ma to′sis
chro″ma to dys o′pi a
chro″ma tog′e nous
chro mat′o gram
chro″ma to graph′ic
chro″ma tog′ra phy
chro″ma tol′o gy
chro″ma tol′y sis
chro″ma to lyt′ic
chro mat′o mere
chro″ma tom′e ter
chro″ma tom′e try
chro″ma top′a thy
chro′ma to phil
chro″ma to pho′bi a
chro′ma to phore″
chro″ma toph′o rous
chro′ma to plasm
chro′ma to plast
chro″ma top′si a
chro″ma top tom′e try

chro″ma to′sis
chrome
chrom″hi dro′sis
chro′mic
chro′mi cize
chro mid′i um
chro′mi um
Chro″mo bac te′ri um
chro′mo blast
chro″mo blas″to my co′sis
chro′mo cen″ter
chro″mo crin′i a
chro″mo cys tos′co py
chro′mo cyte
chro″mo dac″ry or rhe′a
chro′mo gen
chro″mo gen′e sis
chro″mo gen′ic
chro′mo mere
chro″mo ne′ma
chro″mo par′ic
chro′mo phane
chro′mo phil
chro′mo phobe
chro″mo pho′bi a
chro″mo pho′bic
chro′mo phore
chro″mo phor′ic
chro′mo phose
chro″mo phy to′sis
chro′mo plasm
chro′mo plast
chro″mo pro′te in
chro mop′si a
chro″mop tom′e ter
chro mos′co py
chro″mo so′mal
chro′mo some
chro′nax ie
chron″ax im′e ter
chron′ic
chron ic′i ty
chron′o graph
chro nom′e try
chron″o pho′bi a
chron′o scope
chron″o trop′ic
chrys′a lis
chry′sene
chry si′a sis
chrys″o cy″a no′sis
Chry′sops
chry″so ther′a py
chrys″o tox′in
Chvostek's sign
chyl an″gi o′ma
chyle
chy le′mi a
chy″li dro′sis
chy′lo cele
chy″lo der′ma
chy′loid
chy″lo mi′crons
chy″lor rhe′a
chy″lo tho′rax
chy′lous
chy lu′ri a
chyme
chy′mo sin
chy″mo sin′o gen
chy″mo tryp′sin
chy″mo tryp sin′o gen
chy′mous
ci bis′o tome
ci″bo pho′bi a
cic″a tric′ial
cic′a trix
ci cat′ri zant
cic″a tri za′tion
cic′a trize
cic′er ism
cil′i a

cil″i ar′i scope
cil″i ar ot′o my
cil′i ary
cil″i ate′
cil″i at′ed
cil″i o scle′ral
cil lo′sis
ci met′ i dine
cin cho′na
cin chon′ic
ci″ne an′gi o gram
cin″e flu″o rog′ra phy
ci ni′re a
cin″e roent″gen og′ra phy
cin′gu late
cin″gu lec′to my
cin″gu lo trac′to my
cin′gu lum
cin nam′ic
cin′na mon
cir′ci nate
cir′cle
cir′cuit
cir′cu lar
cir″cu la′tion
cir′cu la to″ry
cir′cu lin
cir′cu lus
cir″cum a′nal
cir″cum ar tic′u lar
cir″cum ci′sion
cir″cum cor′ne al
cir″cum duc′tion
cir′cum flex
cir″cum in′su lar
cir″cum len′tal
cir″cum nu′cle ar
cir″cum o′ral
cir″cum po″lar i za′tion
cir″cum scribed′
cir″cum stan″ti al′i ty
cir″cum val′late
cir″cum vas′cu lar
cir rho′sis
cir rhot′ic
cir′rus
cir sec′to my
cir′soid
cir som′pha los
cir″soph thal′mi a
cir sot′o my
cis′sa
cis′tern
cis ter′na
cis ter′ no gram
cis ves′ti tism
cit′rate
cit′ric ac′id
cit′rin
cit″ron el′la oil
cit rul′line
ci″trul li ne′mi a
cit″rul lin u′ria
cit′rus
cit to′sis
clair voy′ance
clamp
cla′po
clap′ping
cla rif′i cant
clar″i fi ca′tion
clas mat′o cyte
clas″mo cy to′ma
clas′tic
clau″di ca′tion
claus″tro phil′i a
claus″tro pho′bi a
claus′trum
cla′va
clav′a cin
cla′val
cla′vate

clav″e li za′tion
clav′i cle
clav″i cot′o my
cla vic′u lar
cla vic′u late
cla vic″u lec′to my
cla′vus
claw′foot″
claw′hand″
clear′ance
cleav′age
cleft
clei′dal
clei″do cos′tal
clei″do cra′ni al
clei″do hu′mer al
clei″do hy′oid
clei′do ic
clei″do mas′toid
clei″do-oc cip′i tal
clei″do scap′u lar
clei″do ster′nal
clei dot′o my
clei″thro pho′bi a
cle′oid
cli′er
cli″ma co pho′bi a
cli mac′ter ic
cli′mate
cli″ma tol′o gy
cli″ma to ther′a py
cli′max
clin′ic
clin′i cal
cli ni′cian
clin″i co hem″a to log′ic
clin″i co pa thol′o gy
clin″i co roent″gen o log′ic
Cli′ni stix
cli″no ceph′a lus
cli″no ceph′a ly
cli″no dac′ty ly
cli′noid
cli nom′e ter
cli′no scope
clip
clis″e om′e ter
clit′i on
clit″o ral′gi a
clit″o ri daux′e
cli″to rid e′an
clit″o ri dec′to my
clit″o ri di′tis
clit″o ri dot′o my
clit′o ris
clit′o rism
clit″o ri′tis
clit″o ro ma′ni a
clit″or rha′gi a
cli′vus
clo a′ca
clo a′cal
clo fi′brate
clo′mi phene
clone
clon′ic
clo nic′i ty
clon″i co ton′ic
clon′ism
clon′o graph
clo″nor chi′a sis
Clos trid′i um
clo′sure
clot
clove
clown′ism
club′foot″
club′hand″
clump′ing
clu′ne al
clut′ter ing
Clutton's joint

cly′sis
co″a cer′vate
co″ad ap ta′tion
co ag′u la ble
co ag′u lant
co ag′u lase
co ag′u late
co ag″u la′tion
co″ag u lop′athy
co ag′u lum
co″a les′cence
coal tar
co″ap ta′tion
co arc′tate
co″arc ta′tion
co″arc tot′o my
co″ar tic″u la′tion
coat
co bal′a min
co′balt
Co′bra
co′bra lec′i thid
co″bra ly′sin
co′ca
co caine′
co cain′ism
co′cain ize
co cain″o ma′ni a
co″car box′yl ase
co″car cin′o gen
coc′cal
Coc cid″i oi′des
coc cid″i oi′din
coc cid″i oi″do my co′sis
coc″co ba cil′lus
coc cog′e nous
coc′coid
coc′cus
coc″cy al′gi a
coc″cy ceph′a lus
coc″cy dyn′i a
coc″cy gec′to my
coc″cy ge″o fem o ral′is
coc cyg′e us
coc″cy go dyn′i a
coc′cyx
coch″i neal′
coch′le a
coch′le ar
coch″le o ves tib′u lar
coc″to pre cip′i tin
coc″to sta′bile
co′de ine
co″ef fi′cient
coe len′ter on
coe′lom
coe lom′ic
coe′no cyte
coe nu ro′sis
co en′zyme
coeur en sab″ot′
co′fac tor
cof′fee
cof′fin
Co′ gen tin
cog ni′tion
cog′wheel″
co hab″i ta′tion
co her′ence
co he′sion
co he′sive
coil
co i′tion
co″i to pho′bi a
co′i tus
co la′tion
col″a to′ri um
col′a ture
col′chi cine
co lec′to my
co″le i′tis
co′le o cele″

co″le o cys ti′tis
co″le op to′sis
co″le ot′o my
co′les
co″li bac″il le′mi a
co″li bac″il lo′sis
co″li bac″il lu′ri a
co″li ba cil′lus
col′ic
co′li ca
col′i form
col′i phage
co″li py u′ri a
co li′tis
co″li u′ri a
col′la cin
col′la gen
col′la ge nase
col″la gen′o sis
col lapse′
col′lar bone″
col lar ette′
col lat′er al
col lec′tor
Colles′ frac′ture
col lic″u li′tis
col lic′u lus
col′li ma″tor
col lin′e ar
col″li qua′tion
col liq′ua tive
col li′sion
col lo′di on
col′loid
col loi′dal
col loi″do cla′sis
col loi″do pex′y
col″loid oph′a gy
col″lo ne′ma
col′lum
col″lu na′ri um
col″lu to′ri um
col lyr′i um
col′ma scope
col″o bo′ma
co″lo co los′to my
co″lo hep′a to pex″y
co′lon
col′o ny
col′o pex″y
col″o proc tos′to my
col″op to′sis
col′or
col″o rec tos′to my
col′or gus ta′tion
col″or im′e ter
col″or i met′ric
col″or im′e try
co lor′rha phy
co″lo sig″moid os′to my
co los′to my
col″os tra′tion
co los″tror rhe′a
co los′trum
co lot′o my
col pal′gi a
col″pa tre′si a
col″pec ta′si a
col pec′to my
col″pe de′ma
col″peu ryn′ter
col″peurys′is
col pi′tis
col′po cele
col″po clei′sis
col″po hy″per pla′si a
col″po per″i ne′o plas″ty
col″po per″i ne or′rha phy
col′po pex″y
col′po plas″ty
col por′rha phy
col″por rhex′is

col′po scope
col po scop′ic
col pot′o my
col″u mel′la
col′umn
co lum′na
col′umn ing
col″um ni za′tion
co′ma
com′atose
comb′ing
Comb′s test
com′e do
com″e do-car″ci no′ma
com″e do′nes
co′mes
com′mi nute
com′mi nut ed
com″mi nu′tion
com″mis su′ra
com miss′u ral
com′mis sure
com″mis sur ot′o my
com mit′ment
com mo′ti o
com mun′ni ca ble
com mu′ni cans
com pan′ion ate
com par′a scope
com pat″i bil′i ty
com pat′i ble
Com′ pa zine
com″pen sa′tion
com pen′sa to″ry
com′pe tence
com plaint′
com′ple ment
com″ple men′ta ry
com″ple men′toid
com″ple men′to phil
com′plex
com plex′ion
com″po si′tion
com po′si tus
com′pos men′tis
com′pound
com′press
com pres′sion
com pres′sor
com pul′sion
com pul′sive
co′mus
co na′tion
con′cave
con cav′i ty
con ceive′
con cen tra′tion
con cen′tric
con cep′tion
con cep′tive
con cep′tus
con′cha
con′chal
con chi′tis
con′cho tome
con com′i tant
con′cre ment
con cres′cence
con cre′tion
con cus′sion
con″den sa′tion
con dens′er
con di′tion ing
con′dom
conduct″i bil′i ty
con duc′tion
con″duc tiv′i ty
con duc′tor
con′dyle
con″dy lec′to my
con dyl′i on
con′dy loid

con″dy lo′ma
con″dy lo′ma tous
con″dy lot′o my
cone
con fab″u la′tion
con fec′tion
con fer′tus
con fine′ment
con′flict
con′flu ence
conflu ent
con fo′cal
con″fron ta′tion
con fu′sion
con″ge la′tion
con′ge ner
con gen′i tal
con ges′tion
con ges′tive
con′gi us
con glo′bate
con glom′er ate
con glu′tin
con glu′ti nant
con glu″ti na′tion
con glu′ti nin
co nid′i um
co′ni ism
co″ni om′e ter
co″ni o′sis
co″ni o spor″i o′sis
co′ni um
con″i za′tion
con′ju gate
con″ju ga′tion
con″junc ti′va
con″junc ti′val
con junc″ti vi′tis
con junc″tiv o′ma
con″junc tiv′o plas″ty
co″no my oi′din
con″san guin′e ous
con″san guin′i ty
con′scious ness
con sen′su al
con sent′
con serv′a tive
con sist′ence
consol′i dant
con sol″i da′tion
con sper′gent
con′stant
con″stel la′tion
con″sti pa′tion
con″sti tu′tion
con stric′tor
con sult′ant
con″sul ta′tion
con sump′tion
con sump′tive
con′tact
con tac′tant
con ta′gion
con tam′i nant
con tam′i nating
con tam″i na′tion
con tem′pla tive
con′tent
con tig′u ous
con′ti nence
con′ti nent
con tin′gen cy
con tor′tion
con′tour
con″tra cep′tion
con″tra cep′tive
con tract′
con trac′tile
con″trac til′i ty
con trac′tion
con trac′ture
con″tra fis su′ra

con″tra in″di ca′tion
con″tra lat′er al
con″tra stim′u lant
con″tre coup′
con″trec ta′tion
con trol′
con trude′
con tuse′
con tu′sion
co′nus
con″va les′cence
con″va les′cent
con vec′tion
con ver′gence
con ver′gent
con ver′sion
con ver′tin
con vex′
con vex′i ty
con vex′o con′cave
con vex′o con′vex
con′vo lu″ted
con″vo lu′tion
con vul′sant
con vul′sion
con vul′sive
Cooley's a ne′mi a
Coomb's test
co or″di na′tion
coot′ie
cop′per
co″pre cip″i ta′tion
cop rem′e sis
cop roc′tic
cop″ro lag′ni a
cop″ro la′li a
cop′ro lith
cop roph′a gy
cop″ro phe′mi a
cop″ro phil′i a
cop roph′i lous
cop″ro pho′bi a
cop″ro phra′si a
cop″ro por phy′ri a
cop″ro por′phy rin
cop″ro por″phy ri nu′ri a
cop″u la′tion
cor″a co a cro′mi al
cor″a co bra″chi a′lis
cor″a co cla vic′u lar
cor″a co hu′mer al
cor′a coid
cord
cor dec′to my
cor′dial
cor′di form
cor di′tis
cor′do pex″y
cor dot′o my
cor″e cli′sis
cor ec′ta sis
cor ec′tome
cor″ec to′pi a
cor″e di al′y sis
co rel′y sis
cor″e mor′pho sis
cor″en cli′sis
cor″e om′e ter
cor″on′ci on
cor′e plas″ty
cor″e ste no′ma
cor″e to me″di al′y sis
co′ri um
corn
cor′ne a
cor′ne al
cor″ne o bleph′a ron
cor″ne o scle′ra
cor′ne ous
cor′ne um
cor nic′u late
cor nic′u lum

cor″ni fi ca′tion
cor′nu
co ro′na
co′ro nar″y
co″ro na vi′rus
co ro′ne
cor′o ner
co ro′ni on
cor″o ni′tis
co ro″no bas′i lar
co ro″no fa′cial
cor′o noid
cor″o pa rel′cy sis
co roph′thi sis
co ros′co py
cor po′re al
cor′po rin
cor″pro por phy rin′o gen
corpse
corps ronds
cor′pu lent
cor pul ma na′le
cor′pus
cor′pus cle
cor pus′cu lar
cor pus′cu lum
cor′pus de lec′ti″
cor rec′tion
cor rec′tive
cor″re la′tion
cor″re spond′ence
cor ro′sion
cor ro sive
cor′ru ga″tor
cor′set
cor′tex
cor′ti cal
cor″ti co bul′bar
cor′ti coid
cor″ti co pon″to cer e bel′lar
cor″ti co spi′nal
cor″ti cos′ter oid
cor″ti cos′te rone
cor″ti co stri′ate
cor″ti co tro′phin
cor″ti co tro′pin
cor′tin
cor′ti sone
cor″us ca′tion
cor ym′bi form
Co ry″ne bac te′ri um
co ry′za
cos met′ic
cos′mo tron
cos′ta
cos′tal
cos tal′gi a
cos tal′is
cos′tate
cos tec′to my
cos″ti car′ti lage
cos′ti form
cos′tive
cos″to car′ti lage
cos″to cer″vi cal′is
cos″to chon′dral
cos″to cla vic′u lar
cos″to cor′a coid
cos″to phren′ic
cos″to scap′u lar
cos′to tome
cos tot′o my
cos″to trans verse′
cos″to trans″ver sec′to my
cos″to ver′te bral
cos″to xiph′oid
cot
cot′a zyn
cot′ton
cot″y le′don
cot′y loid
cough

cou′lomb
cou′ ma din
cou′ma rin
count
count′er
coun″ter ac′tion
coun′ter ex ten″sion
coun″ter ir′ri tant
coun′ter o″pen ing
coun′ter poi″son
coun′ter pres″sure
coun′ter punc″ture
coun′ter shock″
coun′ter stain
coun′ter stroke
coun′ter trac″tion
coun′ter trans fer′ence
cou′ple
Courvoisier, Ludwig
co va′lence
Cowper's glands
cow″per i′tis
cow′pox″
cox al′gi a
cox″ar throc′a ce
cox′a vara
cox i′tis
Cox sack′ie vi′rus
co zy′mase
cra′dle
cramp
cra′ni ad
cra′ni al
cra″ni ec′to my
cra′ni o cele
cra″ni o cer′vi cal
cra″ni oc′la sis
cra′ni o clast
cra″ni o clei″do dys os to′sis
cra″ni o did′y mus
cra″ni o fa′cial
cra″ni o fe nes′tri a
cra′ni o graph
cra″ni og′ra phy
cra″ni o la cu′ni a
cra″ni ol′o gy
cra″ni om′e ter
cra″ni o met′ric
cra″ni om′e try
cra″ni op′a gus
cra″ni op′a thy
cra″ni o pha ryn′ge al
cra″ni o pha ryn″gi o′ma
cra′ni o plas″ty
cra″ni o rha chis′chi sis
cra″ni o sa′cral
cra″ni os′chi sis
cra″ni o spi′nal
cra′ni o stat″
cra″ni o ste no′sis
cra″ni os′to sis
cra″ni o syn″os to′sis
cra″ni o ta′bes
cra′ni o tome
cra″ni ot′o my
cra″ni o trac′tor
cra″ni o trip′so tome
cra″ni o tym pan′ic
cra″ni um
cran′ter
crap′u lent
cra″ter i za′tion
cra vat′
craw′-craw″
cream
crease
cre′a tine
cre″a ti ne′mi a
cre at′i nine
cre″a tinu′ri a
cre″a tor rhe′a
Credé's meth′od

cre mas′ter
cre″mas ter′ic
cre ma′tion
cre′ma to″ry
crem″no pho′bi a
cre′na
cre′nate
crena′tion
cre′o sol
cre′o sote
crep′i tant
crep″i ta′tion
crep′i tus
cres′cent
cre′sol
crest
cres′yl blue
cre′ta
cre′tin
cre′tin ism
cre′tin oid
crev′ice
crib′bing
crib′rate
crib′ri form
crib′rose
crick
cri″co ar″y te′noid
cri′coid
Crigler-Najjar syn′drome
cri″coi dec′to my
cri″co pha ryn′ge al
cri″co phar yn′ge us
cri″co thy′roid
cri cot′o my
cri″co tra′che ot′o my
cri″ co thy rot′ o my
crim″i nol′o gy
crimp′er
crin″o gen′ic
cri′nose
cri′sis
cris pa′tion
cris″pa tu′ra
cris′ta
crit′i cal
Crohn′s dis ease′
Cro tal′i dae
crot′a line
crotch′et
cro′ton ism
cro tox′in
croup
croup′ine
Crouzon′s dis ease′
crown
cru′cial
cru′ci ate
cru′ci ble
cru′ci form
cru′or
crup′per
cru′ral
cru′re us
crus
crush
crust
Crus ta′ce a
crutch
cry
cry″al ge′si a
cry an″es the′si a
cry″es the′si a
cry″mo dyn′i a
cry″mo phil′ic
cry″o cau′ter y
cry′o chem
cry″o glob′u lin
cry″o glob″u li ne′mi a
cry om′e ter
cry″o pro′te in
cry′o scope

cry′o stat
cry″o ther′a py
crypt
cryp″tag glu′tin oid
crypt″an am ne′si a
cryp ti′tis
cryp″to coc co′sis
Cryp″to coc′cus
cryp′to gam
cryp″to gen′ic
cryp′to lith
cryp″to men″or rhe′a
cryp″to mer″o rha chis′chi sis
cryp″tom ne′si a
cryp″toph thal′mos
cryp top′or ous
crypt″or chid ec′to my
crypt or′chid ism
crypt″or chid′o pex y
crypt or′chism
crypt″to zo′ite
crypt toz′y gous
crys′tal
crys″tal bu′min
crys″tal fi′brin
crys′tal lin
crys″tal li za′tion
crys″tal log′ra phy
crys′tal loid
crys″tal lo mag′net ism
crys″tal lo pho′bi a
crys″tal lu′ri a
cryst i cil′lin
cry″to did′y mus
crys toid′
cu′beb
cu′beb ism
cubi form
cu′bi tus
cu′boid
cu boi″de o na vic′u lar
cui rass′
cul′-de-sac′
cul″do cen te′sis
cul′do scope
cul dos′co py
cul″dot′o my
Cu′lex
cu′li cide
cul′men
cult
cul″ti va′tion
cul′ture
cu′mu la″tive
cu′mu lus
cu′ne ate
cu ne′i form
cu″ne o cu′boid
cu″ne o na vic′u lar
cu″ne o scaph′oid
cu′ne us
cu nic′u lar
cu nic′u lus
cun″ni lin′guist
cun″ni lin′gus
cun′nus
cu′po la
cupped
cup′ping
cu″pram mon′ni a
cu′prex
cu′pric
cu′prous
cu′pu la
cu″pu lom′e try
cur′age
cu ra′re
cu ra′ri form
cu″ra ri za′tion
cu′ra tive
curd
cure

cu ret′
cu ret′tage
cu′ric
cu′rie
cu′ri um
curled
cur′rent
cur ric′u lum
cur′va ture
curve
Cushing, Harvey
cush′ing oid″
cush′ion
cusp
cus′pid
cu ta″ne o mu co′sal
c ta′ne ous
cu′ti cle
cu tic′u lar
cu″ti fi ca′tion
cu″ti re ac′tion
cu′tis
cu ti′tis
cu″ti za′tion
cy″an am′ide
cy′a nate
cy′a nide
cy″a no co bal′a mine
cy an′o phil
cy′a nosed
cy″a no′sis
cy″a not′ic
cy as′ma
cy″ber net′ics
cy′cla mate
cy′cle
cy clec′to my
cy″clen ceph′a lus
cy″clen ceph′a ly
cy′clic
cy″cli cot′o my
cy cli′tis
cy″clo ceph′a lus
cy″clo ceph′a ly
cy″clo cho″roid i′tis
cy″clo di al′y sis
cy″clo di′a ther my
cy clog′e ny
cy′cloid
cy″clo phor′ase
cy″clo pho′ri a
cy clo′pi a
cy″clo ple′gi a
cy″clo pro′pane
cy′clops
cy′clo scope
cy″clo thy′mic
cy clo′ti a
cy′clo tome
cy clot′o my
cy′clo tron
cy″clo tro′pi a
cy clo′tus
cy e″si ol′o gy
cy e′sis
cyl′in der
cy lin′dri form
cyl′in droid
cyl″in dro′ma
cyl″in dro′sis
cyl″in dru′ri a
cyl″lo so′ma
cyl″lo so′mus
cym″bo ceph′a ly
cy nan′thro py
cyn″i a′tri a
cyn′ic
cyn″o ceph′a lous
cyn″o don′tes
cyn″o lys′sa
cyn″o pho′bi a
cy″o pho′ria

cy ot′ro phy
cy prid″o pho′bi a
cyr″to ceph′a lus
cyr″to cor′y phus
cyr′to graph
cyr tom′e ter
cyr″to me to′pus
cyr″to pis″tho cra′ni us
cyr to′sis
cyr″tu ran′us
cyst
cyst ad″e no car″ci no′ma
cyst″ad e no′ma
cyst″ad e no sar co′ma
cys tal′gi a
cys″ta thi″o ni nu′ri a
cyst″ec ta′si a
cys tec′to my
cys′te ine
cyst′ic
cys″ti cer′coid
cys″ti cer co′sis
cys″ti cer′cus
cys′ti form
cys′tine
cys″ti ne′mi a
cys″ti no′sis
cys″ti nu′ri a
cys ti′tis
cys tit′o my
cys″to bu bon′o cele
cys′to cele
cys″to fi bro′ma pap″il lar′e
cys″to gen′e sis
cys′to gram
cys tog′ra phy
cyst′oid
cys″to lith ec′to my
cys″to li thi′a sis
cys″to li thot′o my
cys to′ma
cys tom′e ter
cys″to met′ro gram
cys″to mor′phous
cys′to pex″y
cys″to pho tog′ra phy
cys′to plas″ty
cys″to pros ta tec′to my
cys″to py″e li′tis
cys″to py″e lo ne phri′tis
cys tor′rha phy
cys″to sar co ma
cys′to scope
cys tos′co py
cys tos″te a to′ma
cys tos′to my
cys tot′o my
cys″to u re′thro gram
cys″to u″re throg′ra phy
cys″to u re′thro scope
cy″to ar″chi tec ton′ic
cy″to ar′chi tec″ture
cy′to blast
cy″to blas te′ma
cy″to chem′ism
cy′to chrome
cy″to chy le′ma
cy toc′la sis
cy″to crin′i a
cy′tode
cy″to dis′tal
cy to gen′ic
cy″to glob′u lin
cy to log′ic
cy tol′o gy
cy″to ly′sin
cy tol′y sis
cy″to me gal′ic
cy″to meg a″lo vi′rus
cy tom′e ter
cy″to mi′cro some
cy″to mi′tome

cy″to mor′pho sis
cy′ton
cy″to path o gen′ic
cy″to pa thol′o gy
cy top′a thy
cy toph′a gy
cy″to pe′ni a
cy′to phil
cy″to phys″i ol′o gy
cy′to plasm
cy″to plas′tin
cy″to poi e′sis
cy″to prox′i mal
cy″to re tic′u lum
cy″tos cop′ic
cy tos′co py
cy′to some
cy″to spon′gi um
cy′tost
cy′to stome
cy″to tax′is
cy toth′e sis
cy″to tox′ic
cy″to tox′in
cy″to troph′o blast
cy tot′ro phy
cy tot′ro pism
cy′to zyme

D

dac no ma′ni a
Dac′ron
dac″ry ad″e no scir′rhus
dac″ry ag″o ga tre′si a
dac′ry a gogue
dac″ry ge lo′sis
dac″ry o ad″e nal′gi a
dac″ry o ad″e nec′to my
dac″ry o ad e ni′tis
dac″ry o blen″nor rhe′a
dac′ry o cyst″
dac″ry o cys tec′to my
dac″ry o cys ti′tis
dac″ry o cys″to blen′nor rhea
dac″ry o cys′to cele
dac″ry o cys″top to′sis
dac″ry o cys″to rhi nos′to my
dac″ry o cys tos′to my
dac″ry o cys′to tome
dac″ry o cys tot′o my
dac′ry o lin
dac′ry o lith″
dac″ry o li thi′a sis
dac″ry o′ma
dac′ry on
dac′ry ops
dac″ry or rhe′a
dac″ry o so″le ni′tis
dac″ry o ste no′sis
dac″ry o syr′inx
dac tin′o my″cin
dac′tyl
dac″ty lif′er ous
dac tyl′i on
dac″ty li′tis
dac′ty lo gram″
dac″ty lo meg′a ly
dac″ty lo sym′phy sis
dac′ty lus
dah′lin
Dal′ mane
dan′der
dan′druff
Darier′s dis ease′
dar′tos
dar′trous
Dar′ von
dau′er schlaf″
daught′er
dax′o lin
de ac″ti va′tion
de af″fer en ta′tion

deaf′-mute″
deaf′ness
de al′bate
de al″co hol″i za′tion
de al″ler gi za′tion
de am′i dase
de am′i nase
de an″es the′si ant
de″a qua′tion
death
de bil′i tant
de bil′i ty
de bride′ment
de bris′
dec′a gram
de cal″ci fi ca′tion
de cal′ci fy
dec′a lit″er
dec′a me″ter
dec′a normal
de cant′
de cap′i tate
de cap″i ta′tion
de cap′i ta″tor
de cap″su la′tion
de car′bon ate
de car″bon i za′tion
de car box″y la′tion
de ca thec′tion
dec″a vi′ta min
de cay′
de cen′tered
de cer″e bel la′tion
de cer′e brate″
de cer″e bra′tion
de chlo″ri da′tion
de chlo″ru ra′tion
dec′i bel
de cid′u a
de cid′u al
de cid′u ate
de cid″u a′tion
de cid″u i′tis
de cid″u o′ma
de cid″u o′sis
de cid′u ous
dec′i gram
dec′i li″ter
dec′i me″ter
dec″i nor′mal
de cip′a ra
de clive′
De clo my′cin
de coc′tion
de″col la′tion
de′col la″tor
de col′or ant
de col′or ize
de com″pen sa′tion
de″com po si′tion
de″com pres′sion
de″con ges′tant
de″con ges′tive
de con tam′i nate
de″con tam″i na′tion
de cor″ti ca′tion
de″cu ba′tion
de cu bi′tal
de cu′bi tus
de cus′sate
de″cus sa′tion
de″den ti′tion
de″dif fer en″ti a′tion
def″e ca′tion
de fect′
de″fem i na′tion
de fense′
def′er ent
def″er en′tial
def″er en″ti o ves′i cal
def″er en ti′tis
de″fer ves′cence

de fib″ril la′tion
de fi″bri na′tion
def″i ni′tion
def″la gra′tion
de flec′tion
def″lo ra′tion
de″flo res′cence
de form′i ty
de fuse′
de gan′gli on ate
de gas′sing
de gen′er a cy
de gen′er ate
de″gen er a′tion
de″gen er a′tive
de gen″i tal′i ty
de″glu ti′tion
deg″ra da′tion
de grease′
de gree′
de″gus ta′tion
de his′cence
de hy′drate
de″hy dra′tion
de hy″dro cor″ti cos′te rone
de hy′dro gen ase
de hy′dro gen ize
de″hy dro i″so an dros′ter one
de i′on iz″er
Deiter's
  cell
de″ja″vu′
de jec′tion
de″lac ta′tion
de lam″i na′tion
De Lee, Joseph
de lim″i ta′tion
de lim′it ed
de lin′quen cy
de″lip i da′tion
del″i ques′cence
de liq′ui um
de lir″i fa′cient
de lir′i ous
de lir′i um
de liv′er y
de″lo mor′phous
de louse′
del′ta
del′toid
de lu′sion
de″mar ca′tion
dem e clo cy′cline
de ment′
de ment′ed
de men′ti a
de′men tia prae′cox
De′mer ol
de meth″yl chlor″te tra cy′cline
dem″i fac′et
dem′i lune
dem″i mon stros′i ty
de min″er al i za′tion
dem″i pen′ni form
de mog′ra phy
de″mon ol′ a try
de″mon ol′ogy
de″mon o ma′nia
de″mon op′ a thy
de″mon o pho′bi a
de mul′cent
de my′e lin ate
de nar′co tize
de na′tur ant
de na′tured
de na″tur i za′tion
den′drite
den″dro phil′i a
de ner′va ted
de″ner va′tion
den′gue
de ni′al
den″i da′tion
den″i gra′tion

de ni″tro gen a′tion
dens
den sim′e ter
den″sit om′e ter
den′si ty
den′so gram
den tag′ra
den′tal
den tal′gi a
den tal″o ru′ bral
den tar′pa ga
den′tar y
den′tate
den ta′tum
den″te la′tion
den′tes
den′ti a pre′cox
den″ti a ski′a scope
den′ti cle
den tic′u late
den″ti fi ca′tion
den′ti form
den′ti frice
den tig′er ous
den′ti lave
den′tin
den″ti nal′gi a
den″ti no blas to′ma
den″ti no ce men′tal
den″ti no gen′e sis
den′ti noid
den″ti no′ma
den″ti nos′te oid
den tip′a rous
den′ti phone
den′tist
dentis try
den ti′tion
den″to al ve′o lar
den″to al″ve o li′tis
den″to fa′cial
den tog′ra phy
den′toid
den″to le′gal
den ton′o my
den′ture
de nu′cle a″ted
de nude′
de ob′stru ent
de″o′dor ant
de o′dor ize
de″o ral′i ty
de or″sum duc′tion
de or″sum ver′gence
de os″si fi ca′tion
de ox″y cor″ti cos′te rone
de ox″y cor′ti sone
de ox″y gen a′tion
de ox″y ri bo nu cle′ic
de ox″y ri bo nu cle′ic
acid
de per″son al i za′tion
de pig″men ta′tion
dep′i late
de pil′a tory
dep′i lous
de plete′
de ple′tion
de″plu ma′tion
de po″lar i za′tion
de″po lym′er ase
de pol″y mer i za′tion
de pos′it
de′pot
de pres′sant
de pres′sion
de pres′sor
dep′side
de pu″li za′tion
der″an en″ce pha′li a
de re″al i za′tion
de′re ism
der e is′tic
der″en ceph′a lus

der″en ceph′a ly
der″i va′tion
de riv′a tive
der′ma
Der″ma cen′tor
der′ma drome
der′mal
der″ma my i′a sis
der man′a plas″ty
der″ma tag′ra
der″ma tal′gi a
der″ma ta neu′ri a
der″mat he′mi a
der′ma therm
der mat′ic
der″ma ti′tis
der″ma to cel″lu li′tis
der″ma to cha la′sis
der″ma to co″ni o′sis
der′ma to cyst″
der″ma to fi bro′ma
der″ma to fi″bro sar co′ma pro tu′ber ans
der″ma to glyph′ics
der″ma tog′ra phy
der″ma tol′o gist
der″ma tol′o gy
der″ma tol′y sis
der′ma tome
der″ma to my′ces
der″ma to my co′sis
der″ma to my o′ma
der″ma to my″o si′tis
der″ma to neu rol′o gy
der″ma to neu ro′sis
der″ma to pa thol′o gy
der″ma to path″o pho′bi a
der″ma top′a thy
der″ma to phi li′a sis
der′ma to phyte″
der″ma toph′y tid
der″ma to phy to′sis
der′ma to plas″ty
der″ma to pol″y neu ri′tis
der″ma tor rha′gi a
der″ma tos′co py
der″ma to′sis
der′ma to some″
der″ma to stom″a ti′tis
der″ma to ther′a py
der″ma to thia′si a
der″ma tot′o my
der″ma to zo′on
der″ma to zo″on o′sis
der′mis
der″ma ti′tis
der′mo blast
der″mo cy′ma
der″mo ep″i der′mal
der″mo graph′i a
der′moid
der″moid ec′to my
der″mo la′bi al
der mop′a thy
der″mo phle bi′tis
der″mo skel′e ton
der″mo ste no′sis
der″mos to′sis
der″mo syn″o vi′tis
der″mo syph″i lop′a thy
der″o did′y mus
de rom′e lus
der′rid
des″an i ma′ni a
de sat″u ra′tion
Descemet′s mem′brane
des″ce me ti′tis
des″ce met′o cele
de scend′ens
de scen′sus
de scent′
des′e nex″
de sen″si ti za′tion
de sen′si tize

de sex″u al′i ty
de sex″u al i za′tion
des′ic cant
des″ic ca′tion
des′ic ca″tor
des′i vac
des″mi o gnath′us
des mi′tis
des″mo cra′ni um
des′mo cyte
des″mo gly′co gen
des′moid
des′mo lase
des′mone
des″mo pla′si a
des mo pres′sin
des′mo some
des mot′o my
des′o gen
des sorp′tion
de spe″ci a′tion
D'Espine's
sign
des′qua mate
des″qua ma′tion
de stru′do
de tach′ment
de ter′gent
de ter′mi nant
de ter″mi na′tion
de tor′sion
de tox″i ca′tion
de tox″i fi′ca tion
de tox′i fy
de tri′tion
de tri′tus
de″trun ca′tion
de tru′sion
de tru′sor
de″tu mes′cence
deu″ter a no′pi a
deu″ter a′tion
deu ter′i um
deu″ter o gen′ic
deu″ter o plasm′
deu″ter o pro′te ose
deu″ter os′to ma
deu tom′er ite
deu″to plas mol′y sis
de vel′op ment
de″vi a′tion
de″vi om′e ter
de vi′tal ize
dev″o lu′tion
dew′claw″
dew′lap″
Dex′a myl
Dex′e drine
dex′ter
dex′trad
dex′tral
dex tral′i ty
dex″tra li za′tion
Dex′tran
dex trau′ral
dex′trin
dex″tri nu′ri a
dex″tro car′di a
dex″tro car′di o
gram″
dex″tro cer′e bral
dex″tro com′pound
dex″tro con′dyl ism
dex troc′u lar
dex″tro duc′tion
dex″tro man′ual
dex″tro pe′dal
dex″tro pho′bi a
dex″tro pho′ri a
dex″tro po si′tion
dex″tro ro′ta to″ry
dex′trose

dex″tro sin′is tral
dex″tro su′ri a
dex″tro tor′sion
dex″tro ver′sion
di″a bet′es
di″a bet′es in sip′i dus
di″a bet′es mel li′tus
di″a bet′ic
di″a be″to gen′ic
di″a be tog′e nous
di″a be″to pho′bi a
Di″a bin′ese
di ab′o lep″sy
di″a ce te′mi a
di″a ce tu′ria
di ac″e tyl mor′phine
di ac′la sis
di′a clast
di ac″o la′tion
di″a crit′ic
di″ac tin′ic
di′ad
di′a derm
di ad″o cho ki ne′si a
di″ag nos′a ble
di″ag nose′
di″ag·no′sis
di″ag·nos′tic
di″ag nos ti′cian
di″a ki ne′sis
di al′y sate
di al′y sis
di′a lyze
di′a ly″zer
di″a mag net′ic
di am′e ter
di″a mine′
di″a mi nu′ri a
Di a′mox
di″a pa′son
di″a pe de′sis
di′a phane
di aph″a nom′e ter
di aph′a no scope
di aph″e met′ric
di aph′o rase
di″a pho re′sis
di″a pho ret′ic
di′a phragm
di″a phrag mat′o cele
di″a phrag mi′tis
di a phy se′al
di a phy se′al ac la′sis
di″aph y sec′to my
di aph′y sis
di ap′la sis
di″a poph′y sis
di″ar rhe′a
di ar′thric
di″ar thro′sis
di as′chi sis
di″a schis′tic
di′a scope
di′as e pam
di a stal′sis
di′a stase
di as′ta sis
di″a stat′ic
di″a ste′ma
di″a stem″a to my e′li a
di as′to le
di as tol′ic
di″a tax′i a
di″a ther′ma nous
di″a ther′mic
di″a ther″mo co ag″u la′tion
di″a ther mom′e ter
di′a ther″my
di ath′e sis
di″a tom′ic
di az ox′ide
di ba′sic

di cal′ci um
di ceph′a lism
di ceph′a lus
di ceph′a ly
di chei′lus
di chi′rus
di cho′ri al
di chot′o mize
di chot′o my
di chro′ic
di chro′mate
di″chro mat′ic
di chro′ma tism
di chro″ma top′si a
di′chro mism
di chro′mo phil
di″cli dot′o my
di cou′ma rin
di cou′ma rol
di crot′ic notch
di′cro tism
dic′ty o cyte
dic″ty o cy to′ma
dic″ty o ki ne′sis
dic ty′o tene
Di cum′a rol
di dac′tic
di dac′tyl ism
di del′phic
did y mi′tis
did′y mus
di el′drin
di″e lec trol′y sis
di em′bry o ny
di″en ceph al′ic
di″en ceph′a lon
di es′trum
di′et
di′e tar″y
di″e tet′ics
di eth″yl stil bes′trol
di″e ti′tian
dif″fer en′tial
dif″fer en″ti a′tion
dif′flu ence
dif frac′tion
dif fus′ate
dif fuse′
dif fus″i bil′i ty
dif fus″si om′e ter
dif fu′sion
di′ga len
di gas′tric
di gen′e sis
di″ge net′ic
di gen′ic
di gest′ant
di gest′er
di gest′i ble
di ges′tine
di ges′tion
dig″i fol′in
dig″i lan′id
dig′it
dig′i tal
dig″i ta′lin
dig″i tal′is
dig″i tal i za′tion
dig″i ta′tion
dig″i ti form
Dig″i tox′in
dig′i tus
di glos′si a
di glos′sus
di gnath′us
di gox′in
di hy′brid
di hy″dro strep″to my′cin
di″i o′do form
di kar′y on
di lac″er a′tion

Di lan′tin
dil″a ta′tion
di la′tion
di′la tor
dil′u ent
di lute′
di lu′tion
di meg′a ly
di me′li a
di men′sion
di″mer cap′rol
di meth′yl
di me′tri a
di mor′phic
di mor′phism
dim′ple
Di o′do quin″
Di′o drast″
di′o nism
di op′ter
di″op tom′e ter
di op′tric
di op′trics
di″or tho′sis
di o′tic
di ox′ide
di pep′tide
di phal′lus
di phas′ic
di pho′ni a
diph the′ri a
diph the′ric
diph the′ri a phor
diph′the rin
diph″the ri ol′y sin
diph″the ri′tis
diph′the roid
diph thon′gi a
Diph phyl″lo both′ri um
di phy′o dont″
dip″ la cu′sis
di″plas mat′ic
di ple′gi a
dip″lo al bu″mi nu′ri a
dip″lo ba cil′lus
dip″lo blas′tic
dip″lo car′di ac
dip″lo ceph′a lus
dip″lo coc′cin
Dip″lo coc′cus
dip″lo co′ri a
dip′lo e
dip″lo gen″e sis
dip′loid
dip″lo kar′y on
dip′lo mate
dip″lo mel″li tu′ri a
dip″lo my e′li a
dip″lo ne′ma
dip″lo neu′ral
di plop′a gus
di plo′pi a
di plo′sis
dip′lo some
dip″lo strep″to coc′cus
dip′lo tene
di po′lar
di′pole″
dip′pol dism
dip″ro so′pi a
di pro′so pus
dip set′ic
dip″so ma′ni a
dip″so pho′bia
dip″so ther′a py
Dip′ter a
di′pus
di py′gus
Di″py lid′i um
dir rhi′nus
di sac′char i dase
di sac′cha ride

di sac″char i du′ri a
dis ag″gre ga′tion
dis″ar tic″u la′tion
dis″as so″ci a′tion
dis charge′
dis cis′sion
disc i′tis
dis″co blas′tu la
disc′o gram
dis′coid
dis col″or a′tion
dis″com po si′tion
Dis″co my′ces
dis coph′o rous
dis″co pla cen′ta
dis crete′
dis crim″i na′tion
dis′cus
dis cu′tient
dis ease′
dis″en gage′ment
dis e″qui lib′ri um
dis″gre ga′tion
dis″in fect′ant
dis″in fec′tion
dis in″fes ta′tion
dis in″hi bi′tion
dis in′te grate
dis″in vag″i na′tion
dis joint′
disk, disc
dis″lo ca′tion
dis mem′ber
dis″mu ta′tion
dis″oc clude′
dis so′ma
dis ord′er
dis or″gan i za′tion
dis o″ri en ta′tion
dis′pa rate
dis par′ity
dis pen′sa ry
dis pen′sa to″ry
dis pense′
dis per′sion
dis place′ment
dis″po si′tion
dis rup′tive
dis sect′
dis sec′tion
dis sec′tor
dis sem″i na′tion
dis sim″u la′tion
dis so″ci a′tion
dis″soc′i a tive
dis sog′e ny
dis″so lu′tion
dis solve′
dis′tad
dis′tance
dis tem′per
dis ten′tion
dis tich′i a
dis′til land
dis′til late
dis″til la′tion
dis″to buc′cal
dis″to buc″co oc clu′sal
dis″to oc clu′sal
dis″to clu′sion
dis″ to la′bi al
dis″to lin′gual
dis″to lin″guo oc clu′sal
di sto′mi a
dis″to mi′a sis
dis″to mo′lar
di sto′mus
dis tor′tion
dis″to ver′sion
dis″tri bu′tion
dis″tri chi′a sis
dis′trix

di sulf'i ram
di"u re'sis
di"u ret'ic
Di'u ril
di"va ga'tion
di va'lent
di var"i ca'tion
di ver'gence
di"ver tic'u la
di"ver tic'u lar
di"ver tic"u lec'to my
di"ver tic"u li'tis
di"ver tic"u lo'sis
di"ver tic'u lum (a)
di vi'nyl
di vi'sion
di vul'sion
di vul'sor
di"zy got'ic
diz'zi ness
Dobell's so lu'tion
do'ca
dol"i cho ceph'a lus
dol"i cho ce phal'ic
dol"i cho ceph'a ly
dol"i cho cham"ae cra'ni al
dol"i choc ne'mic
dol"i cho co'lon
dol"i cho de'rus
dol"i cho eu"ro mes"o ceph'a lu
dol"i cho eu" ro-o pis"tho ceph'a lus
dol"i cho eu"ro pro ceph'a lus
dol"i cho fa'cial
dol"i cho hi er'ic
dol"i cho lep"to ceph'a lus
dol"i cho mor'phic
dol"i cho pel'lic
dol"i cho plat'y ceph'a lus
dol'i chor rhine
dol"i cho u ran'ic
do'lor
dol"or o gen'ic
do"ma to pho'bi a
dom'in ance
dom'i nant
dom'i na tor
do"nee'
do'nor
Donovan bod'y
do'pa
do'pa mine
dope
do"ra pho'bi a
dor'mant
dor'nase
dor'sa
dor'sad
dor'sal
dor sal'gi a
dor sa'lis
dor"si flex'ion
dor"si ven'tral
dor"so an te'ri or
dor"so ceph'al ad
dor"so ep"i tro chle a'ris
dor"so lat'er al
dor"so lum'bar
dor"so me'di an
dor"so na'sal
dor"so pos te'ri or
dor"so ra'di al
dor"so ul'nar
dor"so ven'tral
dor'sum
do'sage
do sim'e ter
do sim'e try
doub'let
douche
doug"la si'tis
dou rine'
Dover's pow'der

drachm (dram)
dra con″ti so′mus
dra cun″cu lo′sis
Dra cun′cu lus med″i nen′sis
dra gee′
Dragstedt's op″er a′tion
drain
drain′age
dram (drachm)
Dram′a mine
drap″e to ma′ni a
dread
dream
drench
drep′a no cyte
drep″a no cy the′mi a
drep″a no cy to′sis
dress′er
drib′ble
drift
driv′el ing
drom′o graph
drom″o ma′ni a
drom″o pho′bi a
drop′let
drop′si cal
drop′sy
Dro soph′i la
drug′gist
drunk′en ness
drunk om′e ter
dru′sen
du″al is′tic
duct
duct′us
du ip′a ra
dum′my
du″o crin′in
du″o de′nal
du″o de nec′ta sis
du″o de nec′to my
du″o de ni′tis
du″o de″no chlo″an gi′tis
du″o de″no chol″e cys tos′to my
du″o de″no cho led″o chot′o my
du″o de″no col′ic
du″o de″no cys tos′to my
du″o de″no en″ter os′to my
du″o de′no gram
du″o den og′raph y
du″o de″no he pat′ic
du″o de″no il″e os′to my
du″o de″no jej″u nos′to my
du″o de″no pan″cre a tec′to my
du″o de′no plas″ty
du o de″no py″lo rec′to my
du″o de nor′rha phy
du″o de nos′co py
du″o de nos ′to my
du″o de not′o my
du″o de′num
du″o pa ren′tal
du′pli ca″ture
du″pli ca′tus
du plic′i tas
du plic′i ty
Dupuytren, Guillaume
du′ra
du′ra ma′ter
du′ra plas″ty
du ri′tis
du″ro ar″ach ni′tis
dwarf
dwarfism
dye
dy nam′e ter
dy nam′ic
dy′na mo
dy″na mo gen′e sis
dy nam′o graph
dy″na mom′e ter
dy nam′o neure

dy″na moph′a ny
dy nam′o scope
dy′na therm
dyne
dys″a cou′si a
dys ad″ap ta′tion
dys″aes the′si a
dys an″ag no′si a
dys an″ti graph′i a
dys a′phi a
dys″ap ta′tion
dys″ar te″ri ot′o ny
dys ar′thri a
dys″ar thro′sis
dys″au to no′ma
dys′bar ism
dys ba′si a
dys bu′li a
dys chi′ri a
dys chi′zi a
dys chon″dro pla′si a
dys chro″ma to der′mi a
dys″chro ma top′si a
dys chro′mi a
dys′chro nous
dys co′ri a
dys cra′si a
dys cri′nism
dys″di ad″o cho ki ne′si a
dys″e coi′a
dys em″bry o pla′si a
dys″e me′si a
dys e′mi a
dys″en doc′rin ism
dys′en ter″y
dys″er ga′si a
dys″es the′si a
dys″fi brin o″ge ne′mi a
dys func′tion
dys″ga lac′ti a
dys″gam ma glob u lin em′ia
dys gen′ic
dys″ger mi no′ma
dys geu′si a
dys glan′du lar
dys gnath′ic
dys gno′si a
dys gon′ic
dys gram′ma tism
dys graph′i a
dys hem″a to poi et′ic
dys″hi dro′sis
dys″ker a to′sis
dys″ki ne′si a
dys la′li a
dys lex′i a
dys″li po pro tein e′mi a
dys lo′gi a
dys″ma se′ sis
dys″men or rhe′a
dys″mer o gen′e sis
dys me′tri a
dys mim′i a
dys mne′si a
dys mor′phi a
dys mor′phic
dys mor″pho pho′bi a
dys no′mi a
dys″o don ti′a sis
dys o′pi a
dys″o rex′i a
dys os′mi a
dys″os to′sis
dys par″a thy′roid ism
dys″pa reu′ni a
dys pep′si a
dys pep′tic
dys″per i stal′sis
dys pha′gi a
dys pha′si a
dys phe′mi a
dys pho′ni a

dys pho′ri a
dys pho′ti a
dys phra′si a
dys″pi tu′i ta rism
dys pla′si a
dysp ne′a
dys prax′i a
dys′ra phism
dys rhyth′mi a
dys se ba′ci a
dys″se cre to′sis
dys sper′ma tism
dys sta′si a
dys tax′i a
dys tec′tic
dys″tha na′si a
dys the′si a
dys thy′mi a
dys tith′i a
dys to′ci a
dys to′ni a
dys to′pi a
dys tro′phi a
dys′tro phy
dys u′ri a

E

ear
ear′ache″
ear′drum″
ear′wax″
Eaton's a′gent
Ebstein's
  a nom′a ly
e′bur
e″bur na′tion
ec bol′ic
ec cen′tric
ec ceph″a lo′sis
ec″chon dro′ma
ec″chy mo′sis
ec′crine
ec″cy e′sis
ec dem′ic
ec dem″o ma′ni a
ec′der on
ec′dy sis
e chid′nase
e chid′nin
e chin′e none
e chi″no coc co′sis
E chi″no coc′cus
E chi″no der′ma ta
ech″i no′sis
ech′o
ech″o a cou′si a
ech″o car di og′ra phy
ech″o graph′i a
ech″o la′li a
ech″o la′lus
ech op′a thy
ech oph′o ny
ech″o phot′o my
ech″o prax′i a
E′cho vi rus
ec la′bi um
ec lamp′si a
ec lamp′sism
ec lec′ti cism
ec′ly sis
e″ cog no′sis
e col′o gy
e″co ma′ni a
e′co site
e cos′tate
ec pho′ri a
e″cra″seur′
ec′sta sy
ec′tad
ec′tal
ec ta′si a

ec ten'tal
ect eth'moid
ec thy'ma
ec"to bat'ic
ec'to blast
ec"to car'di a
ec"to cho roi'de a
ec"to cor"ne a
ec"to cra'ni al
ec'to derm
ec"to der mo'sis
ec"to en'zyme
ec tog'e nous
ec tog'o ny
ec'to mere
ec"o mes'o derm
ec'to morph
ec top'a gus
ec"to par'a site
ec'to phyte
ec to'pi a
ec top'ic
ec"to pla cen'ta
ec'to plasm
ec"to pot'o my
ec"to ret'i na
ec'to sarc
ec'to thrix
Ec"to tri choph'y ton
ec"to zo'on
ec"tro dac tyl'i a
ec trog'e ny
ec"tro me'li a
ec trom'e lus
ec tro'pi on
ec trop'o dism
ec"tro syn dac'ty ly
ec trot'ic
ec"ty lot'ic
ec'ze ma
ec zem"a ti za'tion
ec zem'a toid
ec zem"a to'sis
ec zem'a tous
e de'ma
e de' ma tous
e den'tate
e den'ti a
e den'tu lous
e"de ol'o gy
ed'i ble
ed"o ceph'al us
ef fect'
ef fec'tor
ef'fer ent
ef"fer ves'cence
ef"fer ves'cent
ef"fleu rage'
ef"flo res'cence
ef'flu ent
ef flu'vi um
ef fuse'
ef fu'sion
e"ga grop'i lus
e ger'sis
e ges'ta
e glan'du lar
e'go
e"go bron choph'o ny
e"go cen'tric
e"go cen'trism
e'go ide'al
e"go ma ni a
e goph'o ny
e'go-syn ton'ic
Ehrlich, Paul
ei det'ic im'age
ei'do gen
ei"dop tom'e try
ein'stein
Einthoven's tri'angle
Eisenmenger's com'plex

e jac″u la′tion
e″jac u la″tio prae′cox
e jec′ta
e jec′tion
e jec′tor
e lab″o ra′tion
el′a cin
e′lase
e las′tase
e las′tic
e las′ti ca
e las′tin
e las tom′e ter
El′a vil
el′bow
e lec″tric′i ty
e lec′tri fy
e lec″tri za′tion
e lec″tro af fin′i ty
e lec″tro an″es the′si a
e lec″tro bi ol′o gy
e lec″tro bi os′co py
e lec″tro cap″il lar′i ty
e lec″tro car′di o gram″
e lec″tro car′di o graph″
e lec″tro car″di og′ra phy
e lec″tro car″di o pho nog′ra phy
e lec″tro ca tal′y sis
e lec″tro cau′ter y
e lec″tro chem′is try
e lec″tro chro″ma tog′ra phy
e lec″tro co ag″u la′tion
e lec″tro co′ma
e lec″tro con″duc tiv′i ty
e lec″tro con″trac til′i ty
e lec″tro con vul′sive
e lec″tro cor ti cog′ra phy
e lec″tro cu′tion
e lec″tro cys′to scope
e lec′trode
e lec′tro dent
e lec″tro der′ma tome
e lec″tro des″ic ca′tion
e lec″tro di″ag no′sis
e lec″tro di al′y sis
e lec″tro di′a phane
e lec″tro dy nam′ics
e lec″tro dy″na mom′e ter
e lec″tro en ceph′a lo gram″
e lec″tro en ceph′a lo graph″
e lec″tro en ceph″a log′ra phy
e lec″tro fit′
e lec″tro form′
e lec″tro gas′tro graph
e lec″tro gen′e sis
e lec′tro gram″
e lec″tro he″mo sta′sis
e lec″tro hys″ter og′ra phy
e lec″tro ki net′ics
e lec″tro ky′mo graph″
e lec″tro li thot′rity
e lec″trol′o gy
e lec″trol′y sis
e lec′tro lyte
e lec′tro ly″zer
e lec″tro mag′net
e lec″tro mas sage′
e lec″trom′e ter
e lec″tro mo′tive
e lec″tro my′o gram
e lec″tro my og′ra phy
e lec″tro ny stag mog′ra phy
e lec′tron
e lec″tro nar co′sis
e lec″tro neg′a tive
e lec″tro neu rog′raphy
e lec″tro neu′ro tone
e lec″tro ny stag mog′ram
e lec″tro os mo′sis
e lec″tro pa thol′o gy
e lec″tro pho′bi a
e lec″tro pho re′sis
e lec″troph′o rus

e lec″tro pho″to ther′a py
e lec″tro phren′ic
e lec″tro phys″i ol′o gy
e lec″tro pos′i tive
e lec″tro punc′ture
e lec″tro py rex′i a
e lec″tro re sec′tion
e lec″tro ret′i no gram
e lec″tro scis′sion
e lec′tro scope
e lec″tro sec′tion
e lec″tro shock′
e lec′tro some
e lec″tro steth′o phone
e lec″tro stric′tion
e lec″tro sur′ger y
e lec″tro syn′the sis
e lec″tro tax′is
e lec″tro thal′a mo gram
e lec″tro tha na′si a
e lec″tro ther″a peu′tics
e lec″tro ther′a py
e lec′tro therm
e lec′tro tome
e lec″trot′o nus
e lec″tro tur″bi nom′e ter
e lec″tro va′go gram
e lec″tro va′lence
e lec′tu ar″y
el′e ment
el″e o′ma
el″e om′e ter
el″e o my en′chy sis
el″e phan ti′a sis
el′e va″tor.
e lim′i nant
e lim″na′tion
e lin gua′tion
e lix′ir
el lip′soid
el lip′to cyte
el lip″to cy to′sis
e lon″ga′tion
el′u ate
e ma″ci a′tion
e mac″u la′tion
em″a na′tion
e man″ci pa′tion
em″a no ther′a py
e mas″cu la′tion
em balm′ing
em bed′
em″bo lec′to my
em″bo le′mi a
embol′ic
em′bo lism
em″bo lo la′li a
em′bo lus
em′bo ly
em bra′sure
em″bro ca′tion
em″bry ec′to my
em′bry o
em′bry o blast″
em″bry oc′to ny
em′bry oid
em″bry o lem′ma
em″bry o log′ic
em″bry ol′o gist
em″bry ol′o gy
em″bry o mor′phous
em′bry o tome″
em″bry ot′o my
em″bry o tox′on
em′bry o trophe
em″bry ul′ci a
em″bry ul′cus
em′e sis
e met″a tro′phi a
e met′ic
em′e tine
em″e to ca thar′sis

em″e to ma′ni a
em″e to pho′bi a
e mic′tion
em″i gra′tion
em′i nence
em″i nen′ti a
em′is sar″y
e mis′sion
em men′a gogue
em men′i a
em men″i op′a thy
em″me nol′o gy
em″me tro′pi a
e mol′li ent
e mo″ti o met″a bol′ic
e mo″ti o mus′cu lar
e mo′tion
e mo″ti o vas′cu lar
em pasm′
em′pa thize
em′pa thy
em′phly sis
em phrac′tic
em phrax′is
em″phy se′ma
em″phy se′ma tous
em pir′ic
Em′pir in
em plas′trum
em″pros thot′o nos
em″pros tho zy go′sis
em″py e′ma
em″py e′sis
em″py reu mat′ic
e mul′si fi″er
e mul′si fy″
e mul′sion
e munc′to ry
en am′el
en am″e lo blas′ma
en am″el o′ma
en″an the′ma
en an″ti o la′li a
en an′ti o morph″
en″ar thro′sis
en can′this
en cap″su la′tion
en cap′suled
en ceph″a lal′gi a
en ceph″a lat′ro phy
en ceph″a lit′ic
en ceph″a li′tis
en ceph″a li to gen′ic
en ceph′a lo cele″
en ceph″a lo dys pla′si a
en ceph′a lo gram″
en ceph″a log′ra phy
en ceph′a loid
en ceph′a lo lith″
en ceph″a lol′o gy
en ceph″a lo′ma
en ceph″a lo ma la′ci a
en ceph″a lo men″in gi′tis
en ceph″a lo me nin′go cele
en ceph″a lo men″in gop′a thy
en ceph′a lo mere″
en ceph″a lom′e ter
en ceph″a lo my″e li′tis
en ceph″a lo my″e lo neu rop′a thy
en ceph″a lo my″e lop′a thy
en ceph″a lo my″e lo ra dic″u li′tis
en ceph″a lo my″e lo ra dic″u lop′a thy
en ceph″a lo my elo′sis
en ceph″a lo my″o car di′tis
en ceph′a lon
en ceph″a lo nar co′sis
en ceph″a lop′a thy
en ceph″a lo punc′ture
en ceph″a lo py o′sis

en ceph″a lo ra chid′i an
en ceph″a lor rha′gi a
en ceph′a lo scope
en ceph″a lo sep′sis
en ceph″a lo′sis
en ceph′a lo tome
en ceph″a lot′o my
en ceph″a lo tri gem′i nal
en″chon dro′ma
en chon″dro ma to′sis
en chon″dro sar co′ma
en″chon dro′sis
en″chy le′ma
en clit′ic
en″co pre′sis
en cra′ni us
en″cy e′sis
en″cys ta′tion
en cyst′ed
en cyst′ment
en″da del′phus
En″da moe′ba
en″dan gi i′tis
en″da or ti′tis
en″dar ter ec′to my
en″dar te′ri al
en″dar te ri′tis
end au′ral
end″ax o neu′ron
end′-bulb″
en dem′ic
end ep″i der′mis
end″er gon′ic
en der′mic
en″der mo′sis
en″do ab dom′i nal
en″do an″eu rys mor′rha phy
en″do an″gi i′tis
en″do a″or ti′tis
en″do bi ot′ic
en″do bron′chi al

en″do car di′al
en″do car di′tis
en″do car′di um
en″do car′do fi bro′sis
en″do ce′li ac
en″do cer″vi ci′tis
en″do cer′vix
en″do cho led′o chal
en″do chon″dral
en″do col pi′tis
en″do cra′ni al
en″do cra ni′tis
en″do cra′ni um
en′do crine
en″do cri nol′o gy
en″do cri nop′a thy
en″do crin″o ther′a py
en″do cy′ma
en′do cyst
en′do derm
en″do der″ma to zo″o no′sis
en″do don′tics
en″do don′tist
en″do en′zyme
en dog′a my
en dog′e nous
en″do gna′thi on
en″do la ryn′ge al
en′do lymph
en′do lym phat′ic
en″do lym phan′gi al
en″do me trec′to my
en″do me″tri o′ma
en″do me″tri o′sis
en″do me tri′tis
en″do me′tri um
en dom′e try
en″do mi to′sis
en′do morph
en′do mor″phy
En″do my′ces

en″do my o car′di al
en″do my″o car di′tis
en″do mys′i um
en″do na′sal
en″do na′sal
en″do neu′ral
en″do neu′ri um
en″do nu cle′o lus
en″do par′a site
en″do pep′ti dase
en″do per″i car di′tis
en″do per″i my″o car di′tis
en″do phle bi′tis
en doph″thal mi′tis
en′do plasm
end or′phrin
en do scope
en″do scop′ic
en″do skel′e ton
en″dos mom′e ter
en″dos mo′sis
en′do sperm
en′do spore
en dos″te o′ma
en dos′te um
en″dos ti′tis
en″dos to′sis
en″do sub til′y sin
en″do ten din′e um
en″do the′li al
en″do the″li o an″gi i′tis
en″do the″li o cho′ri al
en″do the′li oid
en″do the′li o ly′sin
en″do the″li o′ma
en″do the″li o ma to′sis
en″do the″li o′sis
en″do the′li um
en″do ther′mic
en′do thrix
en″do tox″i co′sis
en″do tox′in
en″do tra′che al
en′e ma
en″er get′ics
en″er gom′e ter
en′er gy
en″er va′tion
en gage′ment
en gas′tri us
en globe′ment
en gorge′ment
en′gram
en hem′a to spore
en large′ment
en″oph thal′mos
en″o si ma′ni a
en″os to′sis
en′si form
en som′pha lus
en′stro phe
en″ta cous′tic
en′tad
en′tal
En″ta moe′ba
en ta′si a
en tel′e chy
en′ter al
en″ter al′gi a
en″ter ec′ta sis
en″ter ec′to my
en″ter e pip′lo cele
en ter′ic
en ter′i coid
en″ter i′tis
en″ter o a nas″to mo′sis
en′ter o bac″ter i a′ceae
en″ter o bi′a sis
En″ter o′bi us
en′ter o cele″
en″ter o cen te′sis
en″ter o′cin

en″ter oc′ly sis
en″ter o coc′cus
en′ter o coele″
en″ter o co lec′to my
en″ter o co li′tis
en″ter o co los′to my
en′ter o cyst″
en″ter o cys′to cele
en″ter o cys to plas′ty
en″ter o cys tos′che o cele
en″ter o en ter′ic
en″ter o en″ter os′to my
en″ter o gas′tro cele
en″ter o gas′trone
en″ter og′e nous
en′ter o graph″
en″ter o ki′nase
en′ter o lith
en″ter o li thi′a sis
en″ter ol′o gist
en″ter ol′y sis
en″ter o me′ro cele
en″ter o my co′sis
en″ter o my′ia sis
en ′ter on
en″ter op′a thy
en″ter o pex′y
en′ter o plas″ty
en″ter o ple′gi a
en″ter o proc′ti a
en″ter op to′sis
en″ter or rha′gi a
en″ter or′rha phy
en″ter or rhex′is
en′ter o scope
en″ter o sep′sis
en′ter o spasm
en″ter o sta′sis
en″ter o ste no′sis
en″ter os′to my
en′ter o tome
en″ter ot′o my
en″ter o tox′in
en″ter o vi′rus
en″ter o zo′on
en″the o ma′ni a
en′the sis
en thet′ic
en ti′ris
en′to blast
en′to cele
en″to cho roid′e a
en′to cone
en″to co′nid
en′to derm
en″to derm′al
en′to mere
en to′mi on
en to mog′e nous
en″to mol′o gist
en″to mol′o gy
en″to mo pho′bi a
ent″oph thal′mi a
ent op′tic
ent″op tos′co py
en″to ret′i na
ent″os to′sis
ent o′tic
en″to zo′on
en train′ment
en tro′pi on
en′tro py
en′ty py
e nu′cle ate
en″u re′sis
en vi′ron ment
en″zy mat′ic
en′zyme
en″zy mol′o gy
en″zy mol′y sis
e′on ism
e′o sin

e″o sin″o pe′ni a
e″o sin′o phil
e″o sin″o phil′i a
e″o sin ″o phil′ic
e pac′tal
ep″ar te′ri al
ep ax′i al
ep en′dy ma
ep en″dy mi′tis
ep en″dy mo blas to′ma
ep en′dy mo cyte
e″pen dy mo′ma
ep en″dy mop′a thy
eph″e bo gen′e sis
e phed′rine
eph e′lis
e phem′er al
eph″i dro′sis
ep″i a gnath′us
ep′i blast
ep″i bleph′a ron
e pib′o ly
ep″i bulb′ar
ep″i can′thus
ep″i car′di um
ep″i chor′dal
ep″i cho′ri al
ep″i cho′ri on
ep″i col′ic
ep″i co′mus
ep″i con″dyl al′gi a
ep″i con′dy lar
ep″i con′dyle
ep″i con″dy li′tis
ep″i cra′ni o tem″po ral′is
ep″i cra′ni um
ep″i cra′ni us
ep″i cri′sis
ep″i crit′ic
ep″i cys ti′tis
ep″i cys tot′ o my
ep′i cyte
ep″i dem′ic
ep″i de″mi ol′o gist
ep″i de″mi ol′o gy
ep″i der′mal
ep″i der″ma to plas′ty
ep″i der″ma to′zo″on o sis
ep″i der′mic
ep″i der″mi dal i za′tion
ep″i der′mis
ep″i der mi′tis
ep″i der″mi za′tion
ep″i der″mo dys pla′si a ver ru″ci for′mis
ep″i der′moid
ep″i der mol′y sis
ep″i der″mo my co′sis
ep″i der moph′y tid
Ep″i der moph′y ton
ep″i der″mo phy to′sis
ep″i der mo′sis
ep″i did″y mec′to my
ep″i did′y mis
ep″i did″y mi′tis
ep″i did′y mo-or chi′tis
ep″i did″y mot′o my
ep″i did″y mo vas os′to my
ep″i du′ral
ep″i fas′ci al
ep″i fol lic″u li′tis
ep″i gas tral′gi a
ep″i gas′tric
ep″i gas′tri o cele″
ep″i gas′tri um
ep″i gas′tri us
ep″i gas′tro cele
ep″i gen′e sis
ep″i glot′tic
ep″i glot″ti dec′to my
ep″i glot′tis
ep″i glot ti′tis

e pig′na thus
ep″i hy′oid
ep″i la mel′lar
ep″i la′tion
ep″i lem′ma
ep′i lep″sy
ep″i lep′tic
ep″i lep″to gen′ic
ep″i lep′toid
ep″i loi′a
ep′mere
ep″i my″o car′di um
ep″i mys′i um
ep″i neph′rine
ep″i ne phri′tis
ep″i neu′ral
ep″i neu′ri um
ep″i ot′ic
ep″i pal′a tum
ep″i pas′tic
ep″i phar′ynx
ep″i phe nom′e non
e piph′o ra
ep″i phy lax′is
ep″i phys″e o ne cro′sis
ep″i phys″e op′a thy
ep″i phys″i o de′sis
ep″i phys″i ol′is the′sis
ep″i phys″i ol′y sis
e piph′y sis
e piph″y si′tis
ep″i pi′al
ep″i pleu′ral
e pip′lo cele
ep″i plo ec′to my
e pip″lo en′ter o cele″
epi plo′ic
e pip″lom phal′o cele″
e pip′lo on
e pip′lo pex″y
e p″i plor′rha phy
ep″ip ter′ic
ep″i py′gus
ep″i scle′ra
ep″i scle′ral
ep″i scle ri′tis
e pi″si o cli′si a
e pi″si o el″y tror′rha phy
e pi″si o per″i ne′o plas″ty
e pi″si o per″i ne or′rha phy
e pi″si o plas″ty
e pi″si or rha′gi a
e pi″si or′rha phy
e pi″si o ste no′sis
e pi″si ot′o my
ep′i sode
ep″i spa′di as
ep″i spas′tic
ep″i sphe′noid
ep″i spi′nal
ep″i sta′sis
ep″i stat′ic
ep″i stax′is
ep″i stern′um
ep″i stro′phe us
ep″i sym′pus
ep″i ten din′e um
ep″i thal′″a mus
ep″i tha lax′i a
ep″i the′li a
ep″i the″li o cho′ri al
ep″i the″li o ge net′ic
ep″i the′li oid
ep″i the″li o′ma
ep″i the li′tis
ep″i the′li um
ep″i the″li za′tion
ep′i them
ep″i to′nos
ep″i trich′i um
ep″i troch′le ar
ep″i troch″le ar′is

ep″i trich″le o-ol″e cra no′nis
ep″i tu ber″cu lo′sis
ep″i tym pan′ic
ep″i tym′pa num
ep″i zo′ic
ep″i zo ot′ic
ep″o nych′i um
ep″o nym
ep″o oph′o ron
ep ox′y
Ep′som salt
ep u′lis
ep′u loid
ep″u lo fi bro′ma
e qua′tion
e qua′tor
e″qui ax′i al
e″qui li bra′tion
e″qui lib′ri um
eq′uine
eq″ui no ca′vus
eq″ui no va′rus
e qui′nus
eq″ui se to′sis
e quiv′a lent
e ra′sion
Erb′s pal′sy
e rec′tile
e rec′tion
e rec′tor
er″e mi o pho′bi a
e rep′sin
er′e thism
er″e this′tic
erg
er ga′si a
er ga′si a try
er ga″si o ma′ni a
er ga″si o pho′bi a
er″gas′the′ni a
er gas′to plasm
er′go graph
er gom′e ter
er″go no′vine
er″go pho′bi a
er′go phore
er gos′ter ol
er′got
er got′a mine
er″go ther′a py
er′got ism
Er″go trate′
er′i gens
Erlenmeyer flask
e rog′e nous
eros
e rose′
e ro′si o in″ter dig″i ta′lis blas″to my ce′ti ca
e ro′sion
e rot′ic
e rot′i ca
e rot′i cism
er′o tism
er″o to gen′ic
er″o to ma′ni a
er″o top′a thy
er″o to pho′bi a
e″ruc ta′tion
e ru″ga to″ry
e rup′tion
e rup′tive
er″y sip′e las
er″y sip″e lo coc′cus
er″y sip′e loid
e rys′i phake
er″y the′ma
er″y the′moid
er″y thras′ma
e ryth″re de ma pol″y neu rop′a thy
e ry thre′mi a

er″yth re′mic
e ryth′ o blast
e ryth″ro blas to′ma
e ryth″ro blas″to pe′ni a
e ryth″ro blas to′sis fe tal′is
e ryth″ro chlo ro′pi a
E ryth″ro cin
e ryth″ cy″a no′sis
e ryth′ro cyte
e ryth″ro cy the′mi a
e ryth″ro cyt′ic
e ryth″ro cy″to ly′sin
e ryth″ro cy tol′y sis
e ryth″ro cy tom′e ter
e ryth″ro cy′to-op′so nin
e ryth″ cy″to poi e′sis
e ryth″ro cy″tor rhex′is
e rythro cy tos′chi sis
e ryth″ro cy to′sis
e ryth″ro de gen′er a tive
e ryth″ro der′ma
e ryth″ro dont′i a
e ryth″ro gen′e sis
e ryth″ ro gen′in
e ryth′ro gone
er′y throid
e ryth″ro leu″ko blas to′sis
e ryth″ro leu ko′sis
er″y throl′y sin
er″y throl′y sis
e ryth″ro me lal′gi a
e ryth″ro me′li a
er″y throm′e ter
e ryth″ro my′cin
e ryth″ro my″e lo′sis
er′y thron
e ryth″ro ne″o cy to′sis
e ryth″ro no cla′si a
er″y thro pe′ni a
e ryth′ro phage
e ryth″ro pha″go cy to′sis
e ryth′ro phil
e ryth″ro phle′um
e ryth″ro pho′bi a
eryth′ro phose
e ryth″ro pla′si a
e ryth″ro poi e′sis
e″ryth ro poi e′tic
e ryth″ro sar co′ma
e ryth ro′sis
e ryth″ro sta′sis
er″y thru′ri a
Esbach′s re a′gent
es cape′
es′char
es″cha rot′ic
es cha rot′o my
Esch″er ich′i a co′li
es cutch′eon
es′er ine
E sid′rix
e soph″a gal′gi a
e soph″a ge′al
e soph″a gec ta′si a
e soph″a gec′to my
e soph″a gec′to py
e soph″a gi′tis
e soph″a go du″o de nos′to my
e soph″a go en″ter os′to my
e soph″a go e soph″a gos′to my
e soph″a go gas trec′to my
e soph″a go gas′tro plas″ty
e soph″a go gas′tro scope″
e soph″a go gas tros′to my
e soph″a go je″ju nos′to my
e soph″a gom′e ter
e soph″a go my′o to my
e soph″a gop′ a thy
e soph′a go plas″ty
e soph″a gop to′sis
e soph′a go scope″
e soph a gos′copy
e soph′a go spasm″
e soph″a go ste no′sis

e soph″a gos′to ma
e soph″a gos″to mi′a sis
e soph″a gos′to my
e″so phag′o tome
e soph″a got′o my
e soph′a gus
e soph″o gram
es″o pho′ri a
es″o tro′pi a
es′sence
es sen′tial
es′ter
es′ter ase
es ter″i fi ca′tion
es the′si a
es the″si ol′o gy
es the″si om′e ter
es the″si o phys″i ol′o gy
es thet′ic
es″thi om′e ne
Es′tin yl
es′ti val
es″ti va′tion
es tra di′ol
est′ri ol
es′tro gen
es tro gen′ic
es′trus
es″tu a ri′um
eth′ane
eth′a nol
eth′e noid
e′ther
eth″mo ceph′a lus
eth″mo fron′tal
eth′moid
eth moi′dal
eth″moid ec′to my
eth″moid i′tis
eth″moid ot′o my
eth″mo lac′ri mal
eth″mo max′il lar″y
eth″mo na′sal
eth″mo tur′bi nal
eth′nic
eth nol′o gy
eth′yl
eth′yl ene
eth′y nyl
e″ti o la′tion
e″ti o log′ic
e″ti ol′o gy
e″ti o path″o gen′e sis
eu″ca lyp′tus
eu chol′i a
eu chro′ma tin
eu chro″ma top′si a
eu″di om′e ter
eu″es the′si a
eu gen′ics
eu gnath′ic
eu gon′ic
eu″ki ne′si a
eu mor′phic
eu noi′a
eu′nuch
eu′nuch oid
eu′nuch oid ism
eu pho′ni a
eu pho′ri a
eu phys″i o log′ic
eu prax′i a
eu″ro don′ti a
eu″ro pis″o ceph′a lus
eu″ro pro ceph′a lus
eu″ry ce phal′ic
eu″ry chas′mus
eu″ry gnath′ism
eu″ry mer′ic
eu′ry on
eu″ry ther′mal
eu′scope

eu sta′chi an
eu sys′to le
eu″tha na′si a
eu then′ics
Eu the′ri a
eu thy′roid ism
eu to′ci a
e vac′u ant
e vac″u a′tion
e vac′u a tor″
e vag″i na′tion
ev″a nes′cent
e″ven tra′tion
e ver′sion
ev′i dence
ev″i ra′tion
e vis″cer a′tion
e vis″cer o neu rot′o my
ev″o ca′tion
ev″o lu′tion
e vul′sion
ex ac″er ba′tion
ex″al ta′tion
ex am″i na′tion
ex an′them
ex″an the′ma
ex ar″te ri′tis
ex″ca va′tion
ex′ca va″tor
ex″ce men to′sis
ex cer″e bra′tion
ex cip′i ent
ex ci′sion
ex cit″a bil′i ty
ex ci′tant
ex″ci ta′tion
ex clu′sion
ex″coch le a′tion
ex co′ri ate
ex co″ri a′tion
ex′cre ment
ex cres′cence
ex cre′ta
ex′cre tin
ex cre′tion
ex′cre to ry
ex cur′sion
ex cur′va ture
ex cy″clo pho′ri a
ex cy″clo tro′pi a
ex″cys ta′tion
ex′e dens
ex″en ce pha′li a
ex en″ter a′tion
ex′er cise
ex er′e sis
ex″fe ta′tion
ex fo″li a′tion
ex fo″li a′tive
ex″ha la′tion
ex haust′er
ex haus′tion
ex″hi bi′tion
ex″hi bi′tion ism
ex″hi bi′tion ist
ex hil′a rant
ex″hu ma′tion
ex″is ten′tial ism
ex′i tus
Exner's
area
ex″o car′di a
ex″o car′di ac
ex″o cat″a pho ri a
ex″o ce lom′ic
ex″oc cip′i tal
ex″o cho′ri on
ex″o coe′lom
ex′o crine
ex″o don′ti a
ex″o don′tist
ex og′a my
ex″o gas′tru la
ex og′e nous

ex″o hys′ter o pex″y
ex om′pha los
ex″o pho′ri a
ex″oph thal mom′e ter
ex″oph thal mom′e try
ex″oph thalm′mos
ex″o skel′e ton
ex″os″to sec′to my
ex″os to′sis
ex″o ther′mic
ex″o tox′in
ex″o tro′pi a
ex pan′sive
ex pec′to rant
ex pec′to rate
ex pec″to ra′tion
ex pel′
ex per′i ment
ex pi a′tion
ex″pi ra′tion
ex pi′ra tory
ex pire′
ex″plan ta′tion
ex″plo ra′tion
ex po′sure
ex pres′sion
ex pul′sion
ex san′gui nate
ex san͵gui na′tion
ex sic′cant
ex″sic ca′tion
ex′stro phy
ex″suf fla′tion
ex ten′sion
ex ten′sor
ex te″ri or i za′tion
ex′tern
ex ter′nal ize
ex′ter o cep″tor
ex″ter o fec′tive
ex tinc′tion
ex″tir pa′tion
ex tor′sion
ex″tra ar tic′u lar
ex″tra buc′cal
ex″tra bulb′ar
ex″tra cap′su lar
ex″tra car′pal
ex″tra cel′lu lar
ex″tra cer′e bral
ex″tra cor po′re al
ex″tra cor pus′cu lar
ex″tra cra′ni al
ex′tract
ex trac′tion
ex″tra cyst′ic
ex″tra du′ral
ex″tra em″bry on′ic
ex″tra ep″i phys′e al
ex″tra e soph″a ge′al
ex″tra gen′i tal
ex″tra he pat′ic
ex″tra lig″a men′tous
ex″tra med′ul lar″y
ex″tra mu′ral
ex″tra nu′cle ar
ex″tra oc′u lar
ex″tra pa ren′chy mal
ex″tra pel′vic
ex″tra per″i ne′al
ex″tra per″i to ne′al
ex″tra pla cen′tal
ex″tra pros tat′ic
ex″tra py ram′i dal
ex″tra sen′sor y
ex″tra sys′to le
ex″tra tu′bal
ex″tra u′ter ine
ex″tra vag′i nal
ex trav″a sa′tion
ex″tra vas′cu lar
ex″tra ven tric′u lar

ex″tra vis′u al
ex trem′i ty
ex trin′sic
ex′tro phy
ex′tro vert
ex tru′sion
ex″tu ba′tion
ex′u date
ex″u da′tion
ex u″vi a′tion
eye
eye′lash″

F

fa bel′la
fab″ri ca′tion
face
fac′et
fa′cial
fa′ci es
fa cil″i ta′tion
fac″i o scap″u lo hu′mer al
fac ti′tious
fac′tor
fac′ul ta″tive
fag″o py′rism
Fahrenheit
fail′ure
faint
fal′ci form
fal′cu la
fal′cu lar
fal lo′pi an
Fallot, tetral′o gy of
false
falx
fa′mes
fa mil′ial
fa nat′i cism
Fanconi, Guido
fang
fan″go ther′a py
fan′ta sy
far′ad
Faraday, Michael
fa rad′ic
far″a dim′e ter
fa rad″i punc′ture
far′a dism
far″a di za′tion
far″a do con″trac til′i ty
far″a do mus′cu lar
far″i na′ceous
fas′ci a
fas′ci cle
fas cic′u la″ted
fas cic″u la′tion
fas cic′u lar
fas cic′u lus
fas″ci ec′to my
fas ci′num
fas″ci od′e sis
fas ci′o la ci ne′re a
Fas″ci o loi′des
fas′ci o plas″ty
fas″ci or′rha phy
fas″ci o scap″u lo hu′mer al
fas″ci ot′o my
fas ci′tis
fas tig′i um
fa tigue′
fau′ces
fau′na
fa vag′i nous
fa ve′o lus
fa′vi des
fa′vism
fa′vus
fear
fea′ture

feb'ri cant
fe brif'ic
feb'ri fuge
fe'brile
feb"ri pho'bi a
fe'cal
fe'ca lith
fe'cal oid
fe'ces
fec'u lent
fe"cun da'tion
fe cun'di ty
feed'ing
Fehling's re a'gent
fe'line
fel la'ti o
fel"la tor'
fel"la trice'
fel'on
Felty's syn'drome
fe'male
fem'i nism
fem"i ni za'tion
fem'i niz ing
fem'o ral
fem"o ro tib'i al
fe'mur
fe nes'tra
fen"es tra'tion
fen'o mates
Fe'o sol
fer'ment
fer"men ta'tion
fer'ra ted
ferr'ric
fer"ri he"mo glo'bin
fer'rous
fer'tile
fer"ti li za'tion
fer'ti li zin
fes'ter
fes'ti na"ting
fes"ti na'tion
fes toon'
fe'tal ism
fe ta'tion
fe'ti cide
fet'id
fe'tish
fe'tish ism
fet'lock
fe tom'e try
fe"to pel'vic
fe'tor
fe tos'
copy
fe'tus
fe'ver
fi'ber
fi'bril
fi'bril lat ed
fi"bril la'tion
fi bril"lo gen'e sis
fi'brin
fi brin'o gen
fi brin"o gen"o pe'ni a
fi"brin o glob'u lin
fi'bri noid
fi"bri no ly'sin
fi"brin ol'y sis
bi"brin o ly'tic
fi'brin ous
fi"bro ad"e no'ma
fi"bro ad'i pose
fi"bro an"gi o'ma
fi"bro a re'o lar
fi'bro blast
fi"bro blas'tic
fi"bro blas to'ma
fi"bro bron chi'tis
fi"bro cal car'e ous
fi"bro car"ci no'ma
fi"bro car'ti lage
fi"bro cel'lu lar

fi″bro chon dro′ma
fi″bro chon dro-os″te o′ma
fi″bro cys′tic
fi″bro cys to′ma
fi′bro cyte
fi″bro dys pla′si a
fi″bro e las′tic
fi″bro e las to′sis
fi″bro en″chon dro′ma
fi′bro gen
fi″bro gli o′ma
fi′broid
fi″broid ec′to my
fi″bro lam′i nar
fi″bro lei″o my o′ma
fi″bro li po′ma
fi″bro li po sar co′ma
fi″bro ly′sin
fi bro′ma
fi bro′ma toid
fi bro″ma to′sis
fi″bro mus′cu lar
fi″bro my o′ma
fi″bro my″o mec′to my
fi″bro my″o si′tis
fi″bro myx″o en do the″li o′ma
fi″bro myx″o li po′ma
fi″bro myx o′ma
fi″bro myx″o sar co′ma
fi″bro neu ro′ma
fi″bro-os″te o chon dro′ma
fi″bro-os te o′ ma
fi″bro-os″te o sar co′ma
fi″bro pla′si a
fi″bro plas′tic
fi′bro plate″
fi″bro psam mo′ma
fi″bro pu′ru lent
fi″bro sar co′ma
fi″bro ser′rous
fi bro′sis
fi″bro si′tis
fi brot′ic
fi′brous
fib′u la
fib″u lo cal ca′ne al
Fielder′s
    my″o car di′tis
fig′ure
fi la′ceous
fil′a ment
fil″a men ta′tion
fi la′ri a
fi lar′i al
fil″a ri sis
fi lar′i cide
fi lar′i form″
fil′i form″
fil′i punc″ture
fil′let
fil′ter
fil′tra ble
fil′trate
fil tra′tion
fil′trum
fil′lum
fim′bri a
fim′bri al
fin′ger
fis′sion
fis sip′a rous
fis′su la
fis′sure
fis′sure-in-a′no
fis′tu la
fis′tu lar
fis″tu lec′to my
fis″tu li za′tion
fis″tu lo en″ter os′to my
fis″tu lot′o my
fi′th   disease
fix a′tion
fix′a tive
flac′cid

flag′el late
flag″el la′tion
fla gel′li form″
fla gel′lum
flail
Fla′gyl
flap
flare
flat′u lence
flat′u lent
fla′tus
fla′vin
fla″vo bac ter′i a
flex″i bil′i tas
flex′i ble
flex im′e ter
flex′ion
Flexner′s
ba cil′lus
flex′or
flex′u ous
flex′ure
flick′er
floc″cu la′tion
floc′cu lent
floc′cu lus
flor′id
flo ta′tion
flow′me″ter
flu′id
fluke
flu′mi na pi lor′um
fl″o res′ce in
flu′o res′cence
flu″o ri da′tion
flu′o ride
flu″o ri na′tion
flu′o rine
flu′o rite
flu″o ro pho tom′e try
flu′o ro scope″
flu or os′co py
flu″o ro′sis
flu phen′a zine
flut′ter
flux
foam
fo′cal
fo′cus
foil
fold
Foley cath′e ter
fo′lic ac′id
fo lie′a″deux
fo lin′ic
fo′li um
fol′li cle
fol lic′u lar
fol lic″u li′tis
fol lic″u lo′ma
fo″men ta′tion
fo′mes
fo′mi tes
fon″ta nel′
fo ra′men
fo ra′mi na
for″a min′u lum
for′ceps
Forcheimer′s sign
Fordyce′s dis ease′
fore′arm″
fore′brain″
fore′fin″ger
fore′foot″
fore′gut″
fore′head
for′eign
fo ren′sic
fore′pleas″ure
fore′skin″
fore′wa″ters
form al′de hyde
For′ma lin
for ma′tion

form′a tive
for′ma zan
for′mic
for″mi ca′tion
for′mu la
for′mu lar″y
for′ni cate
for″ni ca′tion
for′nix
Foshay′s se′rum
fos′sa
fos sette′
fos′su la
found′ling
four chette′
fo′ve a
fo ve′o la
frac″tion a′tion
fract′ure
fra gil′tas
fra gil′i ty
frag″men ta′tion
fram be′si a
free′mar″tin
Frei test
frem′i tus
fre′nal
fre not′o my
fren′u lum
fre′num
fren′zy
fre′quen cy
Freud, Sigmund
fri′a ble
fric′tion
Friedlander ba cil′li
Friedman test
Friedreich′s a tax′i a
fri gid′i ty
Froehlich′s syn′drome
frole″ment′
fron′tal
fron ta′lis
fron″to ma′lar
fron″to max′il lar
fron″to men′tal
fron″to na′sal
fron″to-oc cip′i tal
fron″to-tem″po ra′le
frost′bite″
frot″tage′
frot″teur′
fruc′tose
frus tra′tion
Fu a′din
fuch′sin
fu′gi tive
fugue
ful′gu ra″ting
ful″gu ra′tion
fu lig′i nous
ful′mi nant
ful′mi na″ting
fu′ma rase
fu″mi ga′tion
fu′ming
func′tion
func′tion al
fun′da ment
fun′di form
fun′dus
fun′du scope
fun″du sec′to my
fun′gate
fun′gi
fun″gi ci′dal
fun′gi cide
fun′gi form
fun″gi stat′ic
Fun gi′zone
fun′goid
fun′gus

fu′ni cle
fu nic′u lar
fu nic″u li′tis
fu nic′u lus
fu′nis
fun′nel
Fu′ra cin
Fu″ra dan′tin
fur′cu la
fur′fur
fur′fur yl
fu′ror
fu ro′se mide
fur′row
fu′run cle
fu″run′cu lar
fu run″cu lo′sis
fus′cin
fu′sel oil
fu′si ble
fu′si form
fu′sion
fu″so cel′lu lar
fu″so spi″ro che′tal
fu″so spi″ro che to′sis

G

gait
ga lac″ta cra′si a
ga lac′ta gogue
ga lac′tase
gal″ac te′mi a
ga lact″hi dro′sis
ga lac′tic
gal″ac tis′chi a
ga lac′to cele
ga lac′to gen
ga lac′toid
gal″ac tom′e ter
gal″ac toph′a gous
gal″ac toph′ly sis
ga lac′to phore
gal″ac toph″o ri′tis
gal″ac toph′y gous
ga lac″to poi et′ic
ga lac″tor rhe′a
gal″ac tos′che sis
ga lac′to scope
ga lac′tose
ga lac″to se′mi a
gal″ac to′sis
gal″ac tos′ta sis
ga lac″to su′ri a
ga lac″to ther′a py
ga lac″to tox′in
gal″ac tot′ro phy
gal″ac tu′ri a
ga′le a
gal″e o phil′i a
gal″e o pho′bi a
gal″e ro′pi a
gall′blad″der
gal′lop
gall′stone
gal van′ic
gal′va nism
gal′van ize
gal″va no con″trac til′i ty
gal″va no far″a di za′tion
gal″va nom′eter
gal″va no mus′cu lar
gal′va no scope″
gal″va no sur′ger y
gal″va no ther′a py
gal′va no ther″my
gam′bi an
gam′ete
ga me′to cyte
gam″e to gen′e sis

ga me′to phyte
gam′ma
gam′ma cism
gam″o ma′ni a
gam″o pho′bi a
gan′gli a″ted
gan′gli o blast″
gan′gli o blas to′ma
gan′gli o cyte″
gan″gli o gli o′ma
gan′gli oid
gan′gli on
gan″gli on ec′to my
gan″gli o neu ro′ma
gan″gli on′ic
gan″gli o ni′tis
gan′gli o side
gan″glio si do′sis
gan″gli o sym path″i co blas to′ma
gan go′sa
gan′grene
gan′gre nous
gan′o blast
Gan ta′nol
Gan′tri sin
gar′get
gar′gle
gar′goyl
gar′goyl ism
gar′lic
gar rot′ing
Gartner's cyst
gasp
Gasserian gan′gli on
Gas″ter oph′i lus
gas tral′gi a
gas″tral go ke no′sis
gas″tras the′ni a
gas″tra tro′phi a
gas trec′ta sis
gas trec′to my
gas′tric
gas′trin
gas tri′tis
gas″tro a ceph′a lus
gas″tro a mor′phus
gas″tro an as″to mo′sis
gas′tro cele
gas″troc ne′mi us
gas″tro col′ic
gas″tro co lot′o my
gas″tro col pot′o my
gas″tro di′a phane
gas″tro di aph″a nos′co py
gas″tro did′y mus
gas″tro du″o de′nal
gas″tro du″o de ni′tis
gas″tro du″o de nos′to my
gas″tro en′ter ic
gas″tro en″ter i′tis
gas″tro en″ter o a nas″to mo′sis
gas″tro en″ter ol′o gist
gas″tro en″ter ol′o gy
gas″tro en″ter op a thy
gas″tro en″ter op to′sis
gas″tro en″ter os′to my
gas″tro ep″i plo′ic
gas″tro e soph′a ge″al
gas″tro e soph″a gi′tis
gas″tro gas tros′to my
gas″tro ga″vage′
gas′tro graph
gas″tro he pat′ic
gas″tro hy″per ton′ic
gas″tro hys″ter ot′o my
gas″tro in tes′ti nal
gas″tro je ju′nal
gas″tro je″ju ni′tis
gas″tro je″ju no col′ic
gas″tro je″ju nos′to my
gas″tro lav′age

gas'tro lith
gas"tro li thi'a sis
gas trol'o gy
gas trol'y sis
gas"tro ma la'ci a
gas"tro meg'a ly
gas trom'e lus
gas"tro my co'sis
gas"tro mu ot'o my
gas trop'a thy
gas'tro pex"y
gas"tro pho'tor
gas"tro phren'ic
gas"tro plas'ty
gas"tro pli ca'tion
gas"trop to'sis
gas troph"lo rec'to my
gas"tror rha'gi a
gas tror'rha phy
gas"tror rhe'a
gas tros'chi sis
gas'tro scope
gas tros'co py
gas'tro spasm
gas"tro splen'ic
gas"tro stax'is
gas tros'to my
gas"tro tho ra cop'a gus
gas trot'o my
gas"tro tym'pa ni'tes
gas'tru la
gat"o phil'i a
gat"o pho'bi a
Gaucher's
dis ease'
gauze
ga'vage
gaze
gel so'ma
ge las'mus
ge lat"i fi ca'tion
gel'a tin
ge lat"i no lyt'ic
ge lat'i nous
geld
geld'ing
Gel'foam
ge lot'o lep"sy
ge mel'lus
gem fib'ro zil
gem'i nate
gem"i na'tion
gem'ma
gem'mule
Gem'o nil
gen"e al'o gy
gene
ge ner'ic
ge ne"si ol'o gy
gen'e sis
ge net'ic
ge net'i cist
ge net'ics
ge net"o troph'ic
ge'ni al
ge nic'u lar
ge nic'u late
ge nic'u lum
ge"ni o glos'sus
ge"ni o hy'oid
ge'ni on
ge"ni o pha ryn'ge us
ge'ni o plas"ty
gen'i tal
gen"i ta'li a
gen'i tal ize
gen'i ta loid
gen"i to cru'ral
gen"i to fem'o ral
gen"i to u'ri nar"y
gen'i us
Gennari's lay'er
gen'o cide
gen'o copy

gen″o der ma to′sis
ge′nome
gen″o pho′bi a
gen ta mi′cin
gen′o type
Gen′ta mi cin
gen′tian
gen′u clast
gen″u cu′bi tal
gen″u fa′cial
gen″u pec′tor al
ge′nus
gen″y chei′lo plas″ty
gen′y plas″ty
ge″o pha′gi a
ge oph′a gy
Ge ot′ri chum
ge phy″ro pho′bi a
ge rat′ic
ger″a tol′o gy
ger″i a tri′ci an
ger″i at′rics
ger″i o psy cho′sis
ger ma′ni um
ger mi ci′dal
ger′mi cide
ger″mi na′tion
ger mi no′ma
ger″o der′ma
ger″o don′ti a
ger″o don′tics
ger″o ma ras′mus
ger″o mor′phism
ge ron′tic
ger″on tol′o gy
ge ron″to phil′ia
ge ron″to pho′bi a
ge ron′to ther′a py
ger″on tox′on
Gerstmann's syn′drome
Gesell, Arnold
ges ta′tion
Ghon tu′ber cle
Gi ar′di a
Gi ar′di a
Lam′blia
gi″ar di′a sis
gib′ber ish
gib bos′i ty
gib′bous
gib′bus
gid′di ness
Giemsa stain
gi gan′tism
gi gan′to blast
gi gan′to cyte
Gigli's saw
gin′gi va
gin′gi val
gin″gi val′gi a
gin″gi vec′to my
gin″gi vi′tis
gin″gi vo glos si′tis
gin″gi vo′sis
gin″gi vo sto″ma ti′tis
gin′gly mus
gi″o tri cho′sis
gir′dle
git′o nin
gi tox′in
giz′zard
gla bel′la
gla′brous
gla′cial
glad″i o′lus
glair′y
gland
glan′ders
gland′u lar
glans
glass′y
Glauber's salt
glau co′ma
gleet

gle″no hu′mer al
gle′noid
gli′a
gli′al
gli′a cyte
gli′a din
gli″o bac te′ri a
gli″o blas to′ma mul″ti for′me
gli″o coc′cus
gli″o fi″bro′sar co′ma
gli o′ma
gli″o ma to′sis
gli o′ma tous
gli″o sar co′ma
gli o′sis
gli′o some
globe
glo′bin
glob′ule
glob′u li cide″
glob u lin
glob″u li nu′ri a
glo′bus
gloe′a
glome
glom′er ate
glo mer′u lar
glo mer″u lo ne phri′tis
glo mer″u lo scle ro′sis
glo mer′u lus
glo′mus
glos′sa
glos′sal
glos sal′gi a
glos san′thrax
glos sec′to my
Glos sin′a
glos si′tis
glos′so cele
glos″so dy″na mom′e ter
glos″so dyn′i a
glos″so ep″i glot′tic
glos′so graph
glos″so hy′al
glos″so kin″es thet′ic
glos″so la′bi al
glos″so la′li a
glos sol′o gy
glos″so man′ti a
glos″so pal′a tine
glos″so pal a ti′nus
glos sop′a thy
glos″so pha ryn′ge al
glos″so pha ryn′ge us
glos′so plas″ty
glos″so ple′gi a
gloss″op to′sis
glos″so py ro′sis
glos sor′rha phy
glos sos′co py
glos′so spasm″
glos sot′o my
glos″so trich′i a
glot′tic
glot′tis
glu′ca gon
glu″co cor′ti coid
glu″co ki′nase
glu″co ne″o gen′e sis
glu″cos′a mine
glu′cose
glu′co side
glu″co su′ri a
glu″co syl cer″bro sid o′sis
glu″cu ron′ic
ac′id
glu″cu ron′i dase
glu tam′ic ac′id
glu″ta thi′one
glu′ten
glu te′us
glu′tin
glut′ton y
gly ce′mi a

glyc′er ide
glyc′er in
glyc′er ol
glyc′er yl
gly′cine
gly′co gen
gly′co ge nase″
gly″co gen′e sis
gly″co gen′ic
gly″co ge nol′y sis
gly″co ge no′sis
gly′col
gly col′ic
gly col′y sis
gly″co me tab′o lism
gly″co ne″o gen′e sis
gly″co phil′i a
gly″co pty′a lism
gly″cor rha′chi a
gly″cor rhe′a
gly″co si al′i a
gly′co side
gly″co su′ri a
gly″co su′ric
glyc″u re′sis
Gmelin's test
gnat
gnath al′gi a
gnath′ic
gna′thi on
gnath i′tis
gnath″o ceph′a lus
gnath″o dy″na mom′e ter
gnath″o dyn′i a
gnath′o plas″ty
gnath os′chi sis
Gnath os′to ma
gno′sis
gnos′tic
Goetsch's test
goi′ter
goi″tro gen′ic
Gołdblatt clamp
Goldthwait's op″e ra′tion
Golgi net′work″
gom phi′a sis
gom pho′sis
gon″a cra′ti a
gon′ad
gon′ad arch″e
gon″a dec′to my
gon″a do cen′tric
gon″a do ther′a py
gon″a do tro′pic
gon″a do tro′pin
gon′a duct
go nag′ra
go nal′gi a
gon″an gi ec′to my
gon″ar thri′tis
gon″ar throc′a ce
gon″a throt′o my
go nat′o cele
gon′e cyst
gon″e cys ti′tis
gon″e cys′to lith
gon″e cys″to py o′sis
gon″e poi e′sis
gon′ic
go″ni o chei los′chi sis
go″ni o cra″ni om′e try
go″ni om′e ter
go′ni on
go′ni o punc′ture
go′ni o scope
go ni ot′o my
go ni′tis
go′ni um
gon′o blast
gon″o coc′cal
gon″o coc ce′mi a
gon″o coc′ci

gon″o coc′cide
gon″o coc′cin
gon″o coc′cus
gon′o cyte
go nom′er y
gon″or rhe′a
gon″y ba′ti a
gon″y camp′sis
gon″y on′cus
gor′get
Gottschalk's op″e ra′tion
gouge
goun′dou
gout
Graafian fol′li cle
grac′i lis
Gradenigo's syn′drome
gra′di ent
grad′u ate
graft
grain′age
gram″i ci′din
gran′di ose
grand″ mal′
gran′u lar
gran′u la″ted
gran″u la′tion
gran′ule
gran′i li form″
gran′u lo blast″
gran′u lo cyte″
gran″u lo cy″to pe′ni a
gran″u lo cy″to poi e′sis
gran″u lo′ma
gran″u lo″ma to′sis
gran″u lo′ma tous
gran″u lo plas′tic
gran″u lo poi e′sis
gran″u lo′sa
graph
graph″e the′si a
graph′ite
graph ol′o gy
graph″o ma′ni a
graph″o mo′tor
graph″o pho′bi a
graph″or rhe′a
grat tage′
grav′el
grav′id
gra′vi da
grav″i do car′di ac
gra vim′e ter
grav″i stat′ic
grav″i ta′tion
grav′i ty
Grawitz's tu′mor
gref′fo tome
gre ga′ri ous ness
grip, grippe
gris′e o ful vin
Grocco's sign
groin
Gruber's test
Grübler stain
gry po′sis
guai′ac
guan′i dine
Guarnieri's bod′ies
gu″ber nac′u lum
Guillain-Barre syn′drome
guil′lo tine
gul′let
gum′boil″
gum′ma
gum′ma tous
gus ta′tion
gus′ta to″ry
Guthrie test
gut′ta
gut′ta-per′cha
gym nas′tics

gym″no pho′bi a
gy nan′der
gy nan″dro blas to′ma
gy nan′dro morph
gy nan″dro mor′phism
gy nan′dro mor″phy
gy nan′drous
gy nan′dry
gyn″a tre′si a
gy ne′cic
gyn″e co gen′ic
gyn″e cog′ra phy
gyn′e coid
gyn″e co log′ic
gyn″e col′o gist
gyn″e col′o gy
gyn″e co ma′ni a
gyn″e co mas′ti a
gyn″e cop′a thy
gyn″e pho′bi a
gyn″e phor′ic
Gy′ner gen
gyn″i at′rics
gyn′o plas ty
gyp′sum
gy ra′tion
gy rec′to my
gyr″en ceph′a late
gy′ro mele
gy′rus

H

ha ben′u la
hab′it
hab′i tat
ha bit″u a′tion
hab′i tus
hack′ing
ha″de pho′bi a
Hagedorn nee′dle
Hageman fac′tor
hair
Hal′a dol
hal′a kone
ha la′tion
ha′la zone
Hal′ci on
hal′ite
hal″i to′sis
hal lu″ci na′tion
hal lu′ci″no gen
hal lu″ci no gen′ic
hal lu″ci no′sis
hal′lux
hal′o gen
hal″lo per′i dol
hal′o thane
Halsted′s op″e ra′tion
ham ar″to blas to′ma
ham″ar to′ma
ham″ar to pho′bi a
ham′ate
ha ma′tum
ham′ster
ham′u lus
hand′ed ness
hang′nail″
Hansen′s dis ease′
haph″al ge′si a
haph″e pho′bi a
hap′lo dont
ha′ ploid
ha plo′pi a
hap′lo scope
hap′ten
hap″te pho′bi a
hap′tics
hap″to dys pho′ri a
hap″to glo′bin
hard′ness

hare′lip″
har″pax o pho′bi a
Hashimoto's stru′ma
hash′ish
ha″shi tox i co′sis
Hassall's cor′pus cle
haunch
haus′trum
Haverhill fe′ver
ha ver′sian sys′tem
head′ache″
heal′ing
hear′ing
heart
he″be phre′ni a
Heberden's nodes
he bet′ic
heb′e tude
hec″a ter o mer′ic
hec′tic
hec′to gram
hec′to li″ter
hec′to me″ter
he do′ni a
he′don ism
he″do no pho′bi a
Hegar's sign
he gem′o ny
heim′lich Procedure
Heinz bod′ies
hel′i cine
hel′i cis
hel′i coid
hel′i co pod
hel″i co tre′ma
he″li en ceph″a li′tis
he″li o phobe″
he″li o pho′bi a
he′li o stat″
he″li o tax′is
he″li o ther′a py
he′li um
he′lix
Heller's test
Helmholtz's the′o ry
hel′minth
hel″min them′e sis
hel″min thi′a sis
hel″min thol′o gist
hel″min tho′ma
hel min″tho pho′bi a
he lo′ma
he lot′o my
he′ma chrome
he″ma dy″na mom′e ter
he″mag glu″ti na′tion
he″mag glu′ti nin
he′mal
he man″gi ec′ta sis
he man″gi o blas to′ma
he man″gi o en″do the″li o′ma
he man″gi o′ma
he man″gi o per i cy to′ma
he man″gi o sar co′ma
he″ma poph′y sis
he″mar thro′sis
he″ma te′in
he″ma tem′e sis
he″mat hi dro′sis
he mat′ic
hem′a tin
hem″a ti ne′mi a
hem″a tin′ic
hem″a to aer om′e ter
hem′a to blast″
hem′a to cele″
hem″a to chy′lo cele
hem″a to chy lu′ri a
hem″a to col′pus
hem a′to crit″
hem′a to cyst″
hem″a to cy tol′y sis
hem″a to dys cra′si a
hem″ a to gen′e sis

he′ma toi′din
he″ma tol′o gist
he″ma tol′o gy
hem″a to lym″phan gi o′oma
hem″a to lym phu′ri a
he″ma tol′y sis
he″ma to′ma
hem″a to me″di a sti′num
he″ma tom′e ter
hem″a to me′tra
hem″a to my e′li a
hem″a to my″e li′tis
hem″a to pa thol′o gy
he″ma top′a thy
hem″a toph′a gus
hem″a to plas′tic
hem″a to poi e′sis
hem″a to poi et′ic
hem″a to por′phy rin
hem″a to por″phy ri ne′mi a
hem″a to por″phy ri nu′ri a
hem″a to pre cip′i tin
hem″a tor rha′chis
hem″a tor rhe′a
hem″a to sal′pinx
hem′a to scope
hem′a tose
hem″a to si phon i′a sis
he″ma to′sis
hem″a to spec′tro scope
hem″a to sper′ma to cele″
hem″a to sper′mi a
hem″a to tym′pa num
he″ma tox′y lin
hem″a tu′ri a
heme
hem″er a lo′pi a
hem″er a pho′ni a
hem′i a car′di us
hem″i a ceph′a lus
hem″i a geu′si a
hem″i an″a cu′si a
hem″i an″al ge′si a
hem″i an″es the′si a
hem″i an op′si a
hem″i a tax′i a
hem″i ath″e to′sis
hem″i at′ro phy
hem″i bal lis′mus
he′mic
hem″i car′di a
hem″i cel′lu lose
hem″i ceph′a lus
hem″i ceph′a ly
hem″i cho re′a
hem″i co lec′to my
hem″i cra′ni a
hem″i cra″ni o′sis
hem″i de cor″ti ca′tion
hem″i di′a phragm
hem′i dys″es the′si a
hem″i fa′cial
hem″i glos sec′to my
hem″i glos″so ple′gi a
hem″i gna′thi a
hem″i hy″pal ge′si a
hem″i hy″per es the′si a
hem″i hy″per hi dro′sis
hem″i hy″per to′ni a
hem″i hy″per′tro phy
hem″i hy″pes the′si a
hem″i hy″po to′ni a
hem″i lab″y rin thec′to my
hem″i lam″i nec′to my
hem″i lar″yn gec′to my
hem″i man″di bu lec′to my
hem″i me′li a
hem″i me′lus
hem″i me tab′o lous
he′min
hem″i ne phrec′to my
he mip′a gus

hem″i pal″a to la ryn″go ple′gi a
hem″i pa re′sis
hem″i pel vect′o my
hem″i ple′gi a
hem″i ra chis′chi sis
hem″i scler o der′ma al′ter nans
hem″i sco to′sis
hem″i sec′tion
hem″i so′mus
hem′i spasm
hem′i sphere
hem″i spher ec′to my
hem″i syn er′gi a
hem″i sys′to le
hem″i thy″roid ec′to my
hem″i ver′te bra
hem″i zy′gote
he″mo al″ka lim′e ter
he″mo bil′i a
he″mo bil″i ru′bin
he′mo blast
he″mo cho′ri al
he″mo chro″ma to′sis
he″mo chro′mo gen
he″mo chro mom′e ter
he″mo cla′si a
he″mo con″cen tra′tion
he″mo co′ni a
he″mo cry os′co py
he″mo cy′a nin
he′mo cyte
he″mo cy′to blast
he″mo cy″to gen′e sis
he″mo cy tol′y sis
he″mo cy tom′e ter
he mo′di a
he″mo di″ag no′sis
he″mo di al′y sis
he″mo di lu′tion
he″mo dy nam′ics
he″mo en″do the′li al
he″mo glo′bin
he″mo glo″bi ne′mi a
he″mo glo″bin if′er ous
he″mo glo″bi nom′e ter
he″mo glo″bin o′path ies
he″mo glo″bi nu′ri a
he′mo gram
he″mo his′ti o blast
he″mo hy per ox′i a
he″mo hy pox′i a
he′mo lith
he′mo lymph
he mol′y sin
he mol′y sis
he mo lyt′ic
he mol″y to poi et′ic
he′mo lyze
he″mo ma nom′e ter
he mom′e ter
he″mo pa thol′o gy
he mop′a thy
he″mo per″i car′di um
he″mo per″i to ne′um
he′mo phage
he′mo phil
he″mo phil′i a
he″mo phil′i ac
he″mo phil′ic
He moph′i lus
he″mo pho′bi a
he″moph thal′mi a
he″moph thi′sis
he″mo pneu″mo tho′rax
he mop per fus′ion
he mop′ty sis
hem′or rhage
hem″or rhag′ic
hem″or rhoi′dal
hem″or rhoid ec′to my
hem′or rhoids
he″mo sid′er in
he″mo sid″er i nu′ri a

he″mo sid″er o′sis
he″mo sta′sis
he′mo stat
he″mo stat′ic
he″mo ta chom′e ter
he″mo ther′a py
he″mo tho′rax
he″mo tox′ic
he″mo tox′in
he′mo trophe
he″mo troph′ic
he″mo tym′pa num
he″mo vil′lous
hen′bane
Henoch's pur′pu ra
he′par
hep′a rin
hep″a rin e′mia
hep′a rin ize
hep a′rin ized
hep″a rin′o cyte
hep″a tal′gi a
hep″a tec′to my
he pat′ic
he pat″i co du″o de nos′to my
he pat″i co en″ter os′to my
he pat″i co gas tros′to my
he pat″i co li thot′o my
he pat″i co pan″cre at′ic
he pat″i cos′to my
he pat″i cot′o my
hep″a tit′i des
hep″a ti′tis
he″pat o bil′i ary
hep″a to cell′u lar
he″pat o ce re′bral
hep″a to cho lan″gi o
du″o de nos′to my
hep″a to cho lan″gi o
en″ter os′to my
hep″a to cho lan″gi o
gas tros′to my
hep″a to cho lan″gi o
je″ju nos′to my
hep″a to col′ic
hep″a to cyst′ic
hep″a to du″o de′nal
hep″a to du″o de nos′to my
hep″a to gen′ic
hep′a to gram
hep″a tog′ra phy
hep″a to len tic′lar
hep″a to li e′nal
hep″a to li″en og′ra phy
hep′a to lith
hep″a to lith ec′to my
hep″a to li thi′a sis
he pat″o ly′sin
hep″a to′ma
hep″a to meg′a ly
hep′a to pex″y
he″pat o phos″phor′y lase
he″pat o por′tal
hep″a top to′sis
hep″a to re′nal
hep″a tor′rha phy
hep″a tor rhex′is
hep″a tos′co py
hep″a to′sis
hep″a to sple″no meg′a ly
hep″a to sple″nop′a thy
hep″a to ther′a py
hep″a tot′o my
hep″a to tox′ic
hep″a to tox′in
Hep′ta chlor
hep to su′ri a
herb
her ba′ceous
her biv′o rous
he red′i ty
her″e do ak″i ne′si a

her″e do fa mil′i al
her″e do path′i a
her′it age
her maph′ro dite
her maph′ro dit ism
he″mar thro′sis
her met′ic
her′nia
her′ni ate
her′ni at″ed
her″ni a′tion
her′ni o plas″ty
her″ni or′rha phy
her′ni o tome
her″ni ot′o my
her′o in
her pan′gin a
her′pes
her′pes vi′rus
her pet′ic
her pet′i form
her″pe tol′o gy
Herxheimer′s re ac′tion
Hesselback′s
tri′an″gle
het″er a de′ni a
het″er a li us
het″er es the′si a
het″er o ag glu′ti nin
het″er o aux′one
het″er o blas′tic
het″er o cel′lu lar
het″er o ceph′a lus
het″er o chro′ma tin
het″er o chro′mi a
het′er o dont″
het″er o dro′mi a
het″er o er′o tism
het″er o fer men′ta tive
het″er o ga met′ic
het″er og′a my
het″er o ge′ne ous
het″er og′o ny
het′er o graft″
het″er o hyp no′sis
het″er o ki ne′si a
het″er o ki ne′sis
het″er ol′o gy
het″er o mer′ic
het″er o met″a pla′si a
het″er o me tro′pi a
het″er o mor′phic
het″er on′y mous
het″er o os′te o plas″ty
het″er op′a thy
het′er o phe″my
het′er o phil
het″er o pho′ni a
het″er o pho′ri a
het″er o pla′si a
het′er o plas″ty
het′er o ploid
het″er op′si a
Het″er op′ter a
het′er op′tics
het′er o scope″
het″er o sex″u al′i ty
het″er o sug ges′tion
het″er o tax′is
het″er o to′ni a
het″er o to′pi a
het″er o trans plan ta′tion
het″er o tro′pi a
het″er o ty′pus
het″er o zy′gote
het″er o zy′gous
hex″a chro′mic
hex′ad
hex″a dac′ty lism
hex″a gen′ic
hex′ane
hex″′o bar′bi tal
hex″o ki′nase
hex′ose

hex"yl res or'cin ol
hi a'tal
hi a'tus
hi"ber na'tion
hi"ber no'ma
hic'cough
hic'cup
hid rad"e ni'tis
hid rad"e car"ci no'ma
hid rad'e no cyte
hid rad"e no'ma
hid ro'a
hid"ro cys to'ma
hid"ro poi e'sis
hid"ror rhe'a
hi"dros ad"e ni'tis
hid ros'che sis
hi dro'sis
hi drot'ic
hid"ro to path'ic
hi"er o pho'bi a
hi'lar
hi'lum
hi'lus
hip pan'thro py
hip"po cam'pus
Hippocrates
hip'po lith
hip"po myx o'ma
hip pu'ri a
hip pu'ric ac'id
hip'pus
Hirschsprung's dis ease'
hir'sute
hir su'ti es
hir'sut ism
hir'u din
his'ta mine
his"ta min'ic
his'ti dine
his"ti di ne'mi a
his'ti o cyte
his"ti o cy to'ma
his"ti o cy"to sar co'ma
his"ti o cy to'sis
his'to blast
his"to chem'is try
his"to di al'y sis
his"to flu"o res'cence
his"to gen'e sis
his'toid
his to log'ic
his tol'o gist
his tol'o gy
his tol'y sis
his"to lyt'ic
his to'ma
his"to met"a plas'tic
his"to mor phol'o gy
his"to pa thol'o gy
his"to phys"i ol'o gy
His"to plas'ma
his"to plas'min
his"to plas mo'sis
his"to spec tros'co py
his"to ther'a py
his"to throm'bin
his'to tome
his tot'o my
his"to tox'ic
his'to trophe
his"tri on'ic
hives
hoarse
hoar'y
hob'ble
Hodgkin's dis ease'
ho"do pho'bi a
Hofmeister-Finsterer op"e ra'tion
hol"er ga'si a
ho' lis tic

hol″o a car′di us
hol″o blas′tic
hol″o ce phal′ic
hol″o cra′ni a
hol′o crine
hol″o di″as tol′ic
hol″o gas tros′chi sis
hol″o gyn′ic
hol″o met″a bol′ic
hol″o ra chis′chi sis
hol″o so mat′ic
hol″o sys tol′ic
hom″a lo ceph′a lus
hom″a lo cor′y phus
hom″a lo″me to′pus
hom″a lo pis″tho cra′ni us
hom″a lu ra′nus
hom at′ro pine
hom ax′i al
ho′me o chrome″
ho″me o ki ne′sis
ho″me o mor′phous
ho″me o path′ic
ho″me op′a thy
ho″me o pla′si a
ho″me o′sis
ho″me os′ta sis
ho″me o ther′mal
ho″mi chol pho′bi a
hom′i cide
ho″mo cen′tric
ho′mo chrome
ho″mo chro″mo i som′er ism
ho″mo clad′ic
ho″mo cys′tin e mia
ho″mo cys tin u′ria
ho′mo dont
ho″mo dy′na my
ho″mo er′o tism
ho″mo ga met′ic
ho mo′ gamy
ho″mo ge′ne ous
ho″mo gen′ic
ho″mo ge″ni za′tion
ho mog′e nous
ho″mo gen tis′ic ac′id
ho′mo graft
ho″mo i other′mic
ho″mo lac′tic
ho mol′o gous
ho mon′o mous
ho″mo mor′phic
ho mon′y mous
ho′mo plas″ty
ho″mo sex″u al′i ty
ho″mo ther′mic
ho″mo trans″plan ta′tion
ho′mo type
ho″mo zy′gote
ho″mo zy′gous
ho mun′cu lus
hor de′o lum
hor″me pho′bi a
hor′mi on
Hor″mo den′drum
hor mo′nal
hor′mone
hor mo″no poi e′sis
hor′mo zone
Horner's syn′drome
horn″i fi ca′tion
ho rop′ter
hos′pi tal
hos″pit al i za′tion
hot flash′es
Houssay, Bernardo Alberto
Hoyne's sign
hu man′o scope
Hu′ma tin
hu mec′tant
hu′mer al
hu″mer o ra′di al

hu″mer o scap′u lar
hu″mer o ul′nar
hu′mer us
hu mid″i fi ca′tion
hu mid′i ty
hu′min
hu′mor
hu′mor al
hu′mu lus
hu′mus
Hurler's dis ease′
hy′a lin
hy′a line
hy″a lin i za′tion
hy″a lin o′sis
hy″a li nu′ri a
hy″a li′tis
hy″a lo cap″su li′tis
hy al′o gen
hy′a loid
hy′a lo mere
hy″a lo mu′coid
hy″a lo nyx′is
hy″a lo pho′bi a
hy′a lo plasm
hy″a lo se″ro si′tis
hy″a lu ron′i dase
hy′brid
by″brid i za′tion
hy dan′to in
hy dat′id
hy da tid′i form″
hy″da tid′o cele
hy dat″i do′sis
hy′dra gogue
hy dral′a zine
hy dram′ni os
hy″drar gyr′i a
hy″drar gyr″o pho′bi a
hy″drar gyr″oph thal″mi a
hy″drar thro′sis
hy′drase
hy′drate
hy dra′tion
hy drau′lics
hy′dra zine
hy″dre lat′ic
hy dre′mi a
hy″dren ceph′a lo cele
hy″dren ceph″a lo me min′go cele
hy dri od′ic ac′id
hy dro′a
hy″dro bil″i ru′bin
hy″dro bro′mic
hy″dro ca′lix
hy″dro car′bon
hy′dro cele
hy″dro ce lec′to my
hy″dro ce phal′ic
hy″dro ceph′a lus
hy″dro ceph′a ly
hy″dro chin″o nu′ri a
hy″dro chlo′ric ac′id
hy″dro chlo′ride
hy″dro col′loid
hy″dro col′pos
hy″dro co′ni on
hy″dro cor′ti sone
hy″dro dip″so ma′ni a
hy″dro dy nam′ics
hy′dro gen
hy″dro gen a′tion
hy″dro gen ly′ase
hy″dro glos′sa
hy″dro gym nas′tics
hy″dro hem″a to ne phro′sis
hy″dro ki net′ic
hy″dro lac tom′e ter
hy′dro lase
hy drol′o gy
hy drol′y sis

hy drol'y zate
hy"dro ma'ni a
hy"dro mas sage'
hy'dro mel
hy"dro me nin'go cele
hy drom'e ter
hy"dro me"tro col'pos
hy"dro mi"cro ceph'a ly
Hy'dro mox
hy"dro my e'li a
hy"dro my'e lo cele"
hy"dro my'rinx
hy"dro ne phro'sis
hy drop'a thy
hy"dro per"i car di'tis
hy"dro per"i car'di um
hy"dro per'i on
hy"dro per"i to ne'um
Hy droph'i dae
hy'dro phil
hy"dro phil'ic
hy'dro phobe
hy"dro pho'bi a
hy'dro phone
hy"droph thal'mos
hy drop'ic
hy'dro plasm
hy"dro pneu"ma to'sis
hy"dro pneu"mo per"i car'di um
hy"dro pneu"mo per"i to ne'um
hy"dro pneu"mo tho'rax
hy'drops
hy"dro py"o ne phro'sis
hy"dror rhe'a
hy"dro sal'pinx
hy"dro sat'ur nism
hy"dro sol'u ble
hy"dro sper'ma to cyst"
hy"dro spi rom'e ter
hy'dro stat
hy"dro sy rin"go my e'li a
hy"dro tax'is
hy"dro ther"a peu'tics
hy"dro ther'a py
hy"dro ther'mal
hy"dro thi"o nu'ri a
hy"dro tho'rax
hy dro'tis
hy drot'ro pism
hy"dro tym'pa num
hy"dro-u re'ter
hy drox'ide
hy drox'yl
hy drox' y lase
hy dru'ri a
hy"e tom'e try
Hygeia
hy'giene
hy'gi en ist
hy"gre che'ma
hy"gro ble phar'ic
hy gro'ma
hy grom'e ter
hy"gro pho'bi a
hy'gro scope
hy"gro scop'ic
hy"gro sto'mi a
Hy'ki none
hy"lo pho'bi a
hy"lo trop'ic
hy"lo zo'ism
hy'men
hy"me nec'to my
hy"me ni'tis
Hy"me nol'e pis
hy"me nol'o gy
Hy"me nop'ter a
hy"me nor'rha phy
hy men'o tome
hy"me not'o my
hy"o ep"i glot'tic
hy"o glos'sal
hy"o glos'sus

hy′oid
hy″o man dib′u lar
hy o′cine
hy″os cy′a mine
hy″o sta pe′di al
hy″o ver″te brot′o my
hyp″a cu′si a
hyp″al bu″min o′sis
hyp″al ge′si a
hyp am′ni on
hy pan″i sog′na thism
hy″par te′ri al
hy″pas the′ni a
hy pax′i al
hy pen″gy o pho′bi a
hy″per ab duc′tion
hy″per a cid′i ty
hy″per a cu′i ty
hy″per a cu′si a
hy″per a cu′sis
hy″per ad″e no′sis
hy″er ad re′nal ism
hy″per ad re′ni a
hy″per ad re″no cor′ti cism
hy″per a″er a′tion
hy″per al dos′ter on ism
hy″per al ge′si a
hy″per al″i men ta′tion
hy″per al″i men to′sis
hy″per am mon e′mi a
hy″per an″a ki ne′si a
hy″per a′phi a
hy″per bar′ic
hy″per bar′ism
hy″per bil″i ru″bi ne′mi a
hy″per brach″y ceph′a ly
hy″per bu′li a
hy″per cal ce′mi a
hy″′per cal ci nu′ri a
hy″per cap′ni a
hy″per car″ o te ne′mi a
hy″per ca thar′sis
hy″per ca thex′is
hy″per ce″men to′sis
hy″per ce″nes the′si a
hy″per cham′aer rhine
hy″per chlo re′mi a
hy″per chlor hy′dri a
hy″per cho les″ter e′mi a
hy″per cho′li a
hy″per chro mat′ic
hy″per chro′ma tism
hy″per chro″ma to′sis
hy″per chy′li a
hy″per chy″lo mi cro ne′mi a
hy″per cor′ti cism
hy″per cry″al ge′si a
hy″per di crot′ic
hy″per dis ten′tion
hy″per dy nam′ic
hy″per e che′ma
hy″per e″las to′sis
hy″per em′e sis
hy″per e′mi a
hy″per en ceph′a lus
hy″per ep″i thy′mi a
hy″per e″qui lib′ri um
hy″per er′gi a
hy′per ergy
hy″per es″o pho′ri a
hy″per es the′si a
hy″per es′trin ism
hy″per es″tro ge ne′mi a
hy″per ex″o pho′ri a
hy″per ex ten′sion
hy″per flex′ion
hy″per func′tion
hy″per gam″ma glob u li ne′mi a
hy″per gen′e sis
hy″per geu′si a
hy″per gi gan″to so′ma
hy″per glob′u li ne′mi a

hy″per gly ce′mi a
hy″per gly ce′mic
hy″per gly cer e′mi a
hy″per gly ci ne′mi a
hy″per gly″co ge nol′y sis
hy″per gly″cor rha′chi a
hy″per gly″co su′ri a
hy″per gon′ad ism
hy″per go′ni a
hy″per he do′ni a
hy″per hi dro′sis
hy″per his″ta mi ne′mi a
hy″per hor mo′nal
hy″per in″o se′mi a
hy″per i no′sis
hy″per in′su lin ism
hy″per in″vo lu′tion
hy″per ka le′mi a
hy″per ker″a to′sis
hy″per ker″a tot′ic
hy″per ke″to nu′ri a
hy″per ki ne′mi a
hy″per ki ne′si a
hy″per ki net′ic
hy″per lac ta′tion
hy″per lep′tor rhine
hy″per ley′dig ism
hy″per li pe′mi a
hy″per li″po pro tein e′mi a
hy″per li sin e′mi a
hy″per li thu′ri a
hy″per lo′gi a
hy″per mac″ro glob u lin e′mi a
hy″per mag ne si′mia
hy″per ma′ni a
hy″per ma′nic
hy″per mas′ti a
hy″per ma ture′
hy″per mel an o′sis
hy″per men″or rhe′a
hy″per me tro′pi a
hy″per mi″cro so′ma
hy″per mim′i a
hy″perm ne′si a
hy″per mo til′i ty
hy″per na tre′mi a
hy″per neph′roid
hy″per ne phro′ma
hy″per noi′a
hy″per nu tri′tion
hy″per on cho′ma
hy″per on′to morph
hy″per o nych′i a
hy″per o′pi a
hy″per o rex′i a
hy″per or′tho gna″thy
hy″per os′mi a
hy″per os″mo lar′i ty
hy″per os″te og′e ny
hy″per os to′sis
hy″per ox a lu′ri a
hy″per ox e′mi a
hy″per ox″y gen a′tion
hy″per par′a site
hy″per par″a thy′roid ism
hy″per path′i a
hy″per pep sin′i a
hy″per per″i stal′sis
hy″per pha′gi a
hy″per pha lan′gism
hy″per pho ne′sis
hy″per pho′ni a
hy″per phos pha tas′i a
hy″per phos″pho li pi de′
mi a
hy″per phos pha te′mi a
hy″per pi e′si a
hy″per pig″men ta′tion
hy″per pi tu′i ta rism
hy″per pla′si a
hy″per plas mi ne′mi a
hy″per plas′tic
hy″per plat″y mer′ic
hy″perp ne′a

hy″per po ro′sis
hy″per pot″as se′mi a
hy″per pra′gi a
hy″per prax′i a
hy″per pres″by o′pi a
hy″per pro″cho re′sis
hy″per pro ges″ter o ne′mia
hy″per pro lin e′mi a
hy″per pro sex′i a
hy″per pro″te in e′mi a
hy″per psy cho′sis
hy″per py rex′i a
hy″per re flex′i a
hy″per res′o nance
hy″per sal″i va′tion
hy″per sar co si ne′mi a
hy″per se cre′tion
hy″per sen″si tiv′i ty
hy″per som′ni a
hy″per sple′nism
hy″per ster″e o roent″gen og′ra phy
hy″per sthe′ni a
hy″per sthen′ic
hy″per sus cep″ti bil′i ty
hy″per syn′chro ny
hy″per tel′or ism
hy″per ten′sin
hy″per ten′sin ase
hy″per ten sin′o gen
hy″per ten′sion
hy″per the′li a
hy′per therm″
hy″per ther″mal ge′si a
hy″per ther′mi a
hy″per ther′my
hy″per thy″mi za′tion
hy″per thy′roid ism
hy″per to′ni a
hy″per ton′ic
hy″per tri cho′sis
hy per tro′phi a
hy″per troph′ic
hy per′tro phy
hy″per tro′pi a
hy″per u″ri ce′mi a
hy″per val in e′mi a
hy″per vas′cu lar
hy″per veg′e ta″tive
hy″per ven″ti la′tion
hy″per vi″ta min o′sis
hy″per vo le′mi a
hyp″es the′si a
hy′pha
hyp″he do′ni a
hy phe′ma
hyp″hi dro′sis
hyp″i no′sis
hyp″na gog′ic
hyp′na gogue
hyp nal′gi a
hyp′nic
hyp″no a nal″y sis
hyp″no gen′ic
hyp″no go′gic
hyp′noid
hyp′no lep″sy
hyp nol′o gy
hyp″no nar co′sis
hyp″no pho′bi a
hyp″no phre no′sis
hyp″no pom′pic
hyp″no si gen′e sis
hyp no′sis
hyp″no ther′a py
hyp not′ic
hyp′no tism
hyp′no tist
hyp′no tize
hyp′no toid
hyp″no tox′in
hy′po

hy″po a cid′i ty
hy″po ac tiv′i ty
hy″po ad ren″i ne′mi a
hy″po ad re′nal ism
hy″po ad re′ni a
hy″po ag′na thus
hy″po al dos′ter on ism
hy″po al″bu min e′mi a
hy″po al ler gen′ic
hy″po az″o tu′ri a
hy″po bar′ic
hy″po bar′ism
hy″po ba rop′a thy
hy″po be ta li″po pro tein e′mi a
hy″po bran′chi al
hy″po bu′li a
hy″po cal ce′mi a
hy″po cal″ci fi ca′tion
hy″po cap′ni a
hy″po ca thex′is
hy″po chlo re′mi a
hy″po chlor hy′dri a
hy″po chlo′rite
hy″po chlor u′ri a
hy″po cho les″ter e′mi a
hy″po chon′dri a
hy″po chon′dri ac
hy″po chon dri′a sis
hy″po chon′dri um
hy″po chor′dal
hy″po chro mat′ic
hy″po chro′mic
hy″po chy′li a
hy″po coe′lom
hy′po cone
hy″po con′id
hy″po con′ule
hy″po con′u lid
hy″po cy clo′sis
hy″po cy the′mi a
hy″po der mi′a sis
hy″po der′mic
hy″po der′mis
hy″po der moc′ly sis
hy″po don′ti a
hy″po er′gy
hy″po es″o pho′ri a
hy″po es′trin ism
hy″po ex″o pho′ri a
hy″po fer re′mi a
hy″po func′tion
hy″po gal ac′ti a
hy″po gam ma glob″u lin e′mi a
hy″po gas′tric
hy″po gas′tri um
hy″po gas trop′a gus
hy″po gas tros′chi sis
hy″po gen′i tal ism
hy″po geu′si a
hy″po glos′sal
hy″po glos si′tis
hy″po glos′sus
hy″po gly ce′mi a
hy″po gly″co ge nol′y sis
hy″po gnath′ous
hy″po gon′ad ism
hy″po gran″u lo cy to′sis
hy″po in′su lin ism
hy′ po kal e′mi a
hy″po ki ne′si a
hy″po lem′mal
hy″po lep″si o ma′ni a
hy″po ley′dig ism
hy″po li po pro″tein e′mi a
hy″po lo′gi a
hy″po mag″ne se′mi a
hy″po ma′ni a
hy″po ma′nic
hy″po mas′ti a
hy″po men″or rhe′a
hy′po mere
hy″po me tab′o lism

hy″po me tro′pi a
hy″po mi″cro gnath′us
hy″po mi′cron
hy″po mi″cro so′ma
hy″pom ne′si a
hy″po mo til′i ty
hy″po nan″o so′ma
hy″po nat re′mi a
hy″po no′ic
hy″po nych′i um
hy″po os to′sis
hy″po par″a thy′roid ism
hy″po per″me a bil′i ty
hy″po pha lan′gism
hy″po phar″yn gos′co py
hy″po phar′ynx
hy″po pho′ni a
hy″po pho′ri a
hy″po phos″pha ta′sia
hy″po phos″pha te′mi a
hy″po phre′ni a
hy poph″y sec′to my
hy poph′y sis
hy″po pi e′si a
hy″po pin′e al ism
hy″po pi tu′i ta rism
hy″po pla′si a
hy pop′nea
hy″po pot″as se′mi a
hy″po prax′i a
hy″po pro sex′i a
hy″po pro″te i ne′mi a
hy″po pro throm″bi ne′mi a
hy″po psel″a phe′si a
hy″po psy cho′sis
hy″po′py on
hy″po sal″i va′tion
hy″po scle′ral
hy″po se cre′tion
hy″po sen″si tiv′i ty
hy pos′mi a
hy″po som′ni a
hy″po spa′di ac
hy″po spa′di as
hy″po sper″ma to gen′e sis
hy″pos phre′si a
hy′po spray
hy pos′ta sis
hy″po stat′ic
hy″pos the′ni a
hy pos″the nu′ri a
hy″po sto′mi a
hy″po syn er′gi a
hy″po tax′i a
hy″po tax′is
hy″po tel′or ism
hy″po ten′sion
sy″po ten′sive
hy″po ten′sor
hy″po thal′a mus
hy″po the′nar
hy″po therm″es the′sia
hy″po ther′mal
hy″po ther′mi a
hy″poth′e sis
hy″po thy′mi a
hy″po thy′roid ism
hy″po thy ro′sis
hy″po to′ni a
hy″po ton′ic
hy″po tri cho′sis
hy″po tro′pi a
hy″po tym′pan um
hy″po veg′e ta″tive
hy po ven′ti la″tion
hy″po vi″ta min o′sis
hy″po vo le′mi a
hy″pox e′mi a
hy pox′i a
hyp″sar rhyth′mia
hyp″si brach″y ce phal′ic
hyp″si ceph′a ly

hyp′si conch″
hyp″si sta phyl′i a
hyp so chro′mic
hyp″so pho′bi a
hys′sop
hys″ter al′gi a
hys″ter ec′to my
hys″ter e′sis
hys″ter eu ryn′ter
hys te′ri a
hys ter′i cism
hys ter′i cal
hys ter′ics
hys ter′i form
hys″ter o bu bon′o cele
hys′ter o cele″
hys″ter o clei′sis
hys″ter o de″mon op′a thy
hys″ter o dyn′i a
hys″ter o ep′i lep″sy
hys″ter o fren′ic
hys″ter og′e ny
hys″ter og′ra phy
hys′ter oid
hys″ter o lap″a rot′o my
hys′ter o lith
hys″ter o li thi′a sis
hys″ter ol′o gy
hys″ter ol′y sis
hys″ter o ma′ni a
hys″ter om′e ter
hys″ter o my o′ma
hys″ter o my″o mec′to my
hys″ter o my ot′o my
hys″ter o-o″pho rec′to my
hys″ter op′a thy
hys′ter a pex″y
hys″ter o phil′i a
hys″ter o plas′ty
hys″ter op to′sis
hys″ter or′rha phy
hys″ter or rhex′is
hys″ter o sal″pin gec′to my
hys″ter o sal″ pin gog′ra phy
hys″ter o sal pin″go o″o pho rec′to my
hys″ter o sal pin″go o″o the cec′to my
hys″ter o sal″pin gos′to my
hys′ter o scope″
hys″ter os to ma′ to my
hys′ter o tome″
hys″ter ot′o my
hys″ter o tra″che lec′to my
hys″ter o tra′che lo plas″ty
hys″ter o tra″che lor′rha phy
hys″ter o tra″che lot′o my
hys″ter o trau′ma tism
hy′ther

I

i am″a tol′o gy
i at″ro chem′is try
i at″ro gen′ic
i at″ro phys′ics
ich′no gram
i′chor
i″chor rhe′a
i″chor rhe′mi a
ich′tham mol
ich″thy is′mus
ich″thy o col′la
ich′thy oid
ich″thy ol′o gy
ich″thy oph′a gous
ich″thy o pho′bi a
ich″thy o′sis
ich″thy o tox′i con
ich″thy o tox is′mus

i′con
i″co nog′ra phy
i con″o lag′ny
i con″o ma′ni a
ic′tal
ic ter′ic
ic″ter o gen′ic
ic′ter oid
ic′ter us
ic′tus
id
i de′a
i de″al i za′tion
i″de a′tion
id″e o ge net′ic
id″e o glan′du lar
id″e ol′o gy
id″e o me tab′o lism
id″e o mo′tor
id″e o pho′bi a
id′e o plas″ty
id″e o syn chy′si a
id″e o vas′cu lar
id″i o chro′mo some
id″i oc′ra sy
id″i oc to′ni a
id′io cy
id″i og′a mist
id″i o gen′e sis
id″i o glos′si a
id″i o hyp′no tism
id″i ol′o gism
id″i o me tri′tis
id″i o mus′cu lar
id″i o path′ic
id″i op′a thy
id′i o phone
id′i o plasm
id″i o psy chol′o gy
id″i o re′flex
id″i o ret′i nal
id′i o some″
id′i o syn′cra sy
id″i o syn crat′ic
id′i ot
id″i o ven tric′u lar
i dol″o ma′ni a
i dro′sis
ig′ni punc″ture
ig ni′tion
il′e ac
il″e ec′to my
il″e i′tis
il″e o ce cos′to my
il″e o ce′cal
il″e o ce′cum
il″e o col′ic
il″e o co li′tis
il″e o co los′to my
il″e o il″e os′to my
il″e or′rha phy
il″e o sig″moid os′to my
il″e os′to my
il″e ot′o my
il′e um
il′e us
il′i a
il′i ac
i li′a cus
il″i o cap″su lar′is
il″i o cap″ su lo tro″chan ter′i cus
il″i o coc cyg′e al
il″i o coc cyg′e us
il″i o cos tal′is
il″i o cos″to cer″vi cal′is
il″i o fem′o ral
il″i o hy″po gas′tric
il″i o in′gui nal
il″i op′a gus
il″i o par″a si′tus
il″i o pec tin′e al

il″i o pso′as
il″i o sac ral′is
il″i o tho″ra cop′a gus
il″i o xi phop′a gus
il′i um
il laq″ue a′tion
il″le git′i mate
il″li ni′tion
il lin′i um
ill′ness
il lu′mi nance
il lu″mi na′tion
il lu′mi nism
il lu′sion
I lo ty′cin
i′ma
im′age
im ag″i na′tion
i ma′go
im bal′ance
im′be cile
im″be cil′i ty
im″bi bi′tion
im′bri ca″ted
Imhotep
I mip′ ra mine
im″i ta′tion
im″ma ture′
im med′i ca ble
im mer′sion
im mis′ci ble
im mo″bi li za′tion
im″mor tal′i ty
im mune″
im mu′ni ty
im″mu ni za′tion
im′mu nize
im mu′no blasts
im mu″no chem′is try
im mu′no cytes
im″ mu no de fi′cien cy
imm″u no flu o res′cense
im mu″no gen′ic
im″mu no glob′u lin
im mu′no he″ma tol′o gy
im mu″no log′ic
im″mu nol′o gist
im″ mu nol′o gy
imm″u no sup pres′sive
imm″u no ther′a py
im mu″no trans fu′sion
im pac′tion
im pal′pa ble
im′par
im par″i dig′i tate
im passe′
im pe′dance
im per′a tive
im″per cep′tion
im per′fo rate
im per′me a ble
im per′vi ous
im″pe tig″i ni za′tion
im″pe ti′go
im pin′ger
im″plan ta′tion
im′plants
im pon′der a ble
im′po tence
im′po tent
im preg′nate
im pres′sion
im pro′cre ant
im pu′ber al
im′pulse
im pul′sion
im″ pul siv′ i ty
im pu″ta bil′i ty
in″a cid′i ty
in ac′ti vate
in ad′e qua cy
in al″i men′tal
in an′i mate
in″a ni′tion

in ap′pe tence
in″ar tic′u late
in ar tic′u lo mor′tis
in″as sim′i la ble
in′born
in′breed″ing
in car″cer a′tion
in ca′ri al
in car′nant
in′cest
in′ci dence
in′ci dent
in cin″er a′tion
in cip i ent
in ci′sal
in cised′
in ci′sion
in ci′sive
in ci si′vis la′bi i in″fer i or′is
in ci si′vis la′bi i
su″per i or′is
in ci′sor
in″ci su′ra
in″ci sur′ae he′li cis
in ci′sure
in″cli na′tion
in″cli nom′e ter
in clu′sion
in″co ag′u la ble
in″co her′ence
in″co her′ent
in″com bus′ti ble
in″com pat′i ble
in″com pen sa′tion
in com′pe tence
in con′gru ence
in″con gru′i ty
in con′ti nence
in con′ti nent
in con tin en′ti a pig men′ti
in″co or″di na′tion
in cor″po ra′tion
in′crement
in cre′tion
in″crus ta′tion
in″cu ba′tion
in′cu ba″tor
in′cu bus
in″cu dec′to my
in″cu do mal′le al
in″cu do sta pe′di al
in cur′a ble
in′cus
in cy″clo pho′ri a
in cy″clo tro′pi a
in de′cent
in″de ci′sion
in″den ta′tion
In′ de ral
in′dex
in′di can
in′di cant
in″di ca nu′ri a
in″di ca′tion
in′di ca″tor
in′di ces
in dig′e nous
in″di ges′tion
in dig″i ta′tion
in′di go
in′dole
in′do lent
in″ do meth′ a cin
in duction
in″duc to′ri um
in duc′to ther″my
in′du rat″ed
in″du ra′tion
in e′bri ant
in e″bri a′tion
in″e bri′e ty
in ef′fi ca cy
in″e nu′cle a ble
in er′ti a

in′fant
in fan′ti cide
in′fantile
in fan′ti lism
in farct′
in farct′ion
in fec′tion
in fec′tious
in fec′tious ness
in″fe cun′di ty
in fe′ri or
in fe″ri or′i ty
in″fer til′i ty
in″fes ta′tion
in fib u la′tion
in fil′trate
in″fil tra′tion
in fin′i ty
in firm′
in fir′ma ry
in fir′mi ty
in″flam ma′tion
in fla′tion
in flec′tion
in″flo res′cence
in″flu en′za
in″fra car′di ac
in″fra cla vic′u lar
in″fra cla vic u lar′is
in″fra con′dyl ism
in″fra cos′tal
in frac′tion
in″fra di″a phrag mat′ic
in″fra glenoid′
in″fra glot′tic
in″fra hy′oid
in″fra oc clu′sion
in″fra or′bit al
in″fra pa tel′lar
in″fra phys″i o log′ic
in″fra red′
in″fra scap′u lar
in″fra spi na′tus
in″fra spi′nous
in″fra ster′nal
in″fra tem″po ra′le
in″fra ten to′ri al
in″fra troch′le ar
in fric′tion
in″ fun dib′u li form″
in″fun dib u lo′ma
in″fun dib″u lo pel′vic
in″fun dib′u lar
in″fun dib′u lum
in fu′sion
in″fu so′ri a
in ges′ta
in ges′tion
in″gra ves′cent
in gre′di ent
in′grow″ing
in′guen
in′gui nal
in″gui no dyn′i a
in″gui no fem′o ral
in″gui no scro′tal
in ha′lant
in″ha la′tion
in′ha la″tor
in ha′ler
in her′ent
in her′it ance
in her′it ed
in hib′in
in″hi bi′tion
in hib′i tor
in″i en ceph′a lus
in″i od′y mus
in′i on
in″i op′a gus
in′i ops
in ject′

in jec′tion
in′ju ry
in′lay″
in′let
in′nate
in″ner va′tion
in′no cent
in noc′u ous
in nom′nate
in nox′ious
in″oc ci pit′i a
in″o chon dri′tis
in oc″u la′tion
in oc′u la″tor
in oc′u lum
in′o gen
in op′er a ble
in″or gan′ic
in os′cu late
in os″cu la′tion
in″o se′mi a
in′o sine
in o′si tol
in″stil la′tion
in″o trop′ic
in′quest
in″qui si′tion
in sal″i va′tion
in″sa lu′bri ous
in″sa lu′bri ty
in san′i tar″y
in san″i ta′tion
in san′i ty
in scrip′tion
in scrip″ti o′nes
in′sect
in sec′ti cide
in sec′ti fuge
in″se cu′ri ty
in sem″i na′tion
in sen′si ble
in sheathed′
in sid′i ous
in′sight″
in sip′id
in si′tu
in″so la′tion
in sol′u ble
in som′ni a
in spec′tion
in″spi ra′tion
in spi′ra to″ry
in″spi rom′e ter
in spis′sant
in spis′sate
in″spis sat′ed
in″sta bil′i ty
in′step
in″stil la′tion
in′stil la″tor
in′stinct
in stinc′tive
in′stru ment
in″stru men ta′tion
in″suf fi′cien cy
in″suf fla′tion
in′suf fla″tor
in′su la
in′su lin
in″su lin e′mi a
in″su lin o′ma
in″sus cep″ti bil′i ty
in″te gra′tion
in″teg′u ment
in′tel lect
in tel′li gence
in tel′li gent
in tem′per ance
in ten″si fi ca′tion
in″ten sim′e ter
in ten′si ty
in ten′tion

in″ter ac ces′so ry
in″ter ac′i nous
in″ter al ve′o lar
in″ter ar″y te noid′e us
in″ter a′tri al
in ter′ca la″ted
in″ter cap′il lar″y glo mer″u lo scle ro′sis
in″ter car′pal
in″ter cav′ern ous
in″ter cel′lu lar
in″ter chon′dral
in″ter cli′noid
in″ter co lum′nar
in″ter con′dy lar
in″ter cos′tal
in″ter cos″to bra′chi al
in″ter coup′ler
in′ter course
in″ter cri″co thy rot′o my
in″ter cris′tal
in″ter cru′ral
in″ter cur′rent
in″ter cusp′ing
in″ter den′tal
in″ter den′ti um
in″ter dic′tion
in″ter dig′i tal
in″ter dig″i ta′tion
in′ter face
in″ter fere′
in″ter fer′ence
in″ter fer om′e ter
in″ter fer om′e try
in″ter fer′on
in″ter fi′bril lar
in″ter fol lic′u lar
in″ter glob′u lar
in″ter go′ni al
in te′ri or
in″ter kin e′sis
in″ter la′bi al
in″ter la mel′lar
in″ter lam′i nar
in″ter lin′gua
in″ter lo′bar
in″ter lob′u lar
in″ter mar′riage
in″ter max′il lar″y
in″ter me′din
in″ter me″di o lat′er al
in″ter mem′bra nous
in″ter me nin′ge al
in″ter men′stru al
in ter′ment
in″ter mes″o blas′tic
in″ter met″a mer′ic
in″ter mic cel′lar
in″ter mi tot′ic
in″ter mit′tent
in″ter mu′ral
in″ter mus′cu lar
in ter′nal
in″ter na′ri al
in″ter neu′ron
in″ter neu′ro nal
in ter′nist
in′ter node″
in″ter nun′ci al
in″ter o cep′tor
in″ter o fec′tive
in″ter ol′i var″y
in″ter os′se us
in″ter pal′pe bral
in″ter pa ri′e tal
in″ter pe dun′cu lar
in″ter pha lan′ge al
in″ter prox′i mal
in″ter prox′i mate
in″ter pu′pil la″ry
in′ter sex″
in″ter spi nal′es

in″ter spi′nous
in ter′sti ces
in″ter sti′tial
in″ter tar′sal
in″ter trans″ver sa′ri i
in″ter trans verse′
in″ter tri′go
in″ter tro″chan ter′ic
in″ter tu′bu lar
in″ter vas′cu lar
in″ter ven tric′u lar
in″ter ver′te bral
in″ter vil′lous
in″ter zo′nal
in tes′tin al
in tes′tine
in′ti ma
in tol′er ance
in tort′er
in tox′i cant
in tox″i ca′tion
in″tra ab dom′i nal
in″tra ac′i nar
in″tra ar tic′u lar
in″tra a′tri al
in″tra cap′su lar
in″tra car″ti lag′i nous
in″tra cav′i ta ry
in″tra cel′lu lar
in″tra cer e′bral
in″tra cra′ni al
in tract′able
in″tra cu ta′ne ous
in″tra cys′tic
in″tra der′mal
in″tra du′ral
in″tra e soph′a geal
in″tra fu′sal
in″tra gem′mal
in″tra he pat′ic
in″tra lig″a men′tous
in″tra lo′bar
in″tra lob′u lar
in″tra lu′mi nal
in″tra med′ul lar y
in″tra mem′bra nous
in″tra mu′ral
in″tra mus′cu lar
in″tra na′sal
in″tra nu′cle ar
in″tra oc′u lar
in″tra o′ral
in″tra or′bit al
in″tra pa ri′e tal
in″tra pel′vic
in″tra per i to ne′al
in″tra pleu′ral
in″tra scro′tal
in″tra spi′nal
in″tra stro′mal
in″tra the′cal
in″tra tra′che al
in″tra tu′bal
in″tra u re′thral
in″ta u′ter ine
in″tra vas′cu lar
in″tra ve′nous
in″tra ven tric′u lar
in″tra ves′i cal
in″tra vi′tal
in trin′sic
in″tro ces′sion
in″tro flex′ion
in tro′i tus
in″tro jec′tion
in′tro mis′sion
in″tro mit′tent
in″tro spec′tion
in″tro ver′sion
in′tro vert″
in″tu ba′tion
in″tu mes′cence

in″tus sus cep′tion
in″tus sus cep′tum
in″tus sus cip′i ens
in′u lin
in unc′tion
in u′te ro
in vac′u o
in vag′i nate
in vag″i na′tion
in′valid
in va′sion
in ver′sion
in vert′
in ver′tase
in ver′te bral
in ver″te bra′ta
in ver′te brate
in vest′ment
in vet′er ate
in″vi ril′i ty
in″vis ca′tion
in vot′ro
in vi′vo
in″vo lu′crum
in vol′un tar″y
in′vo lute
in″vo lu′tion
i′o dide
i′o dine
i″o din′o phil
i′o dism
i′o dized
i o″do der′ma
i o′do form
i″o dom′e try
i o″do phil′i a
i″o dop′sin
i o″do ther′a py
i″o do thy″ro glub′u lin
i om′e ter
i′on
i o′ni um
i″on i za′tion
i″on om′e ter
i on″to pho re′sis
i″o pho′bi a
ip′e cac
ip″si lat′er al
i ras″ci bil′i ty
ir″i dad″e no′sis
i′ri dal
ir″i dal′gi a
ir″i daux e′sis
ir″i da vul′sion
ir″i dec′tome
ir″i dec′to mize
ir″i dec′to my
ir″i dec tro′pi um
ir″i de′mi a
ir″i den clei′sis
ir″i den tro′pi um
i rid″e re′mi a
ir′i des
ir″i des′cence
i rid′ic
i rid′i um
ir″i di za′tion
ir″i do a vul′sion
ir″i do cap″su li′tis
ir″i do cap″su lot′o my
i rid′o cele
ir″i do cho″roid i′tis
ir″i do col″o bo′ma
ir″i do cy clec′to my
ir′i do cy cli′tis
ir″i do cy″clo cho″roid i′tis
ir″i do cys tec′to my
ir′i do cyte″
ir′i do di″ag no′sis
ir″i do di al′y sis
ir″i do di la′tor
ir″i do do ne′sis

ir″i do ki ne′si a
ir″i do lep tyn′sis
ir″i do ma la′ci a
ir″i do mo′tor
ir″i don co′sis
ir″i don′cus
ir″i do pa ral′y sis
ir″i do pa rel′ky sis
ir″i do pa re′sis
ir″i do per″i pha ki′tis
ir″i do ple′gi a
ir″i dop to′sis
ir″i do pu′pil lar″y
ir″i do rhex′is
ir″i dos′chi sis
ir″i do scle rot′o my
ir″i dot′a sis
ir′i do tome
ir″i dot′o my
ir″i dot′ro mos
i′ris
i rit′ic
i ri′tis
ir″i to ec′to my
i′ron
ir ra′di ate
ir ra″di a′tion
ir ra′tion al
ir″re du′ci ble
ir reg″u lar′i ty
ir″re sus′ci ta ble
ir″re ver′si ble
ir″ri ga′tion
ir″ri ta bil′i ty
ir′ri ta ble
ir′ri tant
ir″ri ta′tion
i″sa del′phi a
is che′mi a
is che′sis
is″chi al′gi a
is″chi a ti′tis
is″chi dro′sis
is″chi o bul bo′sus
is″chi o cap′su lar
is″chi o cav″er no′nous
is″chi o coc cyg′e al
is″chi o coc cyg′e us
is″chi o did′y mus
is″chi o fe mo ra′lis
is chi om′e lus
is″chi o my″e li′tis
is″chi o neu ral′gi a
is chi op′a gus
is″chi o pu′bi cus
is″chi o pu″bi ot′o my
is″chi o pu′bis
is″chi o rec′tal
is′chi um
isch″no pho′ni a
is″cho ga lac′ti a
is″cho gy′ri a
is″cho me′ni a
is chu′ri a
Ishihara (color vision test)
is′let
i″so ag glu′ti nin
i″so an′ti bod″ies
i″so an′ti gen
i″so bar
i″so bar′ic
i″so cel″lo bi′ose
i″so cel′lu lar
i″so chro mat′ic
i soch′ro nal
i″so chro′ni a
i″so co′ri a
i″so cor′tex
i″so cy tol′y sin
i″so dac′ty lism
i″so di″ag no′sis
i′so dont

i″so do′ses
i″so dy nam′ic
i″so e lec′tric
i″so gam′ete
i sog′a mous
i″so gen′e sis
i″sog′na thous
i′so graft
i″so he″mag glu′ti nin
i″so he mol′y sin
i″so he mol′y sis
i″so i co′ni a
i″so im″mu ni za′tion
i″so la′tion
i′so mer
i som′er ism
i″so met′ric
i″so me tro′pi a
i′so morph
i″so mor′phic
i″so ni′a zid
i″so os mot′ic
i sop′a thy
i″so pho′ri a
i so′pi a
i″so plas′tic
i″so pro′pyl
i so pro ter′ e nol
i sop′ters
i′so therm
i′so tope
i″so trop′ic
isth mec′to my
isth′mus
I′ su prol
i su′ri a
itch′ing
i′ter
ix″od′i dac
ix″od′ic
ix″y o my″e li′tis

J

Jacksonian
at tack′
jac″ti ta′tion
jar′gon
jaun′dice
je ju′nal
jej″u nec′to my
jej″u ni′tis
jej″u no ce cos′to my
jej″u no co los′to my
jej″u no il″e i′tis
jej″u no il″e os′to my
jej″u no il′e um
jej″u no jej″u nos′to my
jej″u nor′rha phy
jej″u nos′to my
jej″u not′o my
je ju′num
Jimson weed
Jod bas′e dow phenomen
joint
jug′u lar
jug′ u lar og″ ra phy
ju jit′su
ju men′tous
junc′tion
junc tu′ra
ju″ris pru′dence
jus′to ma′jor
ju′ve nile
jux″ta-ar tic′u lar
jux″to glo mer′u lar
jux″ta po si′tion
jux″ta py lor′ic

K

Kahn test
kai″no pho′bi a
kak″or raph″i o pho′bi a
ka′la-a zar′
kal″li kre′in
ka le′mi a
ka″na my′cin
ka′ o lin
ka″o li no′sis
Ka o pec′tate
Kaposi's dis ease′
Kartagener's syn′drome
ka″ry en′chy ma
ka′ry o blast″
ka′ry o chrome″
ka″ry og′a my
ka″ry o ki ne′sis
ka″ry o lo′bic
ka″ry ol′y sis
ka′ry o mere
ka″ry o mi″cro so′ma
ka″ry o mi′tome
ka″ry o mi to′sis
ka′ry o phage″
ka′ry o plasm
ka″ry or rhex′is
ka′ry o some″
ka″ry os′ta sis
kar″y o the′ca
kar″y o type′
kath″i so pho′bi a
Ke′ flex
Kef′lin
ke′loid
kelp
ken″o pho′bi a
ken″o tox′in
ker″a phyl′lo cele
ker″a phyl′lous
ker′a sin
ler″a tal′gi a
ker″a tec ta′si a
ker″a tec′to my
ke rat′ic
ker′a tin
ker″a tin i za′tion
ker″a tin′o cytes
ke rat′i nous
ker″a ti′tis
ker″a to ac″an tho′ma
ker′a to cele″
ker″a to cen te′sis
ker″a to chro″ma to′sis
ker″a to con junc″ti vi′tis
ker″a to co′nus
ker″a to der′ma
ker″a to gen′e sis
ker″a to glu′bus
ker″a to hel co′sis
ker″a to hy′a lin
ker′a toid
ker″a to ir′i do scope
ker″a to i ri′tis
ker″a to leu ko′ma
ker″a tol′y sis
ker″a to lyt′ic
ker″a to me la′ci a
ker′a tome
ker″a tom′e ter
ker″a to my co′sis
ker″a to nyx′is
ker′a to plas″ty
ker″a tor rhex′is
ker″a to scle ri′tis
ker′a to scope
ker″a tos′co py

ker'a tose
ker"a to'sis
ker a tot'o my
ke rau"no pho'bi a
ke'ri on
ker nic'ter us
Kernig's sign
ker'o cele
ke"to aci do'sis
ke"to gen'i sis
ke'tone
ke"to ne'mi a
ke"to nu'ri a
ke'tose
ke to'sis
ke"to ster'oid
kid'ney
Kiesselbach's tri'angle
kil'o cal"o rie
kil'o gram
kil'o me"ter
Kimmelstiel-Wilson syn'drome
ki'nase
kin"e mat'o graph
kin'e plas"ty
kin"e ra"di o ther'a py
kin'e scope
ki ne'si a
ki ne"si at'rics
ki ne"si es the"si om'e ter
kin"e sim'e ter
ki ne"si ol'o gy
ki ne'sis
ki ne"so pho'bi a
kin"es the'si a
ki net'ic
ki ne'tism
kin"e to car'di o gram
ki ne'to chore
ki"no cen'trum
ki'o tome
Klebs-Loeffler ba cil'lus
Kleb si el'la
klep"to lag'ni a
kelp"to ma'ni a
klep"to pho'bi a
Kline test
Klinfelter's syn'drome
Klippel-Feil syn'drome
knee
knee'cap"
knit'ting
knob
knock'-knee"
knuck'le
knuck'ling
Koch, Robert
koi"lo nych'i a
Kolmer's test
ko"ly phre'ni a
ko'ni me"ter
ko"ni o cor'tex
Koplik's spots
kop"o pho'bi a
Korsakoff psy cho' sis
kra tom'e ter
krau ro'sis
Krukenberg tu'mor
Kupffer cells
Kussmaul's re"spi ra'tion
kwash i or'kor
ky es'te in
ky'mo gram
ky'mo graph
Ky'nex
ky"pho ra chi'tis
ky"pho sco"li o ra chi'tis
ky"pho sco"li o'sis
ky pho'sis
ky phot' ic

L

la′bi a
la′bi al ism
la′bile
la bil′i ty
la″bi o al ve′o lar
la″bi o cer′vi cal
la″bi o den′tal
la″bi o gin′gi val
la″bi o glos′so la ryn′ge al
la″bi o gres′sion
la″bi o men′tal
la″bi o pal′a tine
la′bi o plas″ty
la′bi um
la′bor
lab′o ra to″ry
la′brum
lab′y rinth
lab″y rin thec′to my
lab″ y rin′ thine
lab″y rin thi′tis
lab″y rin thot′o my
lac′er at″ed
lac″er a′tion
la cer′tus
la cin′i ate
lac′ri mal
lac″ri ma′le
lac″ri ma′tion
lac′ri ma″tor
lac′ri mo tome″
lac″ri mot′o my
lac tac″i du′ri a
lac″tal bu′min
lac′tant
lac′tase
lac′tate
lac ta′tion
lac′te al
lac′tic
lac tif′ er ous
lac′ti fuge
Lac′ti gen
lac tig′e nous
lac″ti su′gi um
lac tiv′o rous
Lac″to ba cil′lus
lac′to cele
lac′to crit
lac′to gen
lac″to gen′ic
lac″to glob′u lin
lac tom′e ter
lac′tose
la cu′na
la cu′nu la
la′dre rie″
Laennec′s cir rho′sis
Lafora bo′dies
lag″neu o ma′ni a
lag″oph thal′mos
la′i ty
lal″o pho′bi a
lal la′tion
la lop′a thy
lal″o pho mi′a trist
lal″o ple′gi a
lamb′da cism
lamb′doid
lam bli′a sis
la mel′la
la mel′lar
lame′ness
lam′i na
lam″i na′tion
lam″i nec′to my
lam″i ni′tis
lam″i nog′ra phy

lam″i not′o my
lam′pas
lamp′black″
lam proph′o ny
lan′a to side″
Lancefield group′ing
lan′cet
lan′ci na″ting
Langerhans' is′lets
lan′o lin
Lansing po′lio vi′rus
lan′to cide-C
la nu′go
lan′u lous
lap″a ror′rha phy
lap″a rot′o mist
lap″a rot′o my
lap″a ro tra″che lot′o my
la pros′co py
lap′sus
lar da′ceous
lar′va
lar′val
lar′vate
lar′vi cide
lar″yn gal′gi a
lar″yn ge′al
lar″yn gec′to my
lar″yn gem phrax′is
lar″yn gis′mus
lar″yn gi′tis
la ryn′go cele
la ryn″go cen te′sis
la ryn″go fis′sure
la ryn′ go gram
la ryn′go graph
lar″yn gol′o gist
lar″yn gol′o gy
lar″yn go ma la′ci a
lar″yn gom′e try
la ryn″go pa ral′y sis
lar″yn gop′ athy
la ryn″go phan′tom
la ryn″go pha ryn′ge al
la ryn″go phar″yn gec′to my
la ryn″go pha ryn′ge us
la ryn″go phar″yn gi′tis
la ryn″go phar′ynx
lar″yn goph′o ny
la ryn′go plas″ty
la ryn″go ple′gi a
la ryn″go pto′sis
la ryn″go rhi nol′o gy
la ryn″gor rha′ gi a
lar″yn gor′rha phy
la ryn″gor rhe′a
la ryn″go scle ro′ma
la ryn′go scope
lar″yn go scop′ic
lar″yn gos′co pist
lar″yn gos′co py
la ryn′go spasm″
lar″yn gos′ta sis
lar″yn go ste no′sis
lar″yn gos′to my
la″ryn″go stro′bo scope
la ryn″go syr′inx
la ryn′go tome
lar″yn got′o my
la ryn″go tra′che al
la ryn″go tra″che i′tis
la ryn″go tra″che o bron chi′tis
la ryn″go tra″che ot′o my
la ryn″go xe ro′sis
lar′ynx
las civ′i a
las civ′i ous
Lasegue's sign
La′ six
Lassar's paste
las′ si tude
la′tent

lat′er ad
lat′er al
lat″er o ab dom′i nal
lat″er o duc′tion
lat″er o flex′ion
lat″er o mar′gin al
lat″er o pul′sion
lat″er o tor′sion
lat″er o ver′sion
la′tex
la tis″si mo con″dy lar′is
la tis′si mus
la trine′
Lat″ro dec′tus mac′tans
la′tus
laud′a ble
lau′da num
laugh
laugh′ter
la vage′
la va′tion
lax′a tive
lax′i ty
lay′er
lay ette′
lay′man
leach′ing
lead
lec″a no so″ma top′a gus
lec′i thal
lec′i thin
leech
Leiner′s dis ease′
lei″o der′ma tous
lei″o der′ mi a
lei″o my″o fi bro′ma
lei″o my o′ma
lei″o my″o sar co′ma
lei ot′ri chous
lei″po me′ri a
Leishman-Donovan bod′ies
Leish ma′ni a
leish″man i′a sis
leish′man oid
lem′mo cyte
lem nis′cus
lem′no blast
le″mo ste no′sis
len′i ceps
len′i tive
lens om′e ter
Len′te in′su lin
len″ti co′nus
len tic′u lar
len tic′u late
len tic″u lo stri′ate
len tic″u lo tha lam′ic
len′ti form″
len″ti glo′bus
len ti′go
le″on ti′a sis
lep′er
lep″i do′ma
Lep″i dop′ter a
lep′o thrix
lep′ro lin
lep rol′o gist
lep rol′o gy
lep ro′ma
lep′ro min
lep″ro pho′bi a
lep″ro sar′i um
lep′ro sin
lep′ro sy
lep′rous
lep″to ce pha′li a
lep″to ceph′a lus
lep″to chro mat′ic
lep″to cy′tic
lep″to cy to′sis
lep″to dac′ty lous
lep″to don′tous

lep″ to men′ in ge′ al
lep″to me nin′ges
lep″to me nin″gi o′ma
lep″to men″in gi′tis
lep″to men″in gop′a thy
lep″to me′ninx
lep″to mi″cro gnath′i a
lep″to pel′lic
lep″to pho′ni a
lep″to pro so′pi a
lep′tor rhine″
lep′to scope″
Lep″to spi′ra
Lep″to spi′ra ic″ter o hae mor rha′gi ae
lep″to spi ro′sis
lep′to tene
Lep′to thrix
le re′sis
Les′bi an
le′sion
le′thal
leth′ar gy
le′the
Letterer-Siwe syn′drome
leu cae′thi op
leu′cine
leu″ci no′sis
leu″ci nu′ri a
leu″ka ne′mi a
leu ke′mi a
leu kem′id
leu ke′moid
leu′kin
leu′ko blast″
leu″ko blas to′sis
leu ko′ci din
leu′ko cyte″
leu″ko cy′to blast″
leu″ko cy″to ly′sin
leu″ko cy tol′y sis
leu″ko cy to′ma
leu″ko cy tom′e ter
leu″ko cy to′sis
leu″ko der′ma
leu″ko dys′tro phy
leu″ko en ceph a lop′athy
leu ko′ma
leu″ko nych′i a
leu kop′a thy
leu″ko pe di′sis
leu″ko pe′ni a
leu″ko pe′nic
leu″ko phleg ma′si a
leu″koph thal′mous
leu″ko pla′ki a
leu kop′sin
leu″kor rha′gi a
leu″kor rhe′a
leu″ko sar co′ma
leu″ko sar co″ma to′sis
leu′ko scope″
leu′ko tome″
leu″ko tox′ic
leu″ko tox′in
leu″ko trich′i a
leu″ko u″ro bil′in
leu′kous
lev″ar ter′en ol
le va′tor
le′ver
lev″i ga′tion
lev″i ta′tion
le vo car′di a
le″vo car′di o gram″
le″vo con′dyl ism
le″vo duc′tion
le″vo gy′rous
le″vo pho′bi a
le″vo pho′ri a
le″vo ro ta′tion
le″vo ro′ta to″ry

lev′u lose
lew′is ite
Leydig
cell
lib″er a′tion
li bid′ i nal
li bi′do
Li′bri um
li′cense
li cen′ti ate
li′chen
li″chen if i ca′tion
li″chen i za′tion
lic′o rice
li″e ni′tis
li e′no cele
li″en og′ra phy
li e″no ma la′ci a
li″e nop′a thy
li e″no re′nal
li e″no tox′in
li′en ter″y
li″en un′cu lus
lig′a ment
lig″a men′to pex″y
lig″a men′tum
li′gate
li ga′tion
lig′a ture
lig′ne ous
lig″ni fi ca′tion
lig′num
limb
lim′bic
lim′bus
li′men
li′mes
lim′i na
lim′i nal
lim″i troph′ic
lim nol′o gy
li moph′thi sis
Lin co my′cin
lin′dane
lin′e a
lin′e ar
lin′gua
lin′gual
lin′gu la
lin′gu lar
lin″guo dis′tal
lin″guo gin′gi val
lin′i ment
lin″o le′ic
lin″o le′nic
lin″o no pho′bi a
lin′seed
li′pa
lip″a ro trich′i a
li′a rous
li′pase
lip ec′to my
li pe′mi a
lip′id
li pi′o dol
lip″o blas to′sis
lip″o cal″ci no gran″u lo ma
to′sis
lip″o chon″dro dys′tro phy
lip″o chon dro′ma
lip′o chrome″
lip′o cyte″
lip″o dys′tro phy
lip″o fi″bro myx o′ma
lip″o fi″bro sar co′ma
lip″o gen′e sis
li pog′e nous
lip″o gran″u lo′ma
lip″o gran u lo ma to′sis
lip″o he″mar thro′sis
lip′oid
lip″oi do′sis
li pol′y sis
li po′ma

lip o′ma toid
li po″ma to′sis
lip″o me tab′o lism
li pom′pha lus
lip″o my o hem an″gi o′ma
lip″o my o′ma
lip″o my o sar co′ma
lip″o pe′ni a
lip″o pha′gic
lip′o phil
lip″o phre′ni a
lip″o pro′te in
lip″o sar co′ma
li po′sis
lip″o sol′u ble
li pos′to my
lip″o tro′pic
lip″o vac′cine
Lip′pes loop
lip″pi tu′do
li pu′ri a
liq″ue fac′tion
liq′uid
liq′uor
lisp
lis″sen ce pha′li a
lis″sen ceph′a lous
Lis te′ri a
li′ter
lith′a gogue
lith′arge
lith ec′to my
li the′mi a
li thi′a sis
lith″i co′sis
lith′i um
lith″o di al′y sis
lith″o gen′e sis
lith′oid
lith″o kel″y pho pe′di on
lith′o labe
li thol′a pax″y
lith″o ne phri′tis
lith″o ne phrot′o my
lith″o pe′di on
lith′o phone″
lith′o scope″
li tho′sis
li thot′o mist
li thot′o my
lith′o trip″sy
lith′o trite
lith′ous
lith″u re′sis
li thu′ri a
lit′mus
Litten′s sign
lit′ter
Littré, glands of
liv′er
liv′id
lo″a i′a sis
lo′bar
lobe
lo bec′to my
lo be′li a
lo bot′o my
lob′u lar
lob′u le
lob′u lus
lo′bus
lo″cal i za′tion
lo′cal ized
lo′chia
lo″chi o col′pos
lo′chi o cyte
lo″chi o me′tra
lo″chi o me tri′tis
lo″chi or rha′gi a
lo″chi or rhe′a
lo″chi os′che sis
lo″cho me tri′tis
lo″cho per″i to ni′tis
lo′ci

lock'jaw"
lo"co mo'tion
loc"u la'tion
loc'u li
loc'u lus
lo'cum te'nens
lo'cus
Loeffler's syn'drome
log"a dec'to my
log"a di'tis
log"a do blen"nor rhe'a
log"ag no'si a
log"a graph'i a
log"am ne'si a
log"a pha'si a
log"o ko pho'sis
log"o ma'ni a
log"o neu ro'sis
log op'a thy
log"o pe'dics
log"o pha'si a
log"o ple'gi a
log'o spasm
lo" go ther' a py
lo i'a sis
loin
lon gev'i ty
lon"gi lin'e al
lon"gi ma'nous
lon"gi ped'ate
lon gis'si mus
lon"gi tu'di nal
lon"gi tu"di na'lis
lon"gi typ'i cal
lon'gus
lo'pho dont
lo quac'i ty
lo raz'e pam
lor do'sis
lor dot'ic
lo'ti o
lo'tion
loupe
louse
lous'y
lox a'pine
Lox'i tane
lu cid'i ty
lu cif'u gal
lu'dic
lu'es
lu e'tic
Lugol's so lu'tion
lum ba'go
lum'bar
lum"bo co los'to my
lum"bo co lot'o my
lum"bo cos'tal
lu"bo dor'sal
lum"bo in'gui nal
lum"bo is'chi al
lum"bo sa'cral
lum'bri cal
lu'men
lu'mi nal
lu'mi nance
lu"mi nes'cence
lu"mi nif'er ous
lu"mi nos'i ty
lu'na cy
lu'nar
lu'nate
lu'na tic
lung
lu'nu la
lu po'ma
lu'pus
lu'pus er"y thy ma to'sis
lu'sus na tu'rae
lu'te al
lu'te in
lu"te in iz'ing
lu"te o'ma
lu"te o tro'pic

lux a'tion
lux u'ri ant
lux'us
ly'cine
ly"co rex'i a
ly"go phil'i a
ly"ing-in'
lymph
lym phad"e nec'to my
lym phad"e ni'tis
lym phad"e no'ma
lym phad"e no ma to'sis
lym phad"e nop'a thy
lym phad"e no'sis
lym phad"e not'o my
lym'pha gogue
lym"phan gi ec tas'i a
lym phan"gi ec'ta sis
lym phan"gi ec'to my
lym phan"gi o en"do the"li o'ma
lym phan"gi o'gram
lym phan"gi og'ra phy
lym phan"gi o'ma
lym phan'gi o plas"ty
lym phan"gi o sar co'ma
lym phan"gi ot'o my
lym"phan gi'tis
lym phat'ic
lym phat"i cos'to my
lym"phe de'ma
lym'pho blast
lym"pho blas to'ma
lym"pho car'ci no ma
lym'pho cyte
lym"pho cy'tic
lym"pho cy to'ma
lym"pho cy"to pe'ni a
lym"pho cyto poi e' sis
lym"pho cy to'sis
lym"pho der'mi a
lym"pho ep'i the"li o'ma
lym phog'en ous
lym"pho go'ni a
lym"pho gran"u lo'ma
lym"pho gran"u lo ma to'sis
lym'phoid
lym'pho kines
lym pho'ma
lym"pho ma to'sis
lym"pho path'i a ve ne're um
lym"pho pe'ni a
lym"pho poi e'sis
lym"pho re tic'u lar
lym"pho re tic"u lo'ma
lym"pho re tic"u lo'sis
lym'phor rhage
lym"phor rhe'a
lym"pho sar co'ma
lym"pho sar"co ma to'sis
lym phu'ri a
ly'o phile
ly"o phil i za'tion
ly'o phobe
ly'o sol
ly"o sorp'tion
ly'o trope
lyse
ly ser'gic ac'id
di"eth yl am'ide
ly sim'e ter
ly'sine
ly'sis
ly"so ceph'a lin
Ly'sol
ly'so zyme
lys'sic
lys"so dex'is
lys'soid
lys"so pho'bi a

M

McBurney's in ci'sion
mac'er ate
mac'er a"ter
Macewen, William
mac"ra cu'si a
mac"ren ce phal'ic
mac"ren ceph'a ly
mac"ro bac te'ri um
mac"ro ble phar'i a
mac"ro bra'chi a
mac"ro car'di us
mac"ro ce pha'li a
mac"ro ceph'a lus
mac"ro chei'li a
mac"ro chei'ri a
mac"ro cyte
mac'ro cyt'ic
mac"ro cy to'sis
mac"ro dac tyl'i a
mac"ro don'ti a
mac"ro en ceph'a ly
mac"ro gam'ete
mac"ro glob"u lin e'mi a
mac"ro glos'si a
mac"ro gnath'ic
mac"ro gy'ri a
mac"ro lymph'o cyte
mac"ro mas'ti a
mac"ro me'li a
ma crom'e lus
mac"ro mo lec'u lar
mac"ro mon'o cyte
mac"ro my'e lo blast
mac"ro nor'mo blast
mac"ro nu'cle us
mac"ro nych'i a
mac'ro phage
mac"ro po'di a
mac"ro pol'y cytes
mac"ro pro so'pi a
mac"ro pro'so pus
ma crop'si a
mac"ro scop'ic
mac"ros mat'ic
mac"ro so'mi a
mac'ro spore"
mac"ro sto'mi a
ma cro'ti a
mac'u la
mac'u lar
mac'ule
mac"u lo pap'u lar
mad"a ro'sis
mad'i dans
ma du'ra foot
ma"du ro my co'sis
Maffucci's syn'drome
ma'gen bla se
mag'en stras"se
ma gen'ta
mag'got
mag'is tral
mag'ma
mag ne'si a
mag ne'si um
mag'net
mag'net ism
mag"net i za'tion
mag ne"to e lec"tric'i ty
mag ne'to graph
mag ne'to in duc'tion
mag"ne tom'e ter
mag ne"to-op'tic
mag ne"to ther'a py
mag'ne tron
mag"ni fi ca'tion

mag'num
maid'en head"
ma ieu"si o ma'ni a
ma ieu"si o pho'bi a
ma ieu'tic
maim
mal
mal"ab sorp'tion
ma la'ci a
mal"a co pla'ki a
mal"ad just'ment
mal'a dy
ma laise'
mal'an ders
ma'lar
ma lar'i a
ma lar"i ol'o gist
mal"as sim"i la'tion
Ma la thi'on
mal"di ges'tion
mal"for ma'tion
ma lig'nant
ma lin'ger er
mal"in"ter dig i ta'tion
mal'le a ble
mal"le a'tion
mal"le o in'cu dal
mal le'o lus
mal"le ot'o my
mal'let
mal'le us
mal"nu tri'tion
mal"oc clu'sion
Ma'lo prim
mal"po si'tion
mal pos'ture
mal"prac'tice
mal"pres"en ta'tion
mal"re duc'tion
malt'ase
mal turned'
ma'lum
mal un'ion
mam'e lon
mam'ma
mam'mal
mam mal'gi a
Mam ma'li a
mam'ma plas"ty
mam'ma ry
mam mec'to my
mam'mi form
mam mil'la
mam'mil lar"y
mam'mil la"ted
mam"mil la'tion
mam mil'li form"
mam mil'li plas"ty
mam"mil li'tis
mam"mil lo tha lam'ic
mam mog'ra phy
mam'mose
mam mot'o my
man del'ic ac'id
man'di ble
man dib"u lo glos'sus
man dib"u lo mar"gin al'is
man'drin
man"du ca'tion
man'ga nese
mange
ma'ni a
ma'nic
man'i kin
ma nip"u la'tion
man'ni tol
ma nom'e ter
man om'e try
man'tle
Mantoux test
ma nu'bri um
man"u duc'tion
ma'nus
man"u stu pra'tion

ma ran′tic
ma ras′mus
mar″ble i za′tion
mar che′-a-pet it-pas
Marfan′s syn′drome
mar′gin
mar″gi na′tion
mar′gi no plas″ty
Marie-Strumpell dis ease′
ma″ri hua′na
mar′lex
mar′row
mar su″pi al i za′tion
mas′cu line
mas″cu lin i za′tion
mask′ing
mas′o chism″
mas sage′
mas se′ter
mas seur′
mas seuse′
mas″so ther′a py
mast″ad e ni′tis
mast″ad e no′ma
mas tal′gi a
mast″a tro′phi a
mas tec″chy mo′sis
mas tec′to my
mast″hel co′sis
mas′tic
mas″ti ca′tion
mas″ti ca′tor
mas′ti ca to″ry
mas ti′tis
mas″to car″ci no′ma
mas″to de al′gi a
mas″to dyn′i a
mas′toid
mas″toid ec′to my
mas″toid i′tis
mas″toid ot′o my
mas ton′cus
mas top′a thy
mas′to pex″y
mas″to pla′si a
mas′to plas″ty
mas″tor rha′gi a
mas″to scir′rhus
mas to′sis
mas tos′to my
mas′tous
mas″tur ba′tion
ma ter′nal
ma ter′ni ty
ma′trix
mat′ter
mat′u rate
mat″u ra′tion
ma tu′ri ty
ma tu′ti nel
max ill′la
max′ill ary
max il″lo fa′cial
max il″lo fron ta′le
max′i mal
max′i mum
may′hem
ma zal′gi a
ma′zic
maz″o mor′ro
ma zop′a thy
ma′zo pex″y
mea′sles
meas′ly
me″a ti′tis
me″a tot′o my
me a′tus
mech′a nism
mech″a no ther′a py
me′cism
Meckel′s di′ver tic″u lum
me com′e ter

me″co nal′gi a
mec′on ate
mec″o neu″ro path′i a
mec″o ni or rhe′a
me co′ni um
me cys′ta sis
MEDEX
me′di a
me′di ad
me′di al
me′di an
me″di as ti′nal
me″di as″ti ni′tis
me′di as ti″no per″i car di′tis
me″di as″ti nos′co py
me″di as″ti not′o my
me″di as ti′num
me′di ate
med′i ca ble
me dic′a ment
med″i ca men to′sus
med′i ca″ted
med″i ca′tion
med′i ca″tor
me dic′i nal
med″i co eth′i cal
med″i co le′gal
med″i co psy chol′o gy
me″di o car′pal
me″di o dor′ sal
me″di o fron′tal
me″di o ne cro′sis
me″di o tar′sal
Med″i ter ra′ne an a ne′mi a
me′di um
me′di us
me dul′la
med′ul la″ry
med′ul la″ted
med″ul la′tion
med″ul li za′tion
med′ul lo blast″
med″ul lo blas to′ma
meg″a car′di a
meg″a ce′cum
meg″a coc′cus
meg″a co′lon
meg′a dont
meg″a du″o de′num
meg′a dyne
meg″a e soph′a gus
meg″a gna′thus
meg″a kar′y o blast
meg″a kar′y o cyte
meg″a kar″y oph′thi sis
me gal′gi a
meg′a lo blast
meg″a lo car′di a
meg″a lo ce phal′ic
meg″a lo ceph′a ly
meg″a loc′er us
meg″a lo chei′rous
meg″a lo cor′ne a
meg′a lo cyte
meg″a lo cy to′sis
meg″a lo en′ter on
meg″a lo gas′tri a
meg″a lo he pat′i a
meg″a lo ma′ni a
meg″a lo me′li a
meg″a lo ny cho′sis
meg″a lo pe′nis
meg″a loph thal′mus
meg″a lo po′di a
meg″a lo splanch′nic
meg′a lo spore″
meg″a lo u re′ter
meg′a phone
meg″a pros′o pous
meg″a rec′tum
meg″a sig′moid
meg′a volt″

meg′ohm″
meo o′sis
me la′gra
me lal′gi a
mel″an cho′li a
mel″an chol′ic
mel″a ne′mi a
mel″an id ro′sis
mel″a nif′er ous
mel′a nin
mel′a nism
mel″a no am″e lo blas to′ma
mel′a no blast″
mel′a no cyte″
mel″a no der′ma
mel″a no der″ma ti′tis tox′i ca
mel″a no der″ma to′sis
me lan′o gen
mel″a no gen′e sis
mel″a no glos′si a
mel′a noid
mel″a no′ma
mel″a no ma to′sis
mel″a no nych′i a
mel′a no phage″
mel′a no phore″
mel″a no pla′ki a
mel″a nor rhe′a
mel″a no′sis
me lan′o some
mel″a not′ri chous
mel″a nu′ri a
me las′ma
me le′na
me″li oi do′sis
me lis″so pho′bi a
me li′tis
mel″i tu′ri a
Mel′lar il
mel″o di dy′mi a
mel″o did′y mus
mel″o ma′ni a
me lom′e lus
mel″o rhe″os to′sis
me los′chi sis
me lo′tus
mem′brane
mem″bra no cra′ni um
mem′brum
mem′o ry
me nac′me
men ad′i one
me nar′che
Mendel, Gregor
Ménière's syn′drome
me nin′ge al
me nin″ge or′rha oht
me nin″gi o′ma
me nin″gi o″ma to′sis
me nin″gi o sar co′ma
me nin″gi o the″li o′ma
me nin′gism
men″in gis′mus
men″in git′i des
men″in gi′tis
men″in git″o pho′bi a
me nin″go ar″te ri′tis
me nin′go cele
me nin″go coc′cal
me nin″go coc ce′mi a
me nin″go coc′cic
me nin″go coc′cus
me nin″go cor′ti cal
me nin′go cyte
me nin″go-en ceph″a li′tis
me nin″go-en ceph′a lo cele
me nin″go-en ceph″a lo my″e lil′tis
me nin″go-en ceph″a lop′a thy
me nin″go my″e li′tis
me nin″go my′e lo cele
men″in gop′a thy

me nin″go ra dic′u lar
me nin″go rha chid′i an
me nin″gor rha′gi a
men″in go′sis
me nin″go vas′cu lar
men″in gu′ri a
me′ninx
men″is cec′to my
men″is ci′tis
me nis′co cyte
me nis′cus
men″o ce′lis
men″o lip′sis
men′o pause
men″o pha′ni a
men″o pla′ni a
men″or rha′gi a
men″or rhal′gi a
men″or rhe′a
me nos′che sis
men″o sta′si a
men″o stax′is
men″o xe′ni a
mens
men′sa
men′ses
men′stru al
men′stru ant
men′stru ate
men′stru a′tion
men′stru um
men′su al
men″su ra′tion
men′tal
men ta′lis
men tal′i ty
men ta′tion
men′thol
men″to hy′oid
men″tu lo ma′ni a
me per′i dine
me phit′ic
me pro′ba mate″
me ral′gi a
me ra lo′pi a
mer″a mau ro′sis
mer cap′tan
Mer cre′sin
Mer″cu hy′drin
mer cu′ri al
mer cu′ri al ism
mer cu″ri al i za′tion
mer cu′ric
Mer″cur o′chrome
mer cu′rous
mer′cu ry
mer″er ga′si a
me rid′i an
mer″in tho pho′bi a
mer′i spore
me ris′tic
mer″o a cra′ni a
mer″o gen′e sis
mer″o mi″cro so′mia
me ro′pi a
mer″o ra chis′chi sis
me ros′mi a
mer″o som′a tous
mer′o some
me rot′o my
Mer thio′late
Mes an′to in
mes″a or ti′tis
mes ar″te ri′tis
mes″a ti pel′lic
mes cal′
mes ec′to derm
mes en″ce phal′ic
mes″en ceph″al i′tis
mes″en ceph′a lon
mes″en cepha lot′o my
me sen′chy ma

mes′en chyme
mes″en chy″mo blas to′ma
mes″en chy mo′ma
mes″en ter ec′to my
mes″en ter′ic
mes″en ter″i co mes″o col′ic
mes″en ter″i o′lum
mes″en ter″i or′rha phy
mes″en ter″i pli ca′tion
mes″en ter′ri um
mes′en ter″y
me sen′to derm
mes″en tor′rha phy
me′si al
me″si o buc′cal
me″si o buc″co oc clu′sal
me″si o clu′sion
me″si o dis′tal
me″si o gres′sion
me″si o in ci′sal
me″si o la′bi al
me′si o lin′gual
me″si o lin″guo oc clu′sal
me″si o oc clu′sal
mes′mer ism
mes″o ap pen′dix
mes″o bil″i ru′bin
mes′o blast
mes″o blas te ma
mes″o blas tem′ic
mes″o car′di a
mes″o car′di um
mes′o carp
mes″o ce′cum
mes″o ce phal′ic
mes″oc ne′mic
mes″o co′lon
mes′o conch
mes′o derm
mes″o du″o de′num
mes″o e soph′a gus
mes″o gas′ter
mes″o gle′a
mes″o gnath′ic
mes″o gna′thi on
mes′o mere
mes″o me′tri um
mes′o morph
mes′o mor″phy
mes′on
mes″o ne phro′ma
mes″o neph′ros
mes′o pex″y
mes″o phle bi′tis
mes o′pic
mes″o pul′mo num
me sor′chi um
mes″o rec′tum
mes″o rop′ter
mes or′rha phy
mes′or rhine
mes″o sal′pinx
mes″o sig′moid
mes″o ten′don
mes″o the″li o′ma
mes″o the′li um
me sot′o my
mes′o tron
mes″o var′i um
met″a bi o′sis
met″a bol′ic fail′ure
met″a bo lim′e ter
me tab′o lism
me tab′o lite
me tab′o lize
met″a bol′o gy
met″a car′pal
met″a car pec′to my
met″a car″po pha lan′ge al
met″a car′pus
met″a chro ma′si a
met″a chro′sis

met'a cele
met'a cone
met"a con'id
met'a con'ule
met"a dra'sis
met"a kar'y o cyte
met'al
me tal'lic
met'al loid
met"al lo pho'bi a
met al'o phil
met'a mere
met"a mor'phic
met"a mor phop'si a
met"a mor'pho sis
met"a mor'phous
met"a my'e lo cyte
met"a neph"ro gen'ic
met"a neph'ros
met'a phase
me taph'y sis
met"a phys i'tis
met"a pla'si a
met'a plasm
met"a pneu mon'ic
met"ar te'ri ole
met'a sta ble
me tas'ta sis
me tas'ta size
met a stat'ic
met"a tar sal'gi a
met"a tar sec'to my
met"a tar"so pha lan'ge al
met"a tar'sus
met"a thal'a mus
met"a troph'ic
Met"a zo'a
me"te or'ic
me'te or o graph"
me"te or ol'o gy
me"te or o path"o log'ic
me'ter
me tes'trus
meth'a done
Meth"am phe'ta mine
meth'a nol
meth'e drine
met he"mo glo'bin
met he"mo glo"bi ne'mi a
met he"mo glo"bi nu'ria
Meth"i cil'lin
meth i'o nine
Meth"o trex'ate
meth'yl
meth'yl ene blue
meth"yl ep'si a
meth"yl phen'i date
Me ti cort'e lone"
Me ti cort'en
met"my o glo'bin
met"o don ti'a sis
me top'a gus
met"o pan tral'gi a
me top'ic
me to'pi on
met"ra pec'tic
met"ra to'ni a
met"ra tro'phi a
Met'ra zol
me'trec
met"rec ta'si a
met"rec to'pi a
me tre'mi a
met"reu ryn'ter
met reu'ry sis
me'tri a
met'ric
met"ri o ce phal'ic
me tri'tis
me'tro cele
me'tro clyst
me"tro col'po cele
me"tro cys to'sis
me'tro cyte

me″tro dy″na mom′e ter
me″tro dyn′i a
me″tro ec ta′si a
me″tro en″do me tri′tis
met rog′ra phy
me trol′o gy
me″tro lym″phan′gi tis
me″tro ma la′ci a
met′ro nome
me″tro pa ral′y sis
me″tro path′i a
me trop′a thy
me″tro per″i to ni′tis
me″tro phle bi′tis
me″trop to′sis
me″tror rha′gi a
me″tror rhe′a
me″tror rhex′is
me″tro sal″pin gi′tis
me″tro sal″pin gog′ra phy
me′tro scope
me″tro stax′is
me′tro tome
me try″per ci ne′sis
me try″per es the′si a
me try″per tro′phi a
Met′y caine Hy″dro chlo′ride
Meulengracht di′et
mi′ca
mi ca′ce ous
mi celle′
mi″cra cous′tic
mi″cren ceph′a lon
mi″cren ceph′a lous
mi″cren ceph′a ly
mi″cro ab′scess
mi″cro a″er o phil′ic
mi″cro au′di phone
Mi″cro bac te′ri um
mi′crobe
mi cro′bi cide
mi″cro bin ert′ness
mi″cro bi ol′o gist
mi″cro bi ol′o gy
mi″cro bi″o pho′bi a
mi″cro bi ot′ic
mi′cro bism
mi′cro blast″
mi″cro bleph′a ron
mi″cro bra′chi a
mi″cro brach″y ce pha′li a
mi″cro bu ret′
mi″cro cal′o rie
mi″ cro car′di a
mi″cro cen′trum
mi″cro ceph′a lus
mi″cro ceph′a ly
mi″cro chei′li a
mi″cro chem′is try
mi″cro chi′ri a
mi″cro coc′cin
Mi″cro coc′cus
mi″cro co′lon
mi″cro co nid′i um
mi″cro cou′lomb
mi″cro cu′rie
mi′cro cyst
mi′cro cyte
mi″cro cy the′mi a
mi″cro cy to′sis
mi″cro dac tyl′i a
mi″cro de ter″min a′tion
mi″cro dis sec′tion
mi′cro dont
mi″cro don′ti a
mi″cro drep′a no cyt ic dis ease′
mi″cro e lec″tro pho ret′ic
mi″cro e ryth′ro cyte
mi″cro far′ad
mi″cro fi lar′i a
mi″cro frac′ture
mi″cro gam′ete
mi″cro ga me′to cyte

mi crog′a my
mi″cro gas′tri a
mi″cro gen′e sis
mi″cro ge′ni a
mi″cro gen′i tal ism
mi″cro glos′si a
mi″cro gna′thi a
mi″cro go′ni o scope
mi″cro gram
mi″cro graph
mi crog′ra phy
mi″cro gy′ri a
mi′crohm
mi″cro in cin″er a′tion
mi″cro in jec′tion
mi″cro len′ti a
mi″cro leu′ko blast
mi′cro li″ter
mi′cro lith
mi″cro li thi′a sis
mi″cro ma′ni a
mi″cro ma nip′u la″tor
mi″cro mas′ti a
mi″cro ma′zi a
mi″cro me′li a
mi crom′e lus
mi crom′e ter disk
mi″cro mi′cron
mi″cro mil′li me″ter
mic″ro mon″o spo′rin
mi″cro mo′to scope
mi″cro my e′li a
mi″cro my′e lo blast
mi″cro my″e lo lym′pho cyte
mi′cron
mi′cro nee″dles
mi cron′e mous
mi″cro nu′cle us
mi″cro nu′tri ents
mi″cro nych′i a
mi″cro or′chism
mi″cro or′gan ism
mi″cro par′a site
mi″cro pe′nis
mi′cro phage
mi″cro pha′ki a
mi″cro phal′lus
mi″cro pho′bi a
mi′cro phone
mi″cro pho′ni a
mi″cro pho′no graph
mi″cro pho′no scope
mi″cro pho′to graph
mi″cro pho tom′e ter
mi″croph thal′mus
mi″cro phys′ics
mi″cro pi pet′
mi″cro ple thys mog′ra phy
mi″cro po′di a
mi″cro po lar′i scope
mi″cro pro jec′tion
mi″cro pro so′pi a
mi″cro pro′so pus
mi crop′si a
mi″cro psy′chi a
mi′cro pus
mi″cro pyk″nom′e ter
mi′cro pyle
mi″cro ra″di og′ra phy
mi″cro res′pi ra″tor
mi″cro rrhi′ni a
mi″cro scel′ous
mi′cro scope
mi″cro scop′ic
micros′co pist
mi cros′co py
mi″cro mat′ic
mi′cro some
mi″cro so′mi a
mi″cro spec trog′ra phy
mi″cro spec″tro
pho tom′e try
mi″cro spec′tro scope
mi″cro spher′o cyte

mi″cro sphyg′my
mi″cro sphyx′i a
Mi″cro spo′ron
mi″cro spo ro′sis
Mi″cro spo′rum au″dou i′ni
mi″cro steth′o phone
mi″cro steth′o scope
mi″cro sto′mi a
mi″cro sur′ger y
mi″cro the′li a
mi′cro therm
mi cro′ti a
mi′cro tome
mi crot′o my
mi″cro trau′ma
mi″cro u′nit
mi′cro volt
mi′cro wave
mi crox′y cyte
mi″cro zo o sper′mi a
mic′tu rate
mic″tu ri′tion
mid″ax il′la
mid′bod″y
mid′brain″
mid″fron′tal
midge
midg′et
mid′gut
mid′pain″
mid′riff
mid′wife″
mid′wife″ry
mi′graf
mi′graine
mi′grate
mi gra′tion
Mikulicz's dis ease′
mil′dew
mil′i a
mil″i a ri′a
mil′i ar″y
Mi′li bis
mi lieu′
mil′i um
mil″li am′me ″ter
mil″li am′pere
mil″li am′pere me″ter
mil′li bar
mil′li cu″rie
mil″li e quiv′a lent
mil′li gram
mil′li li″ter
mil′li me″ter
mil″li mi′cron
mil′li mol
mil″li nor′mal
mil″li os′mol
mil″li ruth′er ford
mil′li volt
mil pho′sis
Mil′town
mi me′sis
mim ma′tion
min″a mo′ta
min′er al
min″e ral o cor′ti coids
min′im
min′i mal
min′i mum
mi nom′e ter
mi″o car′di a
mi″o did′y mus
mi o′pus
mi o′sis
mi ot′ic
mire
mir′ror
mis an′thro py
mis car′riage
mis car′ry
mis′ce

mis″ce ge na′tion
mis′ci ble
mi sog′a my
mi sog′y ny
mi sol′o gy
mis″o ne′ism
mis″o pe′di a
mis″o psy′chi a
mis′tle toe
mi′tis
mit″o chon′dri a
mit″o chon′dri on
mit″o gen′e sis
mi′tome
mi to′sis
mi tot′ic
mit′o some
mi′tral
mi′troid
mit′tel schmerz
mix″o sco′pi a
mne″mas the′ni a
mne″mo der′mia
mne mon′ics
mne′mo tech″ny
mo bil′i ty
mo″bi li za′tion
Möbius′ sign
mo dal′i ty
mod′el
mod′er a tor
mo di′o lus
mod′u la″tor
mod′u lus
mo′dus
mog″i graph′i a
mog″i la′li a
mog″i pho′ni a
moi′e ty
mo′lal
mo′lar
mo las′ses
mold
mold′ing
mole
mo lec′u lar
mol′e cule
mo li′men
mol li′ti es
mol lus′cum
molt
mo lyb′de num
mo lys″mo pho′bi a
mo men′tum
mon′ad
mon ar′thric
mon″ar thri′tis
mon″ar tic′u lar
mon as′ter
mon″a the to′sis
mon″a tom′ic
Monckeberg′s dis ease′
mo nes′trus
mon′go lism
mon′go loid
Mo nil′i a
mo″ni li′a sis
mo nil′i form
mo nil′i id
mon′i tor ing
mon″o am′ine
mo″no a′mine ox i′dase
mon″o ar tic′u lar
mon″o bas′ic
mon′o blast
mon″o blep′si a
mon″o bra′chi us
mon″o car′di an
mon″o car′di o gram
mon″o cell′u lar
mon″o ceph′a lus
mon′o chord

mon″o cho re′a
mon″o chor i on′ic
mon″o chro′ma sy
mon″o chro′mat
mon″o chro mat′ic
mon″o chro mat′o phil
mon″o chro′ma tor
mon″o clin′ic
mon″o coc′cus
mon″o cra′ni us
mon″o crot′ic
mon oc′u lar
mon oc′u lus
mon″o cy e′sis
mon″o cys′tic
mon′o cyte
mon″o cy te′mic
mon″o cy to′ma
mon″o cy″to pe′ni a
mon″o cy to′sis
mon″o dac′ty lism
mon″o di plo′pi a
mon″o dro′mi a
mo nog′a my
mon″o gas′tric
mon″o ger′mi nal
mo nog′o ny
mon″o hy′brid
mon″o hy′drate
mon″o-i de′ism
mon″o ma′ni a
mon″o mel′ic
mon′o mer
mon″o mer′ic
mon″o mo′ri a
mon″o mor′phic
mon″o mor′phous
mo nom′pha lus
mon″o neph′rous
mon″o neu′ral
mon″o neu ri′tis
mon″o nu′cle ar
mon″o nu cle o′sis
mon″o pha′gi a
mo noph′a gism
mon″o pha′si a
mon″o pha′sic
mon″o pho′bi a
mon″oph thal′mi a
mon″o phy′o dont
mon″o ple′gi a
mon″o po′di a
mon″o psy cho′sis
mon″o pty′chi al
mon′o pus
mon″o ra dic′u lar
mon or′chid
mon″o rrhi′nous
mon″o sac′cha ride
mon″o scel′ous
mon″o som′a tous
mon′o some
mon″o stot′ic
mon″o stra′tal
mon″o symp″to mat′ic
mon″o ther′mi a
mon o′tic
mo not′o cous
mon ox′ide
mon″o zy got′ic
mons
mon′ster
mon′stri cide
mon strip′a ra
mon stros′i ty
mon tic′u lus
mor′bi
mor′bid
mor bid′i ty
mor″cel la′tion
mor da′cious
mor′dant

Morgagni, Giovanni B.
morgue
mor′i bund
Moro re′flex
mo′ron
mo ron′i ty
mor′phine
mor′phin ism
mor″pho gen′e sis
mor phol′gy
Morquio's dis ease′
mor′sal
mor tal′i ty
mor′tar
Mo′trin
mor′tu ar″y
mor′u la
mo sa′ic
mo′tile
mo til′i ty
mou″lage′
mu′cin
mu′co cele
mu″co cu ta′ne ous
mu″co en″ter i′tis
mu″co hem″or rhag′ic
mu′coid
mu″co per″i os′te um
mu″co poly″sac′cha ride
mu″co pro′tein
mu″co pu′ru lent
mu″cor my′co sis
mu co′sa
mu″co san guin′e ous
mu″co se′rous
mu cos′i ty
mu′cous
mu″co vis ci do′sis
mu′cro nate
mu′cus
mu″li eb′ri ty
Müllerian duct
mul tan′gu lum
mul″ti cap′su lar
mul″ti cel′lu lar
mul″ti cos′tate
mul″ti cus′pid
mul″ti den′tate
mul″ti dig′i tate
mul″ti fa mil′i al
mul′ti fid
mul tif′i dus
mul′ti form
mul″ti gan′gli on ate
mul″ti glan′du lar
mul″ti grav′i da
mul″ti in fec′tion
mul″ti lo′bar
mul″ti lob′u lar
mul″ti loc′u lar
mul″ti mam′mae
mul″ti nod′u lar
mul″ti nu′cle ar
mul tip′a ra
mul″ti par′i ty
mul tip′a rous
mul″ti po′lar
mul″ti val′lent
mul ti vi′ta min
mum″mi fi ca′tion
mum′mi fied
mumps
mu′ral
mu″ri at′ic
mu′rine ty′phus
mur′mur
mus′ca rine
mus′cle
mus″cu lar′is
mus″cu lar′i ty
mus′cu la ture
mus″cu lo ap″o neu rot′ic

mus″cu lo cu ta′ne ous
mus″cu lo fas′ci al
mus″cu lo fi′brous
mus″cu lo phren′ic
mus″cu lo skel′e tal
mus″cu lo spi′ral
mus″cu lo ten′di nous
mu″si co ma′ni a
mu″si cop ther′a py
mu′tant
mu ta′tion
mu″ti la′tion
mu′tism
my al′gi a
my″as the′ni a
my″a to′ni a
my ce′li oid
my ce′li um
my ce′tes
my″ce to′ma
My″ci fra′din
my″co an″gi o neu ro′sis
My″co bac te′ri um
my′coid
my col′o gy
my″coph thal′mi a
my co′sis
My″co spo′rum
My″co stat′in
my co′tic
my cot″i za′tion
myc″ter o pho′ni a
my de′sis
my dri′a sis
myd″ri at′ic
my ec′to my
my″e lat′ro phy
my″e len ceph′a lon
my el′ic
my′e lin
my″e li nat′ed
my″e li na′tion
my″e li ni za′tion
my″e lin o cla′sis
my″e li no gen′e sis
my″e lin ol′y sis
my″e li nop′a thy
my″e li no′sis
my″e li′tis
my′e lo blast″
my″e lo blas te′mi a
my″e lo blas′tic
my″e lo blas to′ma
my″e lo blas to′sis
my′e lo cele″
my″e lo cys′to cele
my′e lo cyte″
my″e lo cyt′ic
my″e lo cy to′sis
my″e lo dys pla′si a
my″e lo en ceph″a li′tis
my″e lo fi bro′sis
my″e lo gen′e sis
my″e lo gen′ic
my′e lo gram
my″e log′ra phy
my′e loid
my″e lo lym′pho cyte″
my″e lo′ma
my″e lo ma la′ci a
my″e lo ma to′sis
my″e lo men″in gi′tis
my″e lo me nin′go cele″
my′e lo mere″
my″e lo mon′o cyte″
my′el on
my″e lo neu ri′tis
my″e lo pa ral′y sis
my″e lo path′ic
my″e lop′a thy
my″e lop′e tal
my″e loph′thi sic

my″e loph′thi sis
my′e lo plast″
my″e lo ple′gi a
my″e lo poi e′sis
my′e lo pore″
my″e lo pro lif′er a tive
my″e lo ra dic″u li′tis
my″e lo ra dic″u lo dys pla′si a
my″e lo ra dic″u lop′a thy
my″e lo rrha′gi a
my″e lo sar co′ma
my″e los′chi sis
my″e lo scint′o gram
my″e lo scin tog′ra phy
my″e lo scle ro′sis
my″e lo′sis
my en′ta sis
my″en ter′ic
my en′ter on
my″es the′si a
my′ia sis
my″la ceph′a lus
my lo′dus
my″lo glos′sus
my″lo hy′oid
my″lo phar yn′ge al
my′o blast
my″o blast o′ma
my″o car′di al
my″o car di′tis
my″o car′di um
my″o car do′sis
my″o clo′ni a
my″o clo′nic
my″o clo′nus
my′o cyte
my″o dys to′ni a
my″o dys′tro phy
my″o e de′ma
my″o e las′tic
my″o ep″i the′li al
my″o ep″i the″li o′ma
my″o fas′ci al
my″o fas ci′tis
my″o fi′bril
my″o fi″bro sar co′ma
my″o fi″bro si′tis
my″o ge lo′sis
my′o gen
my″o gen′ic
my″o glo′bin
my″o glo″bin u′ri a
my″o gnath′us
my′o gram
my′o graph
my″o he′ma tin
my″o he″mo glo′bin
my″o ki ne′si o gram″
my″o kin″es i og′ra phy
my″o ky′mi a
my ol′o gy
my o′ma
my″o ma la′ci a
my″o mec′to my
my″o me tri′tis
my″o me′tri um
my″o neu′ral
my″o pal′mus
my″o pa ral′y sis
my″o pa re′sis
my″o path′i a
my op′a thy
my′ope
my″o per″i car di′tis
my o′pi a
my o′pic
my′o plasm
my′o plas″ty
my″o por tho′sis
my″o psy chop′a thy
my or′rha phy
my″o sar co′ma

my″o scle ro′sis
my′o sin
my″o sit′ic
my″o si′tis
my″o stat′ic
my″o su′ture
my″o syn″o vi′tis
my″o tac′tic
my ot′a sis
my″o ten″o si′tis
my″o te not′o my
my′o tome
my ot′o my
my″o to′ni a
my″o ot′ro phy
myr′i a gram
myr″i a li′ter
myr″i a me′ter
my rin′ga
myr″in gec′to my
myr″in gi′tis
my rin″go dec′to my
my rin″go my co′sis
my rin′go plas″ty
my rin′go scle ro′sis
my rin′go tome
myr″in got′o my
myr′ti form
My′so line
my″so pho′bi a
myth″o ma′ni a
myth″o pho′bi a
myx ad″e ni′tis
myx″as the′ni a
myx″e de′ma
myx id′i o cy
myx″i o′sis
myx″o ad″e no′ma
myx″o chon″dro fi″bro sar co′ma
myx″o chon″dro sar co′ma
myx″o fi bro′ma
myx″o fi″bro sar co′ma
myx″o gli o′ma
myx′oid
myx o′ma
myx″o ma to′sis
myx o′ma tous
myx″o neu ro′ma
myx″or rhe′a
myx″o sar co′ma
myx″o vi′rus

N

na bo′thi an
Naf′cil lin
nail
na′ked
Nal′line
Na lox′one
na′nism
na″no ceph′a lus
na′noid
na nom′e lus
nan″oph thal′mi a
na″no so′ma
na″no so′mus
na′nus
nape
na′pex
naph′tha
naph′tha lene
nar′can
nar cis′sism
nar cis′sist
nar″cis sis′tic
nar″co an al′y sis
nar″co hyp′ni a
nar″co hyp no′sis
nar′co lep″sy
nar″co lep′tic
nar co′ma

nar″co ma′ni a
nar co′sis
nar′co spasm
nar cot′ic
nar′co tism
nar′co tize
na res′
na′ris
na′sal
na sa′lis
nas′cent
na″si o al ve′o lar
na′si on
na si′tis
na″so cil′i ar″y
na″so fron′tal
na″so gen′i tal
na″so la′bi al
na″so la bi a′lis
na″so lac′ri mal
na″′so max′il lar y
na″so pal′a tine
na″so phar yn gi′tis
na″so pha ryn′go scope
na″so phar′ynx
na″so-spi na′le
na″so tur′bi nal
na′sus
na′tal
na tal′i ty
na tal′o in
na′tant
nat re′mi a
na″tri u ret′ic
nat′u ar″y
nat′u ral
na′tur o path″
nau pa′thi a
nau′se a
nau′se ant
nau′se ous
Na′vane
na′vel
na vic′u lar
na vic″u lar thri′tis
na vic″u lo cu′boid
na vic″u lo cu ne′i form
ne″ar thro′sis
neb′u la
ne bu′li um
neb″u li za′tion
neb′u lize
neb′u li″zer
Ne ca′ tor
amer″i can′us
nec″ro bi o′sis
nec″ro cy to′sis
nec″ro cy″to tox′in
nec″ro gen′ic
nec″ro ma′ni a
nec″ro mi me′sis
ne croph′a gous
nec′ro phile
nec″ro phil′i a
ne croph′il ism
ne croph′i lous
nec″′ro pho′bi a
nec′rop sy
ne crose′
nec′ro sin
ne cro′sis
nec″ro sper′mi a
nec″ro zo o sper′mi a
nee′dle
ne″en ceph′a lon
ne′frens
neg′a tive
neg′a tiv ism
neg′ a tron
neg′li gence
Negri bo′dies
Neis se′ri a
nem″a thel′minth
Nem″a to′da

nem″a to sper′mi a
Nem′bu tal
ne″o ars″phen a mine′
ne″ar thro′sis
ne″o blas′tic
ne″o cer″e bel′lum
ne″o cor′tex
ne″o cys tos′to my
ne″o gen′e sis
Ne″o hy′drin
ne ol′o gism
ne″o mor′phism
ne″o my′cin
ne′on
ne″o na′tal
ne″o na tol′o gy
ne″o na to′rum
ne″o na′tus
ne″o-ol′ive
ne″o pal′li um
ne oph′il ism
ne′o pho′bi a
ne″o phren′i a
ne″o pla′si a
ne′o plasm
ne″o plas′tic
ne″o stig′mine
ne″o stri a′tum
Ne′o-sy neph′rin
neph″e lom′e ter
ne phral′gi a
ne″phrec ta′si a
ne phrec′to mize
ne phrec′to my
neph′ric
ne phrid′i um
ne phrit′i des
ne phrit′ic
ne phri′tis
neph″ro ab dom′i nal
neph″ro cal″ci no′sis
neph″ro cap sec′to my
neph″ro cap″su lot′o my
neph″ro car′di ac
neph′ro cele
neph″ro col′o pex″y
neph″ro co″lop to′sis
neph″ro cys″tan as″to mo′sis
neph″ro cys ti′tis
neph″ro gen′ic
ne phrog′e nous
neph′roid
neph′ro lith
neph″ro li thi′a sis
neph″ro lith′ic
neph″ro li thot′o my
ne phrol′y sin
ne phrol′y sis
neph ro′ma
neph′ron
neph″ro path′ic
ne phrop′a thy
neph′ro pex″y
neph″ro poi′e tin
neph″rop to′sis
neph″ro py″e li′tis
neph″ro py′e lo plas″ty
neph ror′rha phy
neph′ros
neph″ro scle ro′sis
ne phro′sis
neph′ro stome
ne phros′to my
neph rot′ic
neph′ro tome
ne phrot′o my
neph″ro tox′ic
neph″ro tox′in
neph″ro tro′ pic
neph″ro tu ber″cu lo′sis
neph″ro u″re ter ec′to my
nep″i ol′o gy

nerve
nerv′ine
ner vos′i ty
nerv′ous
nerv′ous ness
ner′vus
nes tei′a
nes″ti at′ri a
nes″ti os′to my
nes′tis
neu′ral
neu ral′gi a
neu ral′gic
neu ral′gi form
neu ram′e bim′e ter
neu″ra poph′y sis
neu″ra prax′i a
neu″ras the′ni a
neu rax′is
neu″rax i′tis
neu″rec ta′si a
neu rec′to my
neu″rec to′pi a
neu″ren ter′ic
neu rer′gic
neur″ex e re′sis
neu ri′a sis
neu ri′a try
neu″ri lem′ma
neu″ri lem mi′tis
neu″ri lem mo′ma
neu″ri lem″mo sar co′ma
neu″ri no′ma
neu rit′ic
neu ri′tis
neu″ro ab″i ot′ro phy
neu″ro a nas″to mo′sis
neu″ro a nat′o my
neu″ro ar′thri tism
neu″ro ar throp′a thy
neu″ro as″tro cy to′ma
neu″ro bio ol′o gy
neu″ro bi″o tax′is
neu′ro blast
neu″ro blas to′ma
neu″ro cal″o rim′e ter
neu″ro ca nal′
neu′ro cele
neu″ro chem′is try
neu″ro cho″ri o ret″i ni′tis
neu″ro cho″roid i′tis
neu″ro cir′cu la to″ry
neu roc′la dism
neu″ro cra′ni um
neu″ro cu ta′ne ous
neu′ro cyte″
neu″ro cy to′ma
neu″ro de al′gi a
neu″ro de″a tro′phi a
neu″ro den′drite
neu″ro der″ma ti′tis
neu″ro der″ma to my″o si′tis
neu″ro der″ma to′sis
neu″ro der″ma tro′phi a
neu″ro di as′ta sis
neu″ro dy nam′i a
neu″ro e lec″tro ther″a peu′tics
neu″ro en′do crine
neu″ro ep″i der′mal
neu″ro ep″i the li o′ma
neu″ro ep″i the′li um
neu″ro fi′bril
neu″ro fi bro′ma
neu″ro fi bro″ma to′sis
neu″ro fi″bro sar co′ma
neu″ro fi″bro si′tis
neu″ro gan gli i′tis
neu″ro gas′tric
neu″ro gen′e sis
neu″ro gen′ic
neu rog′e nous
neurog′li a

neu rog″li a cyte″
neu rog″li o′ma
neu rog″li o′sis
neu′ro gram
neu″ro his tol′o gy
neu″ro hu′mor
neu″ro hu′mor al
neu″ro hyp nol′o gy
neu″ro hy poph′y sis
neu′roid
neu″ro in duc′tion
neu″ro in′su lar
neu″ro ker′a tin
neu rol′o gist
neu rol′o gy
neu″ro lu′es
neu′ro lymph″
neu rol′y sis
neu ro′ma
neu″ro ma la′ci a
neu″ro ma to′sis
neu″ro mech′a nism
neu′ro mere
neu rom′er y
neu″ro mi me′sis
neu″ro mus′cu lar
neu″ro my′al
neu″ro my″e li′tis
neu″ro my′on
neu″ro my″o path′ic
neu″ro my″o si′tis
neu′ron
neu″ro ni′tis
neu″ro nog′ra phy
neu ro″no pha′gi a
neu′ro path
neu″ro path″o gen′e sis
neu″ro pa thol″o gy
neu rop′a thy
neu″ro phleg′mon
neu″ro pho′ni a
neu″ro phys″i ol′o gy
neu′o pil
neu′ro plasm
neu′ro plas″ty
neu″ro po′di um
neu′ro pore
neu″ro psy chi′a try
neu″ro psy chol′o gy
neu″ro psy chop′a thy
neu″ro ra″dic u′lar
neu″ro re lapse′
neu″ro ret″i ni′tis
neu ror′rha phy
neu″ror rhex′is
neu″ror rhyc′tes
neu″ro sar co′ma
neu″ro scle ro′sis
neu″ro se cre′tion
neu ro′sis
neu′ro sism
neu″ro skel′e tal
neu′ro somes
neu′ro spasm
neu″ro spon′gi um
neu″ro ste ar′ic
neu″ro sur′geon
neu″ro sur′ger y
neu″ro su′ture
neu″ro syph′i lis
neu″ro the ci′tis
neu″ro ther′a py
neu rot′ic
neu rot′i ca
neu rot′i cism
neu rot″i za′tion
neu″rot me′sis
neu″ro tol′o gy
neu′ro tome
neu rot′o my
neu″ro ton′ic
neu″ro tox′in

neu′ro trau′ma
neu″ro trip′sy
neu″ro troph′ic
neu″ro trop′ic
neu rot′ro pism
neu″ro var″i co′sis
neu″ro vas′cu lar
neu′ru la
neu′tral
neu″tra li za′tion
neu′tral lize
neut′ro clu″sion
neu′tro cyte
neu′tron
neu″tro pe′ni a
neu′tro phil
neu″tro phil′i a
ne′vose
ne″vo xan″tho en″do the″li o′ma
ne′vus
new′born′
nex′us
ni′a cin
niche
nick′el
nic″o tin am′ide
nic′o tine
nic″o tin′ic ac′id
nic′ti ta″ting
nic″ti ta′ti o
nic″ti ta′tion
ni da′tion
ni′dus
Ni fed i pine
nig′ri cans
ni gri′ti es
ni′hil ism
ni keth′a mide″
niph″a blep′si a
niph″o typh lo′sis
nip′ple
ni′sus
ni′trate
Ni′tra zine
ni′trite
ni″tri tu′ri a
ni′tro gen
ni trog′e nous
ni″tro glyc′er in
ni′trous
Nobel,
Alfred
no″car di o′sis
no″ci cep′tive
no″ci fen′sor
no″ci per cep′tion
noc″tal bu″mi nu′ri a
noc tam″bu la′tion
noc″ti pho′bi a
noc tu′ri a
noc tur′nal
noc′u ous
nod′al
node
no′dose
no dos′i ty
nod′u lar
nod′u le
nod′u lus
no″e gen′e sis
no″e mat″ a chym′e ter
no′ma
no mad′ic
no′men cla ture
nom′o graph
nom″o top′ic
non ac′cess
non″ad he′rent
non″al ler′gic
no′nan
non a′que ous
non com′pos men′tis
non″con duc′tor
non″dis junc′tion

non″e lec′tro lyte
no″ni grav′i da
no nip′a ra
non″lu et′ic
non″ma lig′nant
non med′ul la″ted
non mo′tile
non my el′li na″ted
non par′ous
non″py o gen′ic
non re″a gin′ic
non″re frac′tive
non″re straint′
non sex′u al
non″spe cif′ic
non sup′pu ra″tive
non sur′gi cal
non vi′a ble
no′o psy″che
nor ep″i neph′rine
nor′mo blast
nor″mo chro mat′ic
nor″mo chro′mi a
nor″mo chro′mic
nor′mo cyte
nor″mo cy to′sis
nor″mo gly ce′mi a
nor″mo ten′sive
nor″mo ther′mi a
nor″mo ton′ic
nor″mo to′pi a
nor″ mo vo le′mi a
nos er″es the′si a
nos″o co′mi a
Nos o co′mi al
no sog′e ny
no sol′o gy
nos″o ma′ni a
nos″o par′a sites
nos″o pho′bi a
nos′o phyte
nos″o tax′y
nos tal′gi a
nos″to ma′ni a
nos top′a thy
nos″to pho′bi a
nos′tras
nos′trate
nos′tril
nos′trum
no″tan ce pha′li a
no″tan en″ce pha′li a
no ta′tion
notch
no″ten ceph′a lo cele
no″ten ceph′a lus
no′to chord
no″to gen′e sis
no tom′e lus
No vo bi o′cin
No′vo caine
nox′ious
Ntaya vi′rus
nu′bain
nu′bile
nu cel′lus
nu′ces
nu′cha
nu′cle ar
nu′cle ase
nu′cle a″ted
nu″cle a′tion
nu′cle i
nu′cle i form″
nu″cle o al bu′min
nu″cle o chy le′ma
nu′cle o chyme
nu″cle o cy″to plas′mic
nu″cle of′u gal
nu′cle oid
nu cle′o li form
nu cle′o loid
nu cle′o lus
nu″cle o mi″cro so′ma

nu′cle on
nu″cle on′ics
nu″cle op′e tal
nu′cle o plasm
nu″cle o pro′te in
nu″cle o re tic′u lum
nu′cle o tide
nu″cle o tox′in
nu′cle us
nud′ism
nul lip′a ra
numb
numb′ness
num′mi form
num′mu lar
nun na′tion
Nu′per caine
nurs′ling
nu ta′tion
nu′tri ent
nu′tri ment
nu tri′tion
nu tri′tious
nu′tri tive
nu′tri ture
nyc tal′gi a
nyc′to lope
nyc″to lo′pi a
nyc′ter ine
nyc″to phil′i a
nyc″to pho′bi a
nyc″to pho′ni a
nyc″to typh lo′sis
Ny′dra zid
Ny′lon
nymph
nym′pha
nym phec′to my
nym phi′tis
nym′pho lep′sy
nym″pho ma′ni a
nym″pho ma′ni ac
nym phon′cus
nym phot′o my
nys tag′mic
nys tag′mi form
nys tag′mo graph
nys″tag mog′ra phy
nys tag′moid
nys tag′mus
Ny stat′in
nyx′is

O

oa′kum
o″a ri al′gi a
o a′sis
ob″dor mi′tion
ob duc′tion
o be′li on
Obermayer's re a′gent
o bese′
o be′si ty
o′bex
ob″fus ca′tion
ob jec′tive
ob′li gate
ob lique′
ob liq′uity
ob li′ qu us
ob lit′er a′tion
ob″mu tes′cence
ob nu″bi la′tion
ob ses′sion
ob ses′sive
ob″so les′cence
ob″ste tri′cian
ob stet′trics
ob″sti pa′tion
ob struc′tion

ob′stru ent
ob tund′
ob tund′ent
ob″tu ra′tion
ob′tu ra″tor
ob tuse′
ob tu′sion
oc cip′i tal
oc cip″i ta′lis
oc cip′i tal ize
oc cip″i to an te′ri or
oc cip″i to ax′i al
oc cip″i to fron′tal
oc cip″i to fron ta′lis
oc cip″i to pos te′ri or
oc cip″i to scap″u lar′is
oc′ci put
oc clu′sion
oc clu′sive
oc cult′
oc″cu pa′tion al
och le′sis
och″lo pho′bi a
o chrom′e ter
o″chro no′sis
Ochsner, Alton
oc′tan
oc″ti grav′i da
oc tip′a ra
oc″to roon′
oc′u lar
oc″u len′tum
oc′u list
oc″u lo ce phal′ic
oc″u lo cer re″bro re′nal
oc″u lo gy ra′tion
oc″u lo gy′ric
oc″u lo mo′tor
oc″u lo my co′sis
oc″u lo phar yn ge′al
oc″u lo phren″i co re cur′rent
oc″u lo zy″go mat′ic
oc′u lus
o″cy o din′ic
o″dax es′mus
Oedipus com′plex
o″don tag′ra
o″don tal′gi a
o″don tal′gic
o″don tec′to my
o don′ter ism
o″don tex e′sis
o dont″he mo′di a
o″don thy′a lus
o don′ti a
o″don ti′a sis
o″don ti′a try
o don′tic
on don′tin oid
o″don ti′tis
o don′to blast
o don″to blas to′ma
o don″to bo thri′tis
o don″to ″both′ri um
o don″to to cele
o don″to ce ram′ic
o don″to to′cha lix
o don″to chi rur′gi cal
o don to cla′sis
o don′to clast
o don″toc ne′sis
o don″to dyn′i a
o don″to gen′e sis
o″don tog′e ny
o don′to glyph
o don′to gram
o don′to graph
o″don tog′ra phy
o don″to hy″per es the′si a
o don′toid
o don′to lith
o″don tol′o gist

o″don tol′o gy
o don″to lox′i a
o″don tol′y sis
o″don to′ma
o don″to ne cro′sis
o don″to neu ral′gi a
o don″to par″al lax′is
o″don top′a thy
o don″to pho′bi a
o don′to plast
o don″to pri′sis
o don″top to′si a
o don″to ra′di o graph
o don″tor rha′gi a
o″don tos′chi sis
o don′to schism
o don′to scope
o″don tos′co py
o don″to sei′sis
o″don to′sis
o don″to ste re′sis
o don″to syn″er is′mus
o don″to the′ca
o don″to ther′a py
o″don tot′o my
o don″to trip′sis
o″don tot′ry py
o′dor
o″dor if′er ous
o″do rim′e try
o dyn″a cou′sis
o dyn″o pha′gi a
odyn″o pho′bi a
o″dy nu′ri a
oed′i pal
oes′trus
of′fal
ohm
ohm′me″ter
o id″i o my co′sis
O id′i um
oi″ko pho′bi a
oint′ment
o″le ag′i nous
o″le an do my′cin
o″le cra″nar thri′tis
o″le cra″nar throc′a ce
o″le cra″nar throp′a thy
o lec′ra noid
o lec′ra non
o le′ic ac′id
o″le o mar′ga rine
o″le om′e ter
o″le o res′in
o″le o ther′a py
o″le o tho′rax
ol fac′tion
ol″fac tom′e ter
ol fac′to ry
ol″i ge′mi a
ol″i ger ga′si a
ol″i go hy dru′ri a
ol″i go hy dram′ni os
ol″i go ceph′a lon
ol″i go cho′li a
ol″i go chro ma′si a
ol″i go chro me′mi a
ol″i go chy′li a
ol″i go cy the′mi a
ol″i go dac′ry a
ol″i go dac tyl′i a
ol″i go den″dro blas″ to′ma
ol″i go den drog′li a
ol″i go den″dro gli o′ma
ol″i go den″dro gli o″ma to′sis
ol″i go don′ti a
ol″i go dy nam′ic
ol″i go el′e ment
ol″i go ga lac′ti a
ol″i go gen′ic
ol″i go hy dram′ni os
ol″i go hy dru′ri a

ol″i go ma′ni a
ol″i go me′lus
ol″i go men″or rhe′a
ol″i go phos″pha tu′ri a
ol″i go phre′ni a
ol″i gop noe′a
ol″i go psy′chi a
ol″i gop ty′a lism
ol″i go py′rene
ol″i go′ri a
ol″i go si a′li a
ol″i go sper′mi a
ol″i go trich′i a
ol″i go zo″o sper′mi a
ol″i gu′ri a
o lis″ther o chro′ma tin
o lis″ther o zone′
ol″i vif′u gal
ol″i vip′e tal
ol″i vo pon″to cer e bel′lar
ol″o pho′ni a
o″ma ceph′a lus
o ma′gra
o″mar thral′gi a
o″mar thri′tis
o″mar throc′a ce
o ma′sum
om″bro pho′bi a
ao″men tec′to my
o men′to pex y
o″men tor′rha phy
o men′tum
o men″tum ec′to my
o mi′tis
om″ma tid′i um
Om′ni pen
om niv′o rous
o″mo cer″vi ca′lis
o″mo hy′oid
o″mo ver′te bral
om″pha lec′to my
om phal′ic
om″pha li′tis
om phal′o cele
om″pha lo cho′ri on
om″pha lo cra″ni o did′y mus
om″pha lo did′ymus
om″pha lo gen′e sis
om″pha lo mes″en ter′ic
om″pha lo mon″o did′y mus
om″pha lop′a gus
om phal′o pleure
om″pha lo prop to′sis
om′pha los
om phal′o site
om″pha lo so′tor
om″pha lo tax′is
om phal′o tome
om″pha lot′o my
om″pha lo trip″sy
o′nan ism
o′nan ist
On″cho cer′ca
on″cho cer ci′a sis
on″cho cer co′ma
on″cho der ma ti′tis
on″cho my co′sis
on′to cyte
on″co cy to′ma
on″co gen′e sis
on′co graph
on cog′ra phy
on col′o gy
on com′e ter
on co′sis
o nei″ro dyn′i a
on″nei rog′mus
o″nei rol′o gy
o″nei ron′o sus
o″nei ros′co py
o″ni o ma′ni a
on kin′o cele

on″o mat″o ma′ni a
on″o mat″o pho′bi a
on″o mat″o poi e′sis
on tog′e ny
on″y chal′gi a
on″y cha tro′phi a
on″y chaux′is
on″y chec′to my
on″y chex″al lax′is
o nych′i a
on′y chin
on″y choc′la sis
on″y cho cryp to′sis
on″y cho dys′tro phy
on″y cho gen′ic
on″y cho gry po′sis
on″y cho hel co′sis
on″y cho het″er o to′pi a
on′y choid
on″y chol′y sis
on″y cho′ma
on″y cho ma de′sis
on″y cho ma la′ci a
on″y cho my co′sis
on″y cho pac′i ty
on″y chop′a thy
on″y cho pha′gi a
on″y choph′a gist
on″y cho phy′ma
on″y chop to′sis
on″y chor rhex′is
on″y chor rhi′za
on″y cho schiz′i a
on″y cho stro′ma
on″y chot″il lo ma′ni a
on″y chot′o my
on′yx
o″nix i′tis
o″o ceph′a lus
o′o cyst
o′o cyte
o″o gen′e sis
o″o go′ni um
o″o ki ne′sis
o″o pho rec′to my
o″o pho ri′tis
o oph″o ro cys tec′to my
o oph″o ro cys to′sis
o oph″o ro hys″ter ec′to my
o oph″o ro ma la′ci a
o oph″o ro ma′ni a
o oph′o ron
o oph″o ro path′i a
o oph′o ro pex″y
o oph′o ro plas″ty
o oph″o ro sal″pin gec′to my
o oph″o ro sal″pin gi′tis
o″o pho ros′to my
o″o phor′rha phy
o′o plasm
o′o sperm
o pac″i fi ca′tion
o pac′i ty
o″pal es′cent
o paque′
o pei′do scope
op″er a bil′i ty
op′er a ble
op′er ant
op″e ra′tion
op′er a″tive
o phi′a sis
o phid″i o pho′bi a
o′phid ism
oph′i o phobe″
oph″i o′sis
oph″ry i′tis
oph′ry on
oph″ry o′sis
oph″ryph thei ri′a sis
oph′rys
oph thal″ma cro′sis

oph"thal ma'gra
oph"thal mal'gi a
oph"thal mec"chy mo'sis
oph"thal mec'to my
oph"thal men ceph'a lon
oph thal'mi a
oph thal'mi a"ter
oph thal"mi at'rics
oph thal'mic
oph"thal mi'tis
oph thal"mo blen"nor rhe'a
oph"thal moc'a ce
oph thal'mo cele
oph thal"mo cen te'sis
oph thal"mo co'pi a
oph thal"mo di"ag no'sis
oph thal"mo di"a phan' o scope
oph thal"mo di"a stim'e ter
oph thal"mo do ne'sis
oph thal"mo dy"na mom'e ter
oph thal"mo dyn'i a
oph thal"mo fun'do scope
oph"thal mog'ra phy
oph thal"mo gy'ric
oph thal"mo i"co nom'e ter
oph thal"mo leu'ko scope
oph thal'mo lith"
oph"thal mol'a gist
oph"thal mol'o gy
oph thal"mo ly'ma
oph thal"mo ma cro'sis
oph thal"mo ma la'ci a
oph thal"mo mel"a no'ma
oph thal"mo mel"a no'sis
oph"thal mom'e ter
oph thal"mo my co'sis
oph thal"mo my'ia sis
oph thal"mo my i'tis
oph thal"mo my ot'o my
oph thal"mo neu ri'tis
oph"thal mop'a thy
oph thal"mo pha com'e ter
oph thal"mo phan'tom
oph thal"mo phas"ma tos'co py
oph thal"mo pho'bi a
oph"thal moph'thi sis
oph thal"mo phy' ma
oph thal'mo plas"ty
oph thal"mo ple'gi a
oph thal"mop to'sis
oph thal'mo re ac'tion
oph thal"mor rha'gi a
oph thal"mor rhe'a
oph thal"mor rhex'is
oph thal'mos
oph thal'mo scope
oph"thal mos'co pist
oph"thal mos'co py
oph thal'mo spasm
oph thal"mo spin'ther ism
oph"thal mos'ta sis
oph thal'mo stat
oph thal"mo sta tom'e ter
oph thal"mo sta tom'e try
oph thal"mo ste re'sis
oph thal"mo syn'chy sis
oph thal"mo ther mom'e ter
oph"thal mot'o my
oph thal"mo to nom'e ter
oph thal"mo to nom'e try
oph thal'mo trope
oph thal"mo tro pom'e ter
oph thal"mo tro pom'e try
oph thal"mo vas'cu lar
oph thal"mox y'sis
oph thal"mox y'ster
oph thal'mu la
oph thal'mus
o'pi ate
o"pi o ma'ni a
o"pi o pha'gi a
o'pi o phile

o pis′the nar
o pis′thi on
o pis″tho cra′ni on
op″is thog′na thism
o pis″tho neph′ros
o pis″tho po rei′a
op″is thot′o nos
o′pi um
op″o ceph′a lus
op″o del′doc
op″o did′y mus
op″pi la′tion
op po′nens
op por tu′nist
op sig′e nes
op″si o no′sis
op″si u′ri a
op so clo′nus
op″so ma′ni a
op′so nin
op son″i za′tion
op″so no cy″to pha′gic
op″so nom′e try
op son″o ther′a py
op″tes the′si a
op′tic
op′ti cal
op ti′cian
op ti′cian ry
op″ti co chi″as mat′ic
op″ti co cil′i ar″y
op′ti cele
op″ti co pu′pil lar″y
op′tics
op tim′e ter
op′ti mum
op′to gram
op tom′e ter
op tom′e trist
op tom′e try
op″to my om′e ter
op′to type
o′ra
o′rad
o′ral
o ra′le
or bic′u lar
or bic″u la′re
or bic″u lar′is
or′bit
or′bi tal
or″bi ta′le
or″ bi to′gram
or″bi to na′sal
or″bi to nom′e ter
or″bi to nom′e try
or″bi to sphe′noid
or″bi tot′o my
or′chic
or″chi dop′a thy
or chid′o plas″ty
or″chi dot′o my
or″chi ec′to my
or″chi en ceph″a lo′ma
or″chi ep″i did″y mi′tis
or″chi o ca tab′a sis
or′chi o cele
or″chi op′a thy
or′chi o pex″y
or′chi o plas″ty
or′chis
or chi′tis
or′der ly
or′di nate
o rex′is
or′gan
or gan′ic
or′gan ism
or″gan i za′tion
or′gan i″zer
or″ga no gen′e sis
or″ga nog′e ny

or′gan oid
or″ga nol′o gy
or″ga nos′co py
or″ga no ther′a py
or″ga no troph′ic
or″ga no trop′ic
or″gan ot′ro pism
or′gasm
or gas′mo lep″sy
o″ri en ta′tion
or′i fice
or″i fi′ci um
Or″ni tho do′ra
or″ni tho′sis
O ro′ya
o″ro phar′ynx
or″rho men″in gi′tis
or′ris
or″thi auch′e nus
or″thi o chor′dus
or″thi o cor′y phus
or′thi o don′tus
or″thi o me to′pus
or″thi o pis′thi us
or″thi o pis tho cra′ni us
or″thi o pro so′pus
or″thi op′y lus
or″thi or rhi′nus
or″thi u ra nis′cus
or″tho ceph′a ly
or″tho cho re′a
or″tho chro mat′ic
or″tho cra′si a
or″tho dac′ty lous
or″tho di′a gram
or″tho di′a graph
or″tho di ag′ra phy
or″tho dol″i cho ceph′a lous
or″tho don′ti a
or″tho don′tics
or″tho dont′ist
or″tho gen′e sis
or″thog nath′ic
or′tho grade
or″tho mes″o ceph′a lous
or thom′e ter
or″tho pe′dic
or″tho pe′dist
or″tho per cus′sion
or″tho pho′ri a
or″thop ne′a
or″tho prax′is
or″tho psy chi′a try
Or thop′ter a
or″thop′tic
or thop′to scope
or″tho roent″gen og′ra phy
or′tho scope
or″tho scop′ic
or thos′co py
or tho′sis
or″tho stat′ic
or′tho tast
or″tho ter′i on
or thot′o nus
or thot′ro pism
os
o′sa zone
os′che a
os″cil la′tion
os′cil la″tor
os′cil lo graph″
os″cil lom′e ter
os″cil lom′e try
os″cil lop′si a
os cil′lo scope
os′ci tan cy
os″ci ta tion
os′cu lum
Osler, William
os mat′ic
os me′sis

os″mes the′si a
os″mo dys pho′ri a
os′mol
os″mo lar′i ty
os mol′o gy
os mom′e ter
os″mo pho′bi a
os′mo phor
os″mo re cep′tors
os″mo reg″u lar′i ty
os mo′sis
os mot′ic
os phre″si ol′o gy
os phre″si om′e ter
os phre′sis
os″phy al′gi a
os″phy o my″e li′tis
os′sa
os′se in
os′se let
os″se o al bu′mi noid
os″se o car″ti lag′i nous
os″se o fi′brous
os″se o mu′coid
os′se ous
os′si cle
os sic′ u lar
os″si cu lec′to my
os″si cu lot′o my
os sif′er ous
os sif′ic
os″si fi ca′tion
os sif′lu ence
os sif′lu ent
os′si form
os′si fy
os tal′gi a
os″tal gi′tis
os′te al
os″te al″le o′sis
os″te an″a gen′e sis
os″te a naph′y sis
os tec′to my
os tec′to py
os″te i′tis
os″tem py e′sis
os″te o an″a gen′e sis
os″te o an′eu rysm
os″te o ar threc′to my
os″te o ar thri′tis
os″te o ar throp′a thy
os″te o ar thro′sis
os″te o ar throt′o my
os′te o blast
os″te o camp′si a
os″te o car″ci no′ma
os″te o car″ti lag′i nous
os″te o chon′dral
os″te o chon dri′tis
os″te o chon″dro dys pla′si a
os″te o chon″dro dys tro′phi a
os″te o chon dro′ma
os″te o chon″dro ma to′sis
os″te o chon″dro myx o′ma
os″te o chon″dro myx″o sar co′ma
os″te o chon″dro sar co′ma
os″te o chon dro′sis
os″te o chon′drous
os″te oc′la sis
os′te o clast″
os″te o clas to′ma
os″te o cra′ni um
os″te o cys to′ma
os′te o cyte″
os″te o den′tin
os″te o der″ma to plas′tic
os″te o der′mi a
os″te o di as′ta sis
os″te o dyn′i a
os″te o dys tro′phi a
os″te o dys′tro phy

os″te o fi″bro chon dro′ma
os″te o fi″bro li po′ma
os″te o fi bro′ma
os″te o fi″bro sar co′ma
os″te o fi bro′sis
os′te o gen
os″te o gen′e sis
os″te o gen′ic
os″te og′e nous
os″te o ha lis″ter e′sis
os″te o hy″per troph′ic
os′te oid
os″te o lip″o chon dro′ma
os′te o lith
os″te ol′o gy
os″te ol′y sis
os″te o′ma
os″te o ma la′ci a
os″te om′e try
os″te o my″e li′tis
os″te o my″e log′ra phy
os″te o my″e lo scle ro′sis
os″te o myx″o chon dro′ma
os′te on
os″te o ne cro′sis
os″te o neph rop′a thy
os″te o neu ral′gi a
os″te o ny″cho dys pla′sia
os′te o path
os″te o path′i a
os″te o pe′di on
os″te o per″i os ti′tis
os″te o pe tro′sis
os′te o phage
os″te oph′o ny
os′te o phyte″
os′te o plaque″
os″te o plas′tic
os′te o plas″ty
os″te o poi″ki lo′sis
os″te o po ro′sis
os″te o ra″di o ne cro′sis
os″te or rha′gi a
os″te or′rha phy
os″te o sar co′ma
os″te o scle ro′sis
os″te o′sis
os″te o spon″gi o′ma
os″te o stix′is
os″te o su′ture
os″te o syn″o vi′tis
os″te o syn′the sis
os″te o ta′bes
os″te o throm bo′sis
os′te o tome″
os″te o to″mo cla′si a
os″te ot′o my
os′te o tribe
os″te ot′ro phy
os′ ti a
os′ti um
os″tre o tox is′mus
o tal′gi a
o″tan tri′tis
o″thel co′sis
o the″ma to′ma
ot″hem or rha′gi a
ot″hem or rhe′a
o′tic
o″ti co din′i a
o ti′tis
o″to blen″or rhe′a
o″to ca tarrh′
o″to ceph′a lus
o″to clei′sis
o″to co′ni um
o′to cyst
o″to dyn′i a
o″to gen′ic
o″to hem″i neur″as the′ni a
o″to lar″yn gol′o gist
o″to lar″yn gol′o gy

o′to lith
o tol′o gist
o tol′o gy
o″to my″as the′ni a
O″to my′ces
o″to my co′sis
o″to neur″as the′ni a
o″to pha ryn′ge al
o′to pol′y pus
o″to py″or rhe′a
o″to py o′sis
o″to rhi nol′o gy
o″tor rha′gi a
o″tor rhe′a
o″to sal′pinx
o″to scle ro′sis
o″to scle rot′ic
o′to scope
o tos′co py
o tot′o my
oua ba′in
ou′loid
ou″lor rha′gi a
ounce
out′let
out′pa″tient
o′va
o′val
o val′o cyte
o″va lo cy to′sis
o va′ri a
o″va ri al′gi a
o va′ri an
o va″ri ec′to my
o va′ri o cele″
o va″ri o cen te′sis
o va″ri o cy e′sis
o va″ri o dys neu′ri a
o va″ri o gen′ic
o var″ri o hys″ter ec′to my
o va″ri o lyt′ic
o va″ri on′cus
o va″ri or rhex′is
o va″ri o ste re′sis
o va″ri ot′o my
o va″ri o tu′bal
o va′ri um
o′va ry
o″va tes′tis
o′ver bite″
o″ver cor rec′tion
o′ver de pen′den cy
o′ver de ter″mi na′tion
o″ver ex ten′sion
o″ver max′i mal
o′ver tone″
o″vi cap′sule
o′vi duct
o vif′er ous
o″vi fi ca′tion
o′vi form
o″vi gen′e sis
o vig′e nous
o′vi germ
o vig′er ous
o vip′a rous
o″vi po si′tion
o″vi pos′i tor
o′vi sac
o′vo plasm
o″vo tes′tis
ov′u lar
ov″u la′tion
ov′ule
o′vum
ox′a late
ox al′ic
ox″al o′sis
ox″a lu′ri a
ox′i dase
ox″i da′tion
ox′ide

ox′i dize
om im′e ter
ox″y a′phi a
ox″y blep′si a
ox″y ceph′a ly
ox″y ci ne′sis
ox″y es the′si a
ox′y gen
ox′y gen ase″
ox″y ge na′tion
ox″y geu′si a
ox″y hem′a tin
ox″y hem″a to por′phy rin
ox″y he″mo glo′bin
ox″y o′pi a
ox″y op′ter
ox″y os phre′si a
ox″y pho′ni a
ox″y tet″ra cy′cline
ox″y to′ci a
ox″y to′cic
ox″y to′cin
Ox″y u′ris ver mic″u la′ris
ox za′ e pam
o ze′na
o′zone
o″zos to′mi a

P

pab′u lum
pace′mak″er
pach″y ac′ri a
pach″y bleph′a ron
pach″y bleph″a ro′sis
pach″y ceph′a ly
pach″y chi′li a
pach″y chro mat′ic
pach″y dac tyl′i a
pach″y der′ma tous
pach″y der′mi a
pach″y der mo per″i os ti′tis
pach″y glos′si a
pach″y gy′ri a
pach″y hem′a tous
pach″y hy men′ic
pach″y lep″to men″in gi′tis
pach″y lo′sis
pach″y men″in gi′tis
pach″y mem″in gop′a thy
pach″y me′ninx
pa chyn′sis
pach″y o nych′i a
pach″y o′ti a
pach″y pel″vi per″i to ni′tis
pach″y per″i os to′sis
pach″y per″i to ni′tis
pa chyp′o dous
pach″y rhi′nic
pach″y sal pin′go-o″va ri′tis
pach′y tes
pa chyt′ic
pach″y vag″i ni′tis
pac′i fi″er
pack′er
Paget′s dis ease′
pa″go plex′i a
pai dol′o gy
pain
pal′a dang″
pal′a tal
pal′ate
pa lat′ic
pa lat′i form
pal′a tine
pal″a ti′tis
pal″a to glos′sal
pal″a to glos′sus
pal′a to graph″
pal″a to max′il lar″y

pal″a to na′sal
pal″a to pha ryn′ge al
pal″a to pha ryn′ge us
pal′a to plas″ty
pal″a to ple′gi a
pal″a to pter′y goid
pal″a tor′rha phy
pal″a to sal pin′ge us
pal″a tos′chi sis
pal′a tum
pa″le en ceph′a lon
pa″le o cer″e bel′lum
pa″le o ki net′ic
pa″le on tol′o gy
pa″le o-ol′ive
pa″le o pal′li um
pa″le o pa thol′o gy
pa″le o stri a′tum
pa″le o thal′a mus
pal″i ki ne′si a
pal″i la′li a
pal″in dro′mi a
pal″in gen′e sis
pal″i op′si a
pal″i phra′si a
pal″ir rhe′a
pal la′di um
pal″lan es the′si a
pal″les the′si a
pal′li ate
pal″li a′tion
pal′li a″tive
pal′li dum
pal′lor
pal′mar
pal ma′ris
pal′ma ture
pal′mi ped
pal′mi tate
pal mit′ic
pal′mi tin
pal mod′ic
pal″mo plan′tar
pal′mus
pal′pa ble
pal′pate
pal pa′tion
pal″pa to per cus′sion
pal′pe bra
pal′pe brae
pal′pe bral
pal′pe brate
pal″pe bra′tion
pal′pi tate
pal′pi ta′tion
pal′sy
pal′u dal
pan″a ce′a
pan′a quat
pan″ar te ri′tis
pan″ar thri′tis
pan at′ro phy
pan″car di′tis
Pancoast
syn′drome
pan″co lec′to my
pan′cre as
pan″cre a tec′to my
pan″cre at′ic
pan″cre at″i co du″o de′nal
pan″cre at″i co en″ter os′to my
pan″cre at″i co gas tros′to my
pan″cre at″i co je″ju nos′to my
pan″cre at″i co li thot′o my
pan″cre at″i co splen′ic
pan′cre a tin
pan″cre a ti′tis
pan″cre a to du″o de nec′to my
pan″cre a to du″o de nos′to my
pan″cre a to en″ter os′to my
pan″cre a tog′e nous
pan″cre a to li′pase
pan″cre at′o lith
pan″cre a to li thec′to my

pan″cre a to lit thot′o my
pan″cre a tol′y sis
pan″cre a tot′o my
pan″cre op′a thy
pan″cre o zy′min
pan″cy to pe′ni a
pan de′mi a
pan dem′ic
pan dic″u la′tion
Pandy's test
pan″e lec′tro scope
pan″ en ceph a lop″ a thy
pan en′do scope
pan en dos′co py
pan″es the′si a
pan gen′e sis
pan glos′si a
pan hem″at o pe′ni a
pan″hi dro′sis
pan hy′grous
pan hy″po pi tu′i ta rism
pan″hys ter ec′to my
pan hys″ter o col pec′to my
pan hys″ter o-o″o pho rec′to my
pan hys″ter o sal″pin gec′to my
pan hys″ter o sal pin″go-o″o pho rec′to my
pan′ic
pan″im mu′ni ty
pa niv′o rous
pan″me tri′tis
pan mne′si a
Pan my′cin
pan″my e loph′thi sis
pan my″e lo tox″i co′sis
pan nic″u li′tis
pan nic′u lus
pan′nus
pan″oph thal mi′tis
pan″os te i′tis
pan″o ti′tis
pan phar′ma con
pan″phle bi′tis
pan″scle ro′sis
pan sex′ u al ism
pan si′nus i′tis
pan″ta mor′phi a
pan″tan en ce pha′li a
pan″tan en ceph′a lus
pan tan′ky lo bleph′a ron
pan″ta pho′bi a
pan″ta som′a tous
pan″ta tro′phi a
pan′to graph″
Pan to′paque
pan″to pho′bi a
Pan to′pon
pan″top to′sis
pan″to som′a tous
pan″ta tro′phi a
pan′to graph″
pan″to then′ic ac′id
pan trop′ic
pa′nus
pan″zo ot′ic
Papanicolau tech nique′
pa pav′er ine
pa pa′ya
pa pes′cent
pa pil′la
pap′il lary
pap′il late
pap″il lec′to my
pa pil″le de′ma
pap″il lif′er ous
pa pil′li form
pap″il li′tis
pap″il lo′ma
pap″il lo″ma to′sis
pa pil″lo ret″i ni′tis
pa″po va vi′rus
pap′pose

pap′pus
pap″u la′tion
pap′ule
pap″u lif′er ous
pap″u lo er″y them′a tous
pap″u lo pus′tu lar
pap″u lo squa′mous
pap″u lo ve sic′u lar
pap″y ra′ce ous
papr″a-a mi″no ben zo′ic ac′id
par″a-an″al ge′si a
par″a-an″es the′si a
par″a-ap pen″di ci′tis
par″a bi o′sis
par″a bi ot′ic
par″a blep′sis
par″a bu′li a
par ac″an tho′ma
par ac″an tho′sis
par″a ca ri′nal
par″a cen te′sis
par″a cen′tral
par″a ceph′a lus
par″a chol′er a
par″a cho′li a
par″a chor′dal
par″a chro′ma
par″a chro′ma tism
par″a chro′mo phore
par ac′me
par″a coc cid″i oi″do my co′sis
par″a co li′tis
par″a co′lon
par″a col pi′tis
par″a col′pi um
par″a con′dy lar
par′a cone
par″a con′id
par″a cu′si a
par″a cy e′sis
par″a cys′tic
par″a cys ti′tis
par″a cy′tic
par″a de ni′tis
par″a den′tal
par″a di″ag no′sis
par″a did′y mis
Par a di′one
par″a dox′i a sex″u al′is
par″a dox′ic
par″a du″o de′nal
par″a dys′en ter″y
par″a ep′i lep″sy
par″a-e ryth′ro blast
par′af fin
par″af fi no′ma
par″a gan″gli o′ma
par″a gan′gli ons
par″a gen″i tal′is
par″a geu′si a
par″a geu′sic
par″ag glu′ti na′tion
par″a glos′sa
par″a glos′si a
par″a gnath′ous
par″a gnath′us
par″a gom pho′sis
par″a go″ni mi′a sis
Par″a gon′i mus
par″a gram′ma tism
par″a graph′i a
par″a he″mo phil′i a
par″a he pat′ic
par″a hep″a ti′tis
par″a hor′mone
par″a hyp no′sis
par″a in″flu en′za
par″a ker″a to′sis
par″a la′li a
par al′de hyde
par″a lep ro′sis
par′a lep″sy

par″a le re′ma
par″a le re′sis
par″a lex′i a
par″al ge′si a
par al′gi a
par′al lax
par′al lei ism
par″al lei om′e ter
par″a lo′gi a
pa ral′y sis
par″a lyt′ic
par′a ly″zant
par′a ly″zer
par″a mag net′ic
par″a mas ti′tis
par″a mas″toid i′tis
Par″a me′ci um
par″a me′di an
par″a me′ni a
par″a met′ric
par″a met′rism
par″a me tri′tis
par″a me′tri um
par″a me trop′a thy
par″a mim′i a
par″a mi′tome
par″am ne′si a
par″a mo′lar
par″a mor′phism
par″a mu′si a
par″a my′e lo blast″
par am′y loid
par″a my oc′lo nus mul′ti plex
par″a my″o to′ni a
par″a na′sal
par″a ne phri′tis
par″a neu′ral
par″a noi′a
par″a noi′ac
par′a noid
par′a noid ism
par an′tral
par″a nu′cle us
par″a pan″cre at ic
par″a pa re′sis
par″a per tus′sis
par″a pha ryn′ge al
par″a pha′si a
par″a phe′mi a
pa ra′phi a
par″a phil′i a
par″a phi mo′sis
par″a pho′bi a
par″a pho′ni a
pa raph′o ra
par″a phra′si a
par″a phre ne′sis
par″a phre ni′tis
pa raph′y sis
par′a plasm
par″a plas′tic
par″a plec′tic
par″a ple′gi a
par′a pneu mo′ni a
pa rap′o plex″y
par″a prax′i a
par″a proc ti′tis
par″a proc′ti um
par″a pros″ta ti′tis
pa″ra pro″tein e′mi a
par″a pso ri′a sis
par″a psy chol′o gy
par″a pyk″no mor′phous
par″a rec′tal
par″a sa′cral
par″a sag′it tal
par″a sal″pin gi′tis
par″a se cre′tion
par″a sex u al′i ty
par′a site
par″a sit′ic
par″a sit′i cide

par″a sit ism
par′a sit tize
par″a si″to gen′ic
par″a si tol′o gy
par″a si″to pho′bi a
par″a si to′sis
par″a si″to trop′ic
par″a small′pox
par′a some
par″a spa′di as
par′a spasm
par″a ste″a to′sis
par″a ster′nal
par″a sym″pa thet′ic
par″a sym″pa tho lyt′ic
par″a sym″pa tho mi met′ic
par″a syn ap′sis
par″a syph′i lis
par″a sys′to le
par″a te re″si o ma′ni a
par″a ter′mi nal
par″a the li o′ma
Par″ a thi′one
par″a thor′mone
par″a thy′mi a
par″a thy′roid
par″a thy″roid ec′to my
par″a thy″ro pri′val
par″a thy″ro tro′pic
par″a ton′sil lar
par″a tri cho′sis
par″a trip′sis
par″a troph′ic
pa rat′ro phy
par″a typh li′tis
par″a ty′phoid
par″a u re′thral
par″a u′ter ine
par″a vac cin′i a
par″a vag′i nal
par″a vag″i ni′tis
par″a ver′te bral
par″a ves′i cal
par″a vi″ta min o′sis
par ax′i al
par ec′ta sis
Par′e drine
par″e gor′ic
pa ren′chy ma
pa ren chy′mal
par en′ter al
par″ep i thym′i a
par″e reth′i sis
par″er ga′si a
pa re′sis
par″es the′si a
pa reu′ni a
par fo′cal
par″hi dro′sis
pa′ri es
pa ri′e tal
pa ri″e to fron′tal
pa ri″e to mas′toid
pa ri″e to-oc cip′i tal
pa ri″e to squa mo′sal
Parinaud's syn′drome
par′i ty
par′kin son ism
Parkinson's dis ease′
par″o don ti′tis
par″o don′ti um
par″o dyn′i a
par″ol i var″y
par″o ni′ri a
par″o nych′i a
par″o nych″o my co′sis
par″o ny cho′sis
par″o oph″o ri′tis
par″o oph′o ron
par″oph thal′mi a
par″oph thal mon′cus
pa ro′pi a

pa ro′pi on
par op′si a
par op′tic
par″o ra′sis
par″o rex′i a
par os′mi a
par″os ti′tis
par″os to′tis
pa ro′tic
pa rot′id
pa rot″id ec′to my
pa rot″i do scle ro′sis
par″o ti′tis
par′ous
par″o va′ri an
par″o var″ri ot′o my
par″o va ri′tis
par″o va′ri um
par′ox ysm
par″ox ys′mal
pars′ley
par″the no gen′e sis
par′tial
par′ti cle
par tic′u late
par ti′tion
par tu′ri ency
par tu′ri ent
par tu″ri fa′cient
par tu″ri om′e ter
par″tu ri′tion
par′tus
pa ru′lis
par″um bil′i cal
par″vi cel′lu lar
par′vule
pas′sion
pas′siv ism
Pasteur, Louis
Pas″teur el′la
pas″teur i za′tion
pa tel′la
pa tel′la pex″y
pa tel′lar
pat″el lec′to my
pa′tency
path″er ga′si a
path′er gy
pa thet′ic
path′e tism
path′e tist
path″o don′ti a
path′o gen
path″o gen′e sis
path″o gen′ic
path″o ge nic′ity
pa thog″no mon′ic
path″o le′si a
path″o log′ic
pa thol′o gist
pa thol′o gy
path″o ma′ni a
pa thom′e try
path″o mi me′sis
path″o pho′bi a
path″o psy chol′o gy
pa tho′sis
pat″re lin′e al
pat′u lous
pau″lo car′di a
Pav′a trine
pave′ment ing
Pavlov, I.
pa′vor
noc turn′us
pax′i pam
pec ten
pec′tin
pec tin o′sis
pec′to ral
pec″to ra′lis
pec″to ril′o quy
pec′tus
pe″dar throc′a ce

pe dat′ro phy
ped′er as″ty
pe de′sis
ped″i al′gi a
pe″di at′rics
pe″di at′rist
ped′i at″ry
ped′i cel late
ped′i cle
pe dic′te rus
pe dic′u lar
pe dic″u la′tion
pe dic′u li cide
pe dic″u lo pho′bi a
pe dic″u lo′sis
pe dic′u lous
Pe dic′u lus
ped′i cure
pe di′tis
pe″do bar″o ma crom′e ter
pe″do ba rom′e ter
pe″do don′tics
pe″do don′tist
pe dol′o gist
pe dol′o gy
pe dom′e ter
pe dop′a thy
pe″do phil′i a
pe″do pho′bi a
pe dun′cle
peel′ing
pel′age
pel″i o′sis
pel lag′ra
pel′let
pel′li cle
pel lic′u la
pel ol′o gy
pe lop′si a
pel″o ther′a py
pel′vic
pel″vi en ceph″a lom′e try
pel vim′e ter
pel vim′e try
pel″vi o li thot′o my
pel″vi o ne″o cys tos′to my
pel″vi o ra″di og′ra phy
pel″vi ot′o my
pel″vi rec′tal
pel′vis
pel′vi scope
pel″vi sec′tion
pem′mi can
pem′phi goid
pem′phi gus
pen″al ge′si a
pen′du lous
pen′e tra″ting
pen″e tra′tion
pen″e trom′e ter
pen″i cil′li form
pen″i cil′lin
pen″i cil′lin ase
pen″i cil″li o′sis
Pen″i cil′li um
pe′nis
pen′nate
pen′ni form
pen′ny weight″
pe nol′o gist
pe nol′o gy
pe″no scro′tal
Penrose
drain
pen″ta ba′sic
pen″ta dac′tyl
pen′tane
pen″ta va′lent
pen′tose
pen″to su′ri a
Pen′to thal, so′di um
pe″o til″lo ma′ni a

pep′per mint
pep′si gogue
pep′sin
pep sin′o gen
pep′tic
pep′tide
pep′tone
pep″to ne′mi a
pep′to nize
pep″to nol′y sis
pep″to nu′ri a
per″a ceph′a lus
per″ac′id
per″a cid′i ty
per″a cute′
per″a to dyn′i a
per bo′rate
per cent′
per cen′tile
per cep′tion
per″cep tiv′i ty
per clu′sion
Per′co dan
per′co la″tor
per cus′sion
per cus′sor
per″cu ta′ne ous
per′for ans
per′fo ra″ted
per″fo ra′tion
per′fo ra″tor
per″fo ra to′ri um
per″fri ca′tion
per fu′sion
per″i ad″e ni′tis
per″i a″lien i′tis
per″i a′nal
per″i an″gi i′tis
per″i an″gi o cho li′tis
per″i a″or ti′tis
per″i ap′i cal
per″i ap pen″di ce′al
per″i ap pen″di ci′tis
per″i ap″pen dic′u lar
peri ar te′ri al
per″i ar″te ri′tis
per″i ar thri′tis
per″i ar tic′u lar
per″i a′tri al
per″i au ric′u lar
per″i ax′i al
per″i blep′sis
per″i bron′chi al
per″i bron″chi o′lar
per″i bron″chi o li′tis
per″i bron chi′tis
per″i bro′sis
per″i cap′il lar″y
per″i car′di al
per″i car″di ec′to my
per″i car″di o cen te′sis
per″i car″di ol′ y is
per″i car″di o pleu′ral
per″i car″di or′rha phy
per″i car″di os′to my
per″i car″di ot′o my
per″i car di′tis
per″i car′di um
per″i ce′cal
per″i ce ci′tis
per″i cel′lu lar
per″i ce″men ti′tis
per″i ce men″to cla′si a
per″i ce men′tum
per″i cha rei′a
per″i chol″an gi′tis
per″i chol″e cys ti′tis
per″i chon dri′tis
per″i chon′dri um
per″i chon dro′ma
per′i chord
per″i cho′roid
per″i col′ic
per″i co li′tis

per″i con′chal
per″i con chi′tis
per″i cor′ne al
per″i cor″o ni′tis
per″i cow″per i′tis
per″i cra′ni um
per″i cys′tic
per″i cys ti′tis
per″i cys′ti um
per′i cyte
per″i cy′ti al
per′i del
per″i den drit′ic
per″i den′tal
per″i den ti′tis
per′i derm
per″i di″ver tic″u li′tis
per″i du″o de ni′tis
per″i du′ral
per″i en ceph″a li′tis
per″i en ter′ic
per″i en″ter i′tis
per″i ep en′dy mal
per″i e″so phag′e al
per″i e soph″a gi′tis
per″i fis′tu lar
per″i fol lic′u lar
per″i fol lic″u li′tis
per″i gan″gli i′tis
per″i gan″gli on′ic
per″i gas′tric
per″i glan′du lar
per″i glot′tic
per″i gnath′ic
per″i he pat′ic
per″i her′ni al
per″i hi′lar
per″i hys ter′ic
per″i je″ju ni′tis
per″i kar′y on
per″i ker at′tic
per″i lab″y rin thi′tis
per″i la ryn′ge al
per″i lar″yn gi′tis
per″i lu′nar
per′i lymph
per″i lym phan′ge al
per″i lym′phan gi′tis
per″i lym phat′ic
per″i mas ti′tis
per im′e ter
per″i met′ric
per″i me tri′tis
per″i me′tri um
per″i met″ro sal″pin gi′tis
per im′i trist
per im′i try
per″i my″e li′tis
per″i my″o si′tis
per″i mys′i um
per″i ne″o col″po rec″to my″o
mec′to my
per″i ne om′e ter
per″i ne′o plas″ty
per″i ne or′rha phy
per″i ne″o scro′tal
peri″ne″o syn′the sis
per″i ne ot′o my
per″i ne″o vag′i nal
per″i ne″o va gi″no rec′tal
per″i neph′ric
per″i ne phri′tis
per″i neph′ri um
per″i ne′um
per″i neu′ral
per″i neu ri′tis
per″i neu′ri um
per″i nu′cle ar
per″i oc′u lar
per″ri o dic′i ty
per″i o don′tal
per″i o don′tics

per″i o don′tist
per″i o don ti′tis
per″i o don′ti um
per″i o don″to cla′si a
per″i o don tol′o gy
per″i o don to′sis
pe″ri od′o scope
per″i o dyn′i a
per″i om phal′ic
per″i o nych′i a
per″i o nych′i um
per″i o″o pho ri′tis
per″i o oph″or o sal″pin gi′tis
per′i o″ple
per″i op tom′e try
per″i or′al
per″i or′bit
per″i or′bi tal
per″i or″bi ti′tis
per″i os′te o phyte″
per″i os″te ot′o my
per″i os′te um
per″i os ti′tis
per″i os to′ma
per″i os to′sis
per″i o′tic
per″i o′vu lar
per″i pach″y men″in gi′tis
per″i pan″cre a ti′tis
per″i pap′il lar″y
per″i phak′us
per″i pha ryn′ge al
pe riph′er al
pe riph′er a phose″
pe riph′er y
per″i phle bi′tis
per″i pleu ri′tis
per″i por′tal
per″i proc′tal
per″i proc ti′tis
per″i pro stat′ic
per″i py″e li′tis
per″i py e′ma
per″i py″le phle bi′tis
per″i py lor′ic
per″i rec′tal
per″i re′nal
per″i rhi′nal
per″i sal″pin gi′tis
per″i sal′pinx
per″i sig″moid i′tis
per″i sin′u ous
per″i si″nus i′tis
per″i sper″ma ti′tis
per″i splen′ic
per″i sple ni′tis
per″i spon dyl′ic
per″i spon″dy li′tis
per″i stal′sis
per″i stal′tic
per″i staph′y line
per″i sta′sis
per′i stome
per″i syn o′vi al
per″i tec′to my
per″i ten din′e um
per″i ten″di ni′tis
per″i ten′on
per″i the′li um
per″i thy″roid i′tis
per rit′o my
per″i to ne′al
per″i to ne′a tome
per″i to ne″o cen te′sis
per″i to ne op′a thy
per″i to ne″o per″i car′di al
per″i to ne′o pex″y
per″i to ne′o scope
per″i to ne ot′o my
per″i to ne′um
per″i to ni′tis
per′i to nize

per″i ton′sil lar
per″ì ton″sil li′tis
per″i tra′che al
per″i tra″che i′tis
per″i trich′i al
per″i trun′cal
per″i typh′lic
per″i typh li′tis
per″i um bil′i cal
per″i un′gual
per″i u″re ter′ic
per″i u re″ter i′tis
per″i u re′thral
per″i u″re thri′tis
per″i u′ter ine
per″i u′vu lar
per″i vag′i nal
per″i vas′cu lar
per″i vas″cu li′tis
per″i ve′nous
per″i ves′i cal
per″i ve sic″u li′tis
per″i vis′cer al
per″i vis″cer i′tis
per″i vit′el line
per″i xe ni′tis
per le′
per lèche′
per′ma nent
per man′ga nate
per″me a bil′i ty
per′me a ble
per″me a′tion
per ni′cious
per″ni o′sis
per noc ta′tion
pe″ro bra′chi us
pe″ro chi′rus
pe″ro cor′mus
pe″ro dac tyl′i a
pe″ro dac′ty lus
pe″ro hep″a ti′tis
pe″ro me′li a
pe rom′e lus
pe rom′e ly
per″o ne′al
per″o ne″o cal ca′ne us
per″ o ne″o cu boi′de us
per″o ne″o tib″ia′lis
per″o ne′us
pe ro′ni a
pe″ro pla′si a
pe′ro pus
per o′ral
per os
pe ro′sis
pe″ro so′mus
pe″ro splanch′ni ca
per ox′ide
per″pen dic′u lar
per rec′tum
per sev″er a′tion
per′son al
per″son al′i ty
per″spi ra′tion
per spire′
per″tur ba′tion
per tus′al
per tus′sis
per va′ sive
per ver′sion
pes′sa ry
pes′ti cide
pes′tis
pes′tle
pe te′chi a
pe te′chi al
pe ti′o lus
pe tit′ mal′
pet″ri fac′tion
pe″tris sage′
pet″ro bas′i lar

pet″ro la′tum
pė tro′le um
pet″ro mas′toid
pet″ro-oc cip′i tal
pet″ro pha ryn′ge us
pe tro′sa
pe tro′sal
pet″ro si′tis
pet″ro sphe′noid
pet″ro squa′mous
pet′rous
Peutz-Jeghers syn′drome
Peyer's patch′es
Pfannenstiel's in ci′sion
pha cen′to cele
pha ci′tis
phac″o-an″a phy lax′is
phac′o cyst
phac″o cys tec′to my
phac″o er′i sis
phac″o hy″men i′tis
pha′coid
pha col′y sis
phac″o ma to′sis
phac″o met″a cho re′sis
phac″o met″e ce′sis
pha com′e ter
phac″o pla ne′sis
phac″o scle ro′sis
phac′o scope
phac″o sco tas′mus
phag′o cyte
phag″o cy′to blast
phag″o cy tol′y sis
phag″o cy to′sis
pha gol′y sis
phag″o ma′ni a
phag″o ther′a py
pha″ko ma to′sis
pha lan′ge al
phal″an gec′to my
pha lan′ges
phal″an gi′tis
pha lan″gi za′tion
pha lan″go pha lan′ge al
pha′lanx
phal′lic
phal′lo plas ty
phal′lus
phan″er o ma′ni a
phan″er o′sis
phan′tasm
phan tas″ma to mo′ri a
phan′ta sy
phan′tom
phar′ci dous
phar′ma cal
phar″ma ceu′tic
phar′ma cist
phar″ma co dy nam′ics
phar″ma cog′no sy
phar″ma col′o gist
phar″ ma col′o gy
phar″ma co ma′ni a
phar″ma co pe′ia
phar″ma co pho′bi a
phar″ma co psy cho′sis
phar″ma co ther′a py
phar′ma cy
phar″yn gal′gi a
phar″yn ge′al
phar″yn gec′to my
phar″yn gis′mus
phar″yn gi′tis
pha ryn′go cele
pha ryn″go dyn′i a
pha ryn″go ep″i glot′tic
pha ryn″go ep″i glot′ti cus
pha ryn″go e soph′a ge″al
pha ryn″go e soph′a gus
pha ryn″go glos′sal
pha ryn″go glos′sus

pha ryn″go ker″a to′sis
pha ryn″go la ryn′ge al
pha ryn″go lar″yn gi′tis
pha ryn′go lith
phar″yn gol′y sis
pha ryn″go max′il lar″y
pha ryn″go my co′sis
pha ryn″go na′sal
pha ryn″go pal′a tine
phar″yn gop′a thy
pha ryn′go plas′ty
pha ryn″go ple′gi a
pha ryn″go rhi ni′tis
pha ryn″gor rha′gi a
pha ryn″gor rhe′a
pha ryn″go scle ro′ma
pha ryn′go scope
pha ryn′go spasm
pha ryn″go ste′ni a
pha ryn″go ther′a py
pha ryn′go tome
phar″yn got′o my
pha ryn″go ton″sil li′tis
pha ryn″go xe ro′sis
phar′ynx
phase
phat″nor rha′gi a
phe nac′e tin
phen cy′ cli dine
Phen′ er gan
phen″go pho′bi a
phe″no bar′bi tal
phen′o cop″y
phe′nol
phe″nol phthal′ein
phen″nol sul fon phthal′ein
phe″no lu′ri a
phe′ nom e nol′ ogy
phe nom′e non
phe″no thi′a zine
phe′no type
phen tol′ a mine
phen″yl al′a nine
phen″yl ke″to nu′ri a
phen″yl py ru′vic ac′id
phe″o chro″mo blas to′ma
phe″o chro″mo cy to′ma
phi li′a ter
phil″o ne′ism
phil″o pa trid″o ma′ni a
phil′ter
phil′trum
phi mo′sis
phi mot′ic
phi′so hex
phi so my co′sis
phleb an″gi o′ma
phleb″ar te″ri ec ta′si a
phleb″ar te″ri o di al′y sis
phleb″ec ta′si a
phle bec′to my
phleb″ec to′pi a
phelb″em phrax′is
phleb″ep a ti′tis
phleb″ex ai re′sis
phle bis′mus
phle bi′tis
phleb″o car″ci no′ma
phle boc′ly sis
phleb′o gram
phleb′o graph
phle bog′ra phy
phleb′oid
phleb′o lith
phleb″o li thi′a sis
phleb″o ma nom′e ter
phleb″o phle bos′to my
phleb′o plas″ty
phleb″o ple ro′sis
phleb″or rha′gi a
phle bor′rha phy
phleb″or rhex′is
phleb″o scle ro′sis
phle bos′ta sis

phleb″o ste no′sis
phleb″o strep′sis
phleb″o throm bo′sis
phleb′o tome
Phle bot′o mus
phle bot′o my
phlegm
phleg mat′ic
phleg′mon
phlog″o gen′ic
phlyc te′na
phlyc ten′u lar
phlyc ten′ule
pho′bi a
pho′bic
pho″bo pho′bi a
pho″co me′li a
pho″na the′ni a
pho na′tion
pho′na to″ry
phon au′to gram
pho′neme
pho nen′do scope
pho net′ic
pho′ni ca
phon′ics
pho′nism
pho″no car′di o gram″
pho″no car′di o graph″
pho″no chor′da
pho′no gram
pho′no graph
pho″no ma′ni a
pho″no mas sage″
pho nom′e ter
pho″no my oc′lo nus
pho″no my og′ra phy
pho nop′a thy
pho″no pho′bi a
pho″no pho tog′ra phy
pho nop′si a
phor′o blast
phor′o cyte
pho rom′e ter
phor op′ter
phor′o scope
phos′gene
phos′pha tase
phos′phate
phos″pha te′mi a
phos″pha tu′ri a
phos″pho lip′id
phos″pho res′cence
phos″phor hi dro′sis
phos phor′ic ac′id
phos″phor ol′y sis
phos′pho rus
pho tal′gi a
pho tau″gi o pho′bi a
phote
pho′tech″y
pho″tes the′si a
pho′tic
pho′tism
pho″to ac tin′ic
pho″to bi ot′ic
pho′to chrome
pho″to col″or im′e ter
pho″to con″duc tiv′i ty
pho″to der″ma to′sis
pho″to dy nam′ic
pho″to dyn′i a
pho″to dys pho′ri a
pho″to flu″or os′co py
pho′to gene
pho″to gen′ic
pho″to ki net′ic
pho″to ky′mo graph
pho tol′y sis
pho″to ma′ni a
pho tom′e ter
pho″to mi′cro graph

pho″to mo′tor
pho ton′o sus
pho″to path″o log′ic
pho″to per cep′tive
pho″to phil′ic
pho″to pho′bi a
pho″toph thal′mi a
pho top′si a
pho″top tom′e ter
pho″to ra″di om′e ter
pho″to re cep′tive
pho″to sen′si tive
pho″to shock′
pho″to syn′the sis
pho″to tax′is
pho″to ther′a py
pho′to ti″mer
pho″to to′pi a
pho″to troph′
phre nal′gi a
phren″as the′ni a
phren″a tro′phi a
phren″em phrax′is
phre ne′sis
phren′ic
phren″i cec′to my
phren″i co ex er′e sis
phren″i cot′o my
phren″i co trip′sy
phre ni′tis
phren″o bla′bi a
phren″o car′di a
phren″o col′ic
phren″o gas′tric
phren″o glot′tic
phren″o glot tis′mus
phren″o he pat′ic
phren″o lep′si a
phre nol′o gy
phren′o path
phren″o ple′gi a
phren″o splen′ic
phric″to path′ic
phron″e mo pho′bi a
phro ne′sis
phryn″o der′ma
phthi ri′a sis
phthis″i o pho′bi a
phthi′sis
Phy″co my ce′tes
phy″co my co′sis
phyg″o ga lac′tic
phy lax′is
phy log′e ny
phy′ma
phy″ma tor rhy′sin
phy″ma to′sis
phys co′ni a
phys″i at′rics
phys″i at′rist
phys′ic
phy si′cian
phys′i cist
phys″i co chem′i cal
phys″i co gen′ic
phys″i co py rex′i a
phys′ics
phys″i no′sis
phys″i og′no my
phys″i og no′sis
phys″i o log′ic
phys″i o log″i co an″a tom′ic
phys″i ol′o gist
phys″i ol′o gy
phys″i o pa thol′o gy
phys″i o ther′a py
phy sique′
phy″so he″m a to me′tra
phy″so hy″dro me′tra
phy″so me′tra
phy″so py″o sal′pinx
phy″so stig′ma

phy″so stig′mine
phy′tase
phy′tin
phy″to be′zoar
phy″to chem′is try
phy″to gen′e sis
phy tog′e nous
phy′toid
phy″to path″o gen′ic
phy″to pa thol′o gy
phy toph′a gous
phy″to pho″to der″ma to′sis
phy″to pneu″mo no co″ni o′sis
phy to′sis
phy″to tox′ic
phy″to tox′in
pi′a ma′ter
pi an′
pi″a rach′noid
pi blok′to
pi′ca
pic′e ous
Pickwickian syn′drome
pi cor′na vi′rus
pic′ric ac′id
pic″ro tox′in
pie′bald ism
pie′dra
pig′ment
pig″men ta′tion
pig men′to phage
pig men′tum
pig′weed
pile
pi″le ous
pi″li a′tion
pil′i form
pill
pil′lar
pil′le us
pi″lo car′pine
pi″lo cys′tic
pi″lo e rec′tion
pi″lo mo′tor
pi″lo ni′dal
pi′lose
pi″lo se ba′ceous
pi lo′sis
pil′u la
pi′lus
pim″e li′tis
pim″e lo pte ryg′i um
pim″e lor rhe′a
pim″e lor thop′ne a
pim″e lu′ri a
pim′ple
pin′e al
pin″e a lec′to my
pin′e al ism
pin″e a lo′ma
pin gue′cu la
pin′na
pi′no cyte
pi″no cy to′sis
pin′ta
pin′worm″
pi″or thop ne′a
pe per′a zine
pi pet′
pip″to nych′i a
pir′i form
pir″i for′mis
Pirquet test
pis′i form
pi″si met″a car′pus
pi″si un″ci na′tus
pith′i a tism
pith″i at′ric
Pi to′cin
Pi tres′sin
pi tu′i tar″y
Pi tu′i trin

pit″y ri′a sis
pla ce′bo
pla cen′ta
plac″en ta′tion
pla cen′tin
plac″en ti′tis
plac″en tog′ra phy
plac″en to′ma
plad″a ro′ma
pla″gi o cephal′ic
pla″gi o ceph′a ly
plague
pla′ni ceps
plank′ton
pla″no cel′lu lar
pla″no con′cave
pla″no con′ic
pla″no con′vex
plan′o cyte
pla′no gram
plan″o ma′ni a
plan′ta
plan′tar
plan tar′is
plan′ti grade
pla′num
plaque
plasm
plas′ma
plas′ma blast
plas′ma cyte
plas″ma cy to′sis
plas′ma gel
plas″ma lem′ma
plas″ma pher′e sis
plas′ma some
plas mat′ic
plas″ma to sis
plas″mo cy to′ma
Plas mo′di um
plas mol′y sis
plas′mo lyze
plas′mo some
plas″mo trop′ic
plas′ter
plast′ic
plas″ti ciz′er
plas′tid
plas″to dy na′mi a
pla teau′
plate′let
pal′i num
pla″o nych′i a
plat″y ba′si a
play″y ce′li an
plat″y ce phal′ic
plat″yc ne′mi a
pat″y co′ri a
plat″y hi er′ic
plat″y mer′ic
plat″y mor′phi a
plat″y o′pi a
plat″y o′pic
plat″y pel′lic
pla tys′ma
plat″ys ten″ce pha′li a
pledg′et
ple′gia
ple′gic
ple″o cy to′sis
ple″o mor′phism
ple′o nasm
ple″o nec′tic
ple″o nex′ia
ple″on os″te o′sis
ple″o no′tus
ple op′tics
ple ro′sis
ple″si o gnath′us
ple″si o mor′phism
ple″si o′pi a
pless″es the′si a

pleth′o ra
ple thys′mo graph
pleu′ra
pleu″ra cot′o my
pleu′ral
pleu ral′gi a
pleu ram′ni on
pleu″ra poph′y sis
pleur′a tome
pleu rec′to my
pleu′ri sy
pleu rit′ic
pleu ri′tis
pleu″ro cen te′sis
pleu″ro cen′trum
pleu″ro chol″e cys ti′tis
pleu″ro cu ta′ne ous
pleu′ro dont
pleu″ro dy′ni a
pleu″ro gen′ic
pleu″ro hep a ti′tis
pleu′ro lith
pleu rol′y sis
pleu ro′ma
pleu″ro me′lus
pleu″ro per″i car′di al
pleu″ro per″i car di′tis
pleu″ro pneu mo′ni a
pleu″ro pneu″mo ni′tis
pleu″ro pros″o pos′chi sis
pleu″ro pul′mo nar″y
pleu ros′co py
pleu″ro so′ma
pleu″ro so″ma tos′chi sis
pleu″ro so′mus
pleu′ro spasm
pleu″ro thot′o nos
pleu rot′o my
pleu″ro ty′phoid
pleu″ro vis′cer al
plex′i form
Plex′i glas
plex im′e ter
plex′or
plex′us
pli′ca
pli cot′o my
plomb
plom bage′
plo ra′tion
plum ba′go
plum′bism
plu″ri glan′du lar
plu″ri grav′i da
plu″ri loc′u lar
plu rip′a ra
plu″ri par′i ty
plu″to ma′ni a
plu to′ni um
pne″o dy nam′ics
pne′o graph
pneu″mar thro′sis
pneu mat′ic
pneu″ma ti za′tion
pneu″ma to car′di a
pneu′ma to cele″
pneu″ma to dysp ne′a
pneu′ma to gram″
pneu″ma tol′o gy
pneu″ma tom′e ter
pneu″ma tor′ra chis
pneu″ma to′sis
pneu″ma tu′ri a
pneu′ma type
pneu″mo an″gi og′ra phy
pneu″mo-ar throg′ra phy
pneu″mo ba cil′lus
pneu″mo bul′bar
pneu″mo cen te′sis
pneu″mo ceph′a lus
pneu″mo chol″e cys ti′tis
pneu″mo coc′cal

pneu″mo coc ce′mi a
pneu″mo coc′cus
pneu″mo co′lon
pneu″mo co″ni o′sis
pneu″mo cra′ni um
pneu″mo cys tog′ra phy
pneu″mo der′ma
pneu″mo dy nam′ics
pneu″mo en ceph′a lo gram″
pneu″mo en″ter i′tis
pneu″mo gas′tric
pneu′mo graph
pneu mog′ra phy
pneu″mo he″mo per″i car′di um
pneu″mo he″mo tho′rax
pneu″mo hy″dro per″i car′di um
pneu″mo hy″po der′ma
pneu′mo lith
pneu″mo li thi′a sis
pneu″mo me″di as ti′num
pneu mom′e try
pneu″mo nec′to my
pneu mo′ni a
pneu mon′ic
pneu″mo ni′tis
pneu″mo no coc′cic
pneu″mo nol′y sis
pneu″mo no my co′sis
pneu″mo nop′a thy
pneu mo′no pex″y
pneu″mo nor′rha phy
pneu″mo no′sis
pneu″mo not′o my
pneu mop′a thy
pneu″mo per″i car di′tis
pneu″mo per″i car′di um
pneu″mo per″i to ne′um
pneu″mo per″i to ni′tis
pneu″mo py el′o gram″
pneu″mo py″o per″i car′di um
pneu″mo ra′chis
pneu″mo ra″di og′ra phy
pneu″mo roent″gen og′ra phy
pneu″mo scle ro′sis
pneu″mo tax′is
pneu″mo tho′rax
pneu″mo tox′in
pneu″mo ty′phus
pneu″mo ven′tri cle
pneu″mo ven tric″u log′ra phy
pneu′sis
pnig′ma
pni″go pho′bi a
pock
po dag′ra
podal′gi a
po dal′ic
pod″ar thri′tis
pod″ar throc′a ce
pod″e de′ma
pod″el co′ma
pod″en ceph′a lus
po di′a trist
po di′a try
pod″o brom″hi dro′sis
pod″o derm
pod″o dyn′i a
po dom′e ter
po doph′yl lin
pod″o phyl′lum
po go′ni on
po″i kil o ther′mi a
poi′ki lo blast″
poi′ki lo cyte″
poi″ki lo cy to′sis
poi″ki lo der′ma
poi″ki lo der″ma to my″o si′tis
poi″ki lo throm′bo cyte
poi″ki lo zo o sper′mi a
poi′son
poi′son ous
po′lar

po″lar im′e ter
po lar′i scope
po lar′i ty
po″lar i za′tion
po′lar ize
po lar′o gram
po″lar og′ra phy
Po′la roid
pole
po′li o
po′li o en ceph″a li′tis
po′li o en ceph″a lo me nin″ go my″e li′tis
po′li o en ceph″a lo my″e li′tis
po′li o en ceph″a lop′a thy
po′li o my″e len ceph″a li′tis
po′li o my″e li′tis
po′li o my″e lop′a thy
po′li o′sis
po lit′zer i za″tion
pol″la ki u′ri a
pol′len
pol″le no′sis
pol′lex
pol lu′tion
pol toph′a gy
pol″y ar″te ri′tis
pol″y ar′thric
pol″y ar thri′tis
pol″y ar tic′u lar
pol″y ba′sic
pol′y blast
pol″y bleph′a ron
pol″y cel′lu lar
pol″y cen′tric
pol″y chei′ri a
pol″y cho′li a
pol″y chro mat′ic
pol″y chro″ma to phil′i a
pol″y chro″ma to phil′ic
pol″y chro′mi a
pol″y chy′li a
pol″y clin′ic
pol″y clo′ni a
pol″y co′ri a
pol″y cy′clic
pol″y cy e′sis
pol″y cys′tic
pol″y cy the′mi a
pol″y dac′ty ly
pol″y de fi′cien cy
pol″y dip′si a
pol″y em′bry o ny
pol″y men or rhe′a
pol″y e′mi a
pol″y es the′si a
pol″y es′trus
pol″y ga lac′ti a
po lyg′a mous
polyg′a my
pol″y gas′tri a
pol″y a gen′ic
pol″y glan′du lar
pol″y gnath′us
po lyng′o nal
pol′y graph
pol″y gyr′i a
pol″y he′dral
pol″y hy′brid
pol″y hy dram′ni os
pol″y hy dru′ri a
pol″y in fec′tion
pol″y lep′tic
pol″y mas′ti a
pol″y me′li a
pol″y me′lus
pol″y me′ni a
pol′y mer
pol″y me′ri a
pol″y mer′ic
po lym′er ism
pol″y mer i za′tion

pol″y mi cro′bic
pol′y morph
pol″y mor′phic
pol″y mor″pho cel′lu lar
pol″y mor′pho cyte
pol″y mor″pho nu′cle ar
pol″y my″o si′tis
pol″y myx′in
pol″y ne′sic
pol″y neu′ral
pol″y neu ral′gi a
pol″y neu ri′tis
pol″y neu″ro my″o si′tis
pol″y neu rop′a thy
pol″y o don′ti a
pol″y o nych′i a
pol″y o′pi a
pol″y or′chid ism
pol″y or′chis
pol″y o rex′i a
pol″y o stot′ic
pol″y o′ti a
pol′yp
pol″y pa re′sis
pol″y path′i a
pol″y pep′tide
pol″y pha′gi a
pol″y pha lan′gism
pol″y pho′bi a
pol″y phy let′ic
pol″y phy′o dont
pol″y pif′er ous
pol′y plast
pol′y ploid
pol″yp ne′a
pol″y po′di a
pol′yp oid
po lyp′o rous
pol″y po′sis
pol″y pty′chi al
pol″y ra dic″u li′tis
pol″y sac′cha ride
pol″y sce′li a
po lys′ce lus
pol″y se″ro si′tis
pol″y si″nus i′tis
pol″y som′a tous
pol″y sper′mi a
pol′y sper″my
pol″y sphyg′mo graph
pol″y stich′i a
pol″y stom′a tous
pol″y sty′rene
pol″y symp″to mat′ic
pol″y the′li a
po lyt′o cous
pol″y trich′i a
pol″y trop′ic
pol″y un′gui a
pol″y u′ri a
pol″y va′lent
pom″pho ly he′mi a
pon″o pal mo′sis
pons
pon′tic
pon′tine
pon″to bul′bar
Pont′o caine
pop″li te′al
pop″li te′us
pore
po ren″ce pha′li a
po″ren ceph″a li′tis
po″ren ceph′a lus
po″ri o ma′ni a
po′ri on
por nog′ra phy
por″o ceph″a li′a sis
po ro′ma
po ro′sis
po ros′i ty
po′rous

por″pho bi lin′o gen
por phy′ri a
por′phy rin
por″phy rin′o gen
por″phy ri nu′ri a
por′ta
por ta ca′val
por′tal
por′ti o
po′rus
po″si o ma′ni a
po si′tion
pos′i tive
pos′i tron
po sol′o gy
post a′nal
post″an es thet′ic
post″ap o plec′tic
post au′di to″ry
post ax′i al
post bra′chi al
post cap′il lar″y
post car′di nal
post ca′va
post cen′tral
post ci′bal
post″cla vic′u lar
post co′i tal
post″con nu′bi al
post″con vul′sive
post cor′di al
post″di crot′ic
post″di ges′tive
post″diph the rit′ic
post″em bry on′ic
post″en ceph″a lit′ic
post″ep i lep′tic
pos te′ri ad
pos te′ri or
pos te′ri or ly
pos″ter o an te′ri or
pos″ter o ex ter′nal
pos″ter o in ter′nal
pos″ter o lat′er al
pos″ter o me′di al
pos″ter o me′di an
pos″ter o su pe′ri or
post″e rup′tive
post″e so phag′e al
post fe′brile
post″gan gli on′ic
post″gas trec′to my
post gle′noid
post″hem i pleg′ic
post″hem or rhag′ic
pos thet′o my
pos thi′tis
pos′tho lith
post′hu mous
post″hyp not′ic
post ic ter′ic
post″in flu en′zal
post″ mor′tem
post na′ris
post na′sal
post na′tal
post″ne crot′ic
post″neu rit′ic
post nod′u lar
post oc′u lar
post op′er a″tive
post o′ral
post pal′a tine
post″pa lu′dal
post″par a lyt′ic
post-par′tum
post″ pha ryn′ge al
post″phle bi′tic
post pran′di al
post″pu bes′cent
post″ pyc not′ic
post″py ram′i dal

post ro′ta to″ry
post″ scar la ti′nal
post″ste not′ic
post″ syph i lit′ic
post″ trau mat′ic
post ty′phoid
pos′tu late
pos′tur al
pos′ture
post vac′ci nal
po′ta ble
pot″a mo pho′bi a
pot′ash″
pot as se′mi a
po tas′si um
po′ten cy
po ten′tial
po ten″ti a′tion
po′tion
po″to ma′ni a
pouch
poul′tice
pound
pow′der
pox
prag″mat ag no′si a
prag″ mat am ne′si a
pran′di al
pra tique′
prax in′o scope
prax″i ol′o gy
pre ag′o nal
pre am′pul lar y
pre a′nal
pre″an es thet′ic
pre″an ti sep′tic
pre″a or′tic
pre″a sep′tic
pre″a tax′ic
pre″au ric′u lar
pre ax′i al
pre can′cer ous
pre cap′il lar″y
pre car′di ac
pre car′di al
pre car′ti lage
pre ca′va
pre cen′tral
pre chor′dal
pre cip′i tant
pre cip′i tate
pre cip″i ta′tion
pre cip′i ta″tor
pre cip′i tin
pre clin′i cal
pre co′cious
pre coc′i ty
pre cog ni′tion
pre cons′ cious
pre″con vul′sant
pre″con vul′sive
pre cor′di al
pre cor′di um
pre cos′tal
pre cu′ne us
pre den′tin
pre″di crot′ic
pre″di gest′ed
pre″dis po′sing
pre″dis po si′tion
pred nis′o lone
pred′ni sone
pre″dor mi′tion
pre″ec lamp′si a
pre ep″i glot′tic
pre″e rup′tive
pre fron′tal
pre″gan gli on′ic
pre glob′u lin
preg′nan cy
preg na′no lone
preg′nant

pre hal′lux
pre″hem i pleg′ic
pre hen′sile
pre hen′sion
pre″in farc′tion al
pre″lo co mo′tion
pre′lum
pre″ma lig′nant
pre″ma ni′a cal
Pre′ma rin
pre″ma ture′
pre″max il′la
pre″med i ca′tion
pre men′stru al
pre mo′lar
pre″mo ni′tion
pre mon′i to″ry
pre″mu ni′tion
pre my′e lo blast″
pre my′e lo cyte″
pre″nar co′sis
pre na′tal
pre″ne o plas′tic
pre nid′a to″ry
pre″oc cip′i tal
prep″a ra′tion
pre″pa tel′lar
pre pol′lex
pre pon′der ance
pre po′ten cy
pre po′tent
pre″psy chot′ic
pre pu′ber al
pre″pu bes′cent
pre′puce
pre″pu cot′o my
pre pu′tial
pre″py lor′ic
pre″ra chit′ic
pre rec′tal
pre re′nal
pre″re pro duc′tive
pre ret′i nal
pre sa′cral
pres″by at′rics
pres″by card′ia
pres″by a cu′sis
pres″by der′ma
pres by e soph′a gus
pres″by o phre′ni a
pres″by o′pi a
pres″by o sphac′e lus
pres byt′
pre″schiz o phren′ic
pre″scle ro′sis
pre scribe′
pre scrip′tion
pre″se nil′i ty
pres″en ta′tion
pre sphe′noid
pre sphyg′mic
pres′sor
pres″so re cep′tor
pres″so sen′si tive
pres′sure
pre sta′sis
pre su bic′u lum
pre sup′pu ra″tive
pre sys′to le
pre″sys tol′ic
pre″thy rog′e nous
pre″thy roid′e an
pre″trans fer′ence
pre u″re thri′tis
prev′a lence
pre″ven to′ri um
pre″ven tric″u lo′sis
pre″ver tig′i nous
pre ves′i cal
pre′vi a
pre vil′lous
pre zo′nu lar
pre″zy ga poph′y sis

pri'a pism
pri'ma ry
Pri'mate
pri"mi grav'i da
pri mip'a ra
pri"mi par'i ty
pri mi'ti ae
pri" mi ti va' tion
prim'i tive
pri mor'di al
pri mor'di um
prin'ceps
prin'ci ple
prism
pris mat'ic
pris'moid
pris"mop tom'e ter
pris'mo sphere
pro"ag glu'ti noid
pro'al
pro am'ni on
pro at'las
pro'bang
probe
pro'bit
pro bos'cis
pro'caine
pro cal'lus
pro ce'lous
pro"ce phal'ic
pro cer'coid
pro ce'rus
pro ces"so ma'ni a
pro ces'sus
pro chei'li a
pro chei'lon
pro chon'dral
pro chor'dal
pro"cho re'sis
proc"i den'ti a
pro"con'dy lism
pro"con ver'tin
pro"cre a'tion
proc ta'gra
proc tal'gi a
proc"ta tre'si a
proc"tec ta'si a
proc"tec'to my
proc ten'cli sis
proc"teu ryn'ter
proc ti'tis
proc'to cele
proc toc'ly sis
proc to co li'tis
proc"to co"lon os'co py
proc"to col'po plas"ty
proc"to cys'to plas"ty
proc"to de'um
proc"to dyn'i a
proc tol'o gist
proc tol'o gy
proc"to pa ral'y sis
proc'to pex"y
proc"to pho'bi a
proc'to plas"ty
proc"to ple'gi a
proc"top to'si a
proc tor'rha phy
proc"tor rhe'a
proc'to scope
proc tos'co py
proc"to sig"moid ec'to my
proc"to sig"moid i'tis
proc"to sig"moid os'co py
proc'to spasm
proc tos'ta sis
proc"to ste no'sis
proc tos'to my
proc tot'o my
pro cum'bent
pro cur'sive
pro"cur va'tion

pro cu′tin
prod′ro mal
pro′drome
pro duc′tive
pro″en ceph′a lus
pro en′zyme
pro″e ryth′ro blast
pro es′tro gen
pro es′trus
Proetz′s treat′ment
pro fes′sion al
pro″fi brin″o ly′sin
pro flu′vi um
pro fun′da
pro fun′dus
pro gen′er ate
pro gen′e sis
pro gen′i tor
prog′e ny
pro ge′ri a
pro ges′ter one
Pro ges′tin
pro glot′tid
pro gnath′ic
prog′na thism
prog nose′
prog no′sis
prog nos′ti cate
prog″nos ti′cian
pro″gon o′ma
pro grav′id
pro gres′sion
pro gres′sive
pro″i o sys′to le
pro″i o′ti a
pro jec′tion
pro la′bi um
pro lac′tin
pro′lan A or B
pro lapse′
pro lep′sis
pro leu′ko cyte
pro lif′er ate
pro lif″er a′tion
pro lif′ic
pro lig′er ous
pro lym′pho cyte
pro meg″a kar′y o cyte″
Pro′min
prom′i nence
pro mon′o cyte
prom′on to ry
pro my′e lo cyte
pro′nate
pro na′tion
pro na′tor
prone
pro neph′ros
prong
pro′no grade
pro nor′mo blast
pro nu′cle us
pro o′tic
pro″pae deu′tics
prop′a gate
pro pal′i nal
pro′pane
pro″per i to ne′al
pro′phase
pro″phy lac′tic
pro″phy lax″is
pro plas′ma cyte
pro pri′e tar″y
pro″pri o cep′tion
pro″pri o cep′tor
pro′pri us
prop tom′e ter
prop to′sis
pro pul′sion
pro′pyl
pro′pyl ene
pro″pyl thi″o u′ra cil

pro re na′ta
pro se′cre tin
pro sect′
pro sec′tor
pros″en ceph′a lon
pros″o dem′ic
pros″op ag no′si a
pros″o pal′gi a
pro sop′ic
pros″o po″a nos′chi sis
pros″o po″di ple′gi a
pros″o po dyn′i a
pros″o pop′a gus
pros″o po ple′gi a
pros″o pos′chi sis
pros′o po spasm
pros″o po thor″a cop′a gus
pros″o po to′ci a
pros′o pus va′rus
pros′tate
pros″ta tec′to my
pros′ta tism
pros″ta ti′tis
pros″ta to cys ti′tis
pros tat′o gram
pros″ta tog′ra phy
pros tat′o lith
pros″ta to li thot′o my
pros″ta tor rhe′a
pros″ta tot′o my
pros″ta to ve sic″u lec′to my
pros″ta to ve sic″u li′tis
pro ster′num
pros′the sis
pros thet′ics
pros′the tist
pros′thi on
pros″tho don′ti a
pros″tho don′tist
pro stig′mine
pros″ti tu′tion
pros′trate
pros′trat ed
pros tra′tion
pro′ta mine
pro″tan o′pi a
pro tar′gin
pro′te an
pro′te ase
pro tec′tive
pro te′ic
pro te′i form
pro′ te in
pro′te in ase
pro″te in e′mi a
pro″te in o′sis
pro″te in u′ri a
pro″te ol′ y sis
pro′te ose
Pro′teus
pro throm′bin
pro throm″bi ne′mi a
pro throm″bi no pe′ni a
pro throm″bo ki′nase
pro thy′mi a
pro″tis tol′o gist
pro′to blast
pro′to col
pro″to di″as tol′ic
pro″to gas′ter
pro′to gen
pro″to leu′ko cyte
pro tol′y sis
pro″to met′ro cyte
pro′ton
pro″to path′ic
pro″to pep′si a
pro′to plasm
pro″to plas′mic
pro′to plast
pro″to por phy′ri a
pro″to por phy′rin

pro″to spasm
pro″to troph′ic
pro″to tro′py
Pro″to zo′a
pro″to zo′an
pro″to zo′on
pro″to zo′o phage
pro trude′
pro tru′sion
pro tu′ber ance
pro vi′ta min
pro voc′a tive
prox′i mal
prox′i mate
prox″i mo a tax′i a
prox″i mo buc′cal
prox″i mo la′bi al
prox″i mo lin′gual
pru′i nate
pru ri′go
pru ri′tus
prus′sic ac′id
psam′mism
psam mo′ma
psam″mo sar co′ma
psam′ mous
psel′lism
pseu dac″ro meg′a ly
pseu″da cu′sis
pseu″da graph′i a
pseu″dal bu″mi nu′ri a
pseu″dam ne′si a
pseu″dan ky lo′sis
pseu″dar thro′sis
pseu″den ceph′a lus
pseu″des the′si a
pseu″do a ceph′a lus
pseu″do ag glu″ti na′tion
pseu″ do ag gres′ sion
pseu″do al bu″mi nu′ri a
pseu″do alve′o lar
pseu″do an″a phy lac′tic
pseu″do a ne′mi a
pseu″do an gi′na
pseu″do an″gi o′ma
pseu″do an″o rex′i a
pseu″do a or′tic
pseu″do ap′o plex″y
pseu″do ap pen″di ci′tis
pseu″do ath″er o′ma
pseu″do a tro″pho der′ma col′li
pseu″do blep′si a
pseu″do bulb′ar
pseu″do car′ti lage
pseu′do cast
pseu′do cele
pseu″do chan′cre
pseu″do cho les″te a to′ma
pseu″do cho″li nes′ter ase
pseu″do cho re′a
pseu″do chrom″es the′si a
pseu″do chrom″hi dro′sis
pseu″do chro′mi a
pseu″do cir rho′sis
pseu″do claud i ca′tion
pseu″do col′loid
pseu″do col″o bo′ma
pseu″do cri′sis
pseu′do croup″
pseu″do cryp tor′chid ism
pseu″do cy e′sis
pseu″do cyl′in droid
pseu′do cyst″
pseu″do de men′ti a
pseu″do di″a bet′ic
pseu″do di″ver tic′u lum
pseu″do e de′ma
pseu″do en″do me tri′tis
pseu″do ep′i lep″sy
pseu″do ep″i the li om′a tous
pseu″do fluc″tu a′tion
pseu″do gan′gli on

pseu″do geu″ses the′si a
pseu″do geu′si a
pseu″do gli o′ma
pseu″do glob′u lin
pseu″do gon″or rhe′a
pseu″do hal lu″ci na′tion
pseu″do hem″i car′di us
pseu″do he″mo phil′i a
pseu″do her maph′ro dite
pseu″do her maph′ro dit ism
pseu″do hy″dro ne phro′sis
pseu″do hy″dro pho′bi a
pseu″do hy″per troph′ic
pseu″do hy per′tro phy
pseu″do hy po par″a thy′roid ism
pseu″do il′e us
pseu″do in′ti ma
pseu″do i″so chro mat′ic
pseu″do jaun′dice
pseu″do li thi′a sis
pseu″do lo′gi a fan tas′ti ca
pseu″do lys′sa
pseu″do ma lar′i a
pseu″do mam′ma
pseu′do ma′ni a
pseu″do mel″a no′sis
pseu″do mem′brane
pseu″do men″in gi′tis
pseu″do me′ninx
pseu″do men″stru a′tion
pseu″do mi″ cro ceph′a lus
Pseu″do mo′nas ae″rug i no′sa
pseu″do mu′cin
pseu″do my o to′ni a
pseu″do myx o′ma
pseu″do nar′co tism
pseu″do ne′o plasm
pseu″do neu ri′tis
pseu″do neu ro′ma
pseu″do nu cle′o lus
pseu″do nys tag′mus
pseu″do oph thal″ mo ple′gi a
pseu″do os″te o ma la′ci a
pseu″do pa ral′y sis
pseu″do par″a ple′gi a
pseu″do par′a site
pseu″do pa re′sis
pseu″do pho″tes the′si a
pseu″do ple′gi a
pseu″do po′di um
pseu″do pol y po′sis
pseu″do pseu″do hy″po par a thy′roid ism
pseu dop′si a
pseu″do pte ryg′i um
pseu″dop to′sis
pseu′do pus″
pseu″do re ac′tion
pseu″do rhon′cus
pseu″do scar″la ti′na
pseu″do scle ro′sis
pseu″do small′pox
pseu dos′mi a
pseu″do sto′ma
pseu″do strat′i fied
pseu″do ta′bes
pseu″do tet′a nus
pseu″do tho′rax
pseu″do trun′cus ar ter″i o′sus
pseu″do tu ber″cu lo′sis
pseu″do tu′mor
pseu″do ty′phoid
pseu″do vac′u oles
pseu″do ven′tri cle
pseu″do vom′it ing
pseu″do xan tho′ma e las′ti cum
psil o cy′bin
psi lo′sis
psit″ta co′sis
pso′as

psod′y mus
pso i′tis
pso″mo pha′gi a
pso″ri as′i form
pso ri′a sis
pso″ri at′ic
pso″roph thal′mi a
psy′cha go″gy
psy chal′gi a
psy cha′li a
psy″chas the′ni a
psy″cha tax′i a
psych au′di to″ry
psy′che
psy″che de′lic
psy′che ism
psy″chen to′ni a
psy chi′a ter
psy″chi at′ric
psy chi′a trist
psy chi′a try
psy′chic
psy′chi no′sis
psy chlamp′si a
psy″cho an″al ge′si a
psy″cho a nal′y sis
psy″cho an′a lyst
psy″cho bi ol′o gy
psy″cho co′ma
psy″cho cor′ti cal
psy″cho di″ag nos′tic
psy″cho dom′e ter
psy″cho dra′ma
psy″cho dy nam′ics
psy″cho gal″va nom′e ter
psy″cho gen′e sis
psy″cho gen′ic
psy chog′e ny
psy″cho geu′sic
psy chog′no sis
psy′cho gram
psy″cho ki ne′si a
psy″cho ki ne′sis
psy″cho lag′ny
psy′cho lep″sy
psy″cho log′ic
psy″cho log′i cal
psy chol′o gist
psy chol′o gy
psy cho′ma
psy″cho math″e mat′ics
psy″cho met′rics
psy chom′e try
psy″cho mo′tor
psy″cho neu″ro log′ic
psy″cho neu ro′sis
psy″cho neu rot′ic
psy″cho nom′ics
psy chon′o my
psy″cho no se′ma
psy″cho pa re′sis
psy′cho path
psy″cho pa thol′o gist
psy″cho pa thol′o gy
psy chop′a thy
psy″cho pho″nas the′ni a
psy″cho phys′ics
psy″cho phys″i olog′ic
psy″cho phys″i ol′o gy
psy″cho ple′gi a
psy″cho ryth′mi a
psy″chor rha′gi a
psy″cho sen′so ry
psy″cho sex′u al
psy cho′sis
psy″cho so mat′ic
psy″cho sur′ger y
psy″cho tech′nics
psy″cho ther′a py
psy chot′ic
psy″ cho tro′ pic
psy chral′gi a

psy″chro es the′si a
psy″chro lu′si a
psy chrom′e ter
psy″chro pho′bi a
psy′chro phore
psy″chro ther′a py
ptar′mic
ptar′mus
ptel′e or rhine
pter′i on
pter″o yl glu tam′ic ac′id
pte ryg′i um
pter′y goid
pter″y go man dib′u lar
pter″y go max′il lar″y
pter″y go pal′a tine
pter″y go pha ryn′ge us
pter″y go spi′nous
pti lo′sis
pto′sis
pty al′a gogue
pty″a lec′ta sis
pty′a lin
pty′a lism
pty′a lo cele
pty″a lo gen′ic
pty al′o gogue
pty″a log′ra phy
pty′a lo lith
pty″a lo li thi′a sis
pty″a lor rhe′a
pty′a lose
pty″a lo′sis
pty′sis
ptys′ma
ptys′ma gogue
pu bar′che
pu′ber
pu′ber ty
pu′bes
pu bes′cence
pu bes′cent
pu″be trot′o my
pu′bic
pu″bi ot′o my
pu′bis
pu″bo cap′su lar
pu″bo cav″er no′sus
pu″bo coc cyg′e al
pu″bo coc cyg′e us
pu″bo fem′o ral
pu″bo per″i to ne al′is
pu″bo pro stat′ic
pu″bo rec tal′is
pu″bo ves′i cal
pu″bo ves i cal′is
pu″den dag′ra
pu′den da
pu den′dal
pu den′dum
pu′er i cul″ture
pu′er il ism
pu″er i′ti a
pu er′per a
pu er′per al
pu er′per al ism
pu er′per ant
pu″er pe′ri um
Pu′lex ir′ri tans
pu′li cide
pul′lu late
pul′mo nar″y
pul mon′ic
pul′mo″tor
pulp
pul pal′gi a
pul pa′tion
pul pec′to my
pulp″i fac′tion
pulp′i form
pulp′i fy
pulp i′tis

pulp ot′o my
pulp′y
pul′sate
pul′sa tile
pul sa′tion
pul sa′tor
pulse
pul sim′e ter
pul′sion
pul′sus
pul ta′ceous
pul′ver ize
pul vi′nar
pul′vule
pum′ice
punc′tate
punc tic′u lum
punc′ti form
punc′to graph
punc′tum
punc′ta do″lo ro′sa
pun′gent
pu′pa
pu′pal
pu′pil
pu pil′la
pu′pil la ry
pu″pil lom′e ter
pu″pil lo sta tom′e ter
pur ga′tion
pur′ga tive
purge
pu′ri fied
pu′ri form
pu′rine
pu″ro hep″a ti′tis
pu″ro mu′cous
pu″ro thi′o nin
pur′pu ra
pu′ru lence
pu′ru lent
pu′ru loid
pus
pus′tu lant
pus′tu lar
pus′tule
pus′tu li form″
pus″tu lo der′ma
pus″tu lo′sis
pu ta′men
pu″tre fac′tion
pu″tre fac′tive
pu′tre fy
pu tres′cent
pu′trid
py″ar thro′sis
pyc nom′e ter
pyc″no mor′phous
pyc″no phra′si a
pyc no′sis
pyc not′ic
py ec′chy sis
py″e lec ta′si a
py″e lit′tis
py″e lo cys ti′tis
py′e lo gram″
py″e log′ra phy
py″e lo li thot′my
py′e lo ne phri′tis
py′e lo plas″ty
py″e lo pli ca′tion
py″e los′co py
py″e los′to my
py″e lot′o my
py″e lo ve′nous
py em′e sis
py e′mi a
py″en ceph′a lus
py gal′gi a
pyg ma′li on ism
pyg′my
py″go a mor′phus

py″go did′y mus
py gom′e lus
py gop′a gus
py″go par″a si′tus
py″go ter″a toi′des
py′ic
pyk′nic
pyk′no cy to″sis
pyk′no lep″sy
py″lem phrax′is
py″le phle bec′ta sis
py″le phle bi′tis
py″le throm″bo phle bi′tis
py″le throm bo′sis
py″lo ral′gi a
py″lo rec′to my
py lor′ic
py lor″i ste no′sis
py″lor i′tis
py lor″o col′ic
py lor″o di′lator
py lor″o di o′sis
py lor″o gas trec′to my
py lor″o my ot′o my
py lor′o plas″ty
py lor″op to′sis
py lor″o sche′sis
py″lor os′co py
py lor′o spasm″
py lor″o ste no′sis
py″lor os′to my
py″lor ot′o my
py lo′rus
py″o ceph′a lus
py″o che′zi a
py″o coc′cus
py″o co′po cele
py″o col′pos
py″o cy an′ic
py′o cyst″
py″o der′ma
py″o der″ma ti′tis
py″o der″ma to′sis
py og′e nes
py″o gen′e sis
py″o gen′ic
py″o he″mo tho′rax
py′oid
py″o lab″y rin thi′tis
py″o me′tra
py″o my″o si′tis
py″o ne phri′tis
py″o neph″ro li thi′a sis
py″o ne phro′sis
py″o-o va′ri um
py o pa′gus
py″o per″i car di′tis
py″o per″i car′di um
py″o per″i to ne′um
py″o per″i to ni′tis
py″o pha′gi a
py″oph thal′mi a
py″o phy lac′tic
py″o phy″so me′tra
py″o pneu″mo per″i car di′tis
py″o pneu″mo per″i car′di um
py″o pneu″mo per″i to ne′um
py″o pneu″mo per″i to ni′tis
py″o pneu″mo tho′rax
py″o poi e′sis
py op′ty sis
py″or rhe′a
py″o sal″pin gi′tis
py″o sal pin″go-o″o pho ri′tis
py″o sal′pinx
py o′sis
py″o sper′mi a
py″o stat′ic
py″o ther′a py
py″o tho′rax
py″o u′ra chus
py″o u re′ter

pyr′a mid
py ram″i da′lis
pyr″a mid ot′o my
py re′thrum
py ret′ic
py ret′o gen
pyr″e to ge ne′si a
pyr″e to gen′ic
pyr″e tog′ra phy
pry″e tol′o gist
pyr″e tol′o gy
pyr″e tol′y sis
pyr″e to ther′a py
py rex″e o pho′bi a
py rex′i a
pyr he″li om′e ter
Pyr″i benz′a mine
Py rid′i um
py″ro gal′lol
py′ro gen
py″ro gen′ic
py″ro glob″u li ne′mi a
py″ro glos′si a
py″ro lag′ni a
py″ro lig′ne ous
py rol′y sis
py″ro ma′ni a
py rom′e ter
py″ro pho′bi a
py′ro punc″ture
py′ro scope
py ro′sis
py″ro tox′in
py ru′vic ac′id
py u′ ri a

Q

quack′er y
quad ran′gu lar
quad′rant
quad″ran ta no′pi a
quad′rate
quad ra′tus
quad′ri ceps
quad″ri cus′pid
quad″ri gem′i na
quad″ri gem′i nal
quad rip′a ra
quad″ri ple′gi a
quad″ri tu ber′cu lar
quad″ri va′lent
quad roon′
quad′ru plet
qua lim′e ter
qual′i ta″tive
quan tim′e ter
quan′ti ta″tive
quan′tum
quar′an tine
quar′tan
quar tip′a ra
quartz
Queckenstedt′s test
Quervain′s dis ease′
Qui′ bron
quin′a crine
Quincke′s dis ease′
quin′i dine
qui′nine
quin′o line
qui none′
quin′sy
quin′tan
quin tip′a ra
quin′tu plet
quit′tor
quo tid′i an
quo′tient

R

ra′bi ate
rab′id
rab′ies
ra ce′mic
rac′e mose
ra″chi an″al ge′si a
ra″chi an″es the′si a
ra″chi as′mus
ra′chi cele
ra″chi cen te′sis
ra chil′y sis
ra″chi o camp′sis
ra″chi o dyn′i a
ra″chi om′e ter
ra″chi op′a thy
ra″chi o ple′gi a
ra″chi o sco″li o′sis
ra′chi o tome″
ra″chi ot′o my
ra chip′a gus
ra″chi re sis′tance
ra′chis
ra chis′chi sis
ra″chi ter′a ta
ra chit′ic
ra chi′tis
ra′chi tism
rach″i to gen′ic
ra clage′
ra dec′to my
ra′di al
ra″di a′lis
ra′di an
ra′di ant
ra″di a′tion
rad′i cal
ra dic′u lar
ra dic″u lec′to my
ra dic″u li′tis
ra dic″u lo my″e lop′a thy
ra dic″u lo neu ri′tis
ra dic″u lo neu rop′a thy
ra dic″u lop′a thy
ra″di o ac tin′i um
ra″di o ac′tive
ra″di o ac tiv′i ty
ra″di o au′to graph
ra″di obe
ra″di o bi ol′o gy
ra″di o car′pe us
ra′di o cir″cu log′ra phy
ra″di o co′balt
ra″di o cur a bil′i ty
ra″di o cys ti′tis
ra′di ode
ra′di o der″ma ti′tis
ra′di o di″ag no′sis
ra′di o don′ti a
ra′di o don′tist
ra′di o graph″
ra″di og′ra pher
ra″di og′ra phy
ra″di o hu′mer al
ra″di o i′o dine
ra″di o i′so tope
ra″di o ky mog′ra phy
ra″di ol′o gist
ra″di ol′o gy
ra″di o lu′cent
ra″di o lu″mi nes′cence
ra″di o man om′e try
ra″di o mi crom′e ter
ra′di o mi met′ic
ra′di on
ra″di o ne cro′sis
ra″di o neu ri′tis
ra″di o paque′
ra″di o par′ent
ra″di o pel vim′e try
ra″di o pho to scan′ning

ra″di o prax′is
ra″di o re sist′ance
ra″di o si a log′ra py
ra″di os′co py
ra″di o sen″si tiv′i ty
ra″di o ther″a peu′tic
ra′di o ther′a py
ra″di o ther′my
ra″di o tox e′mi a
ra″di o trans par′ent
ra″di o ul′nar
ra′di um
ra′di us
ra′dix
ra′don
ra′fle
rag′weed″
rale
ra′mi
ram″i fi ca′tion
ram′i fy
ra′mose
ram′u lus
ran′cid
ran′u la
rape
ra pha′ni a
ra′phe
rap′tus
ra″e fac′tion
rar′e fy
rash
ra′tio
ra′tion al
ra″tion al i za′tion
Rau wol′fi a
Raynaud′s dis ease′
re ac′tion
re ac′ti vate
re a′gent
re′a gin
re al′gar
re″am pu ta′tion
re″at tach′ment
re bound′
re cal″ci fi ca′tion
re″ca pit′u la′tion
rec″ep tac′u lum
re cep′tive
re cep′tor
re cess′
re ces′sion
re ces′sive
re cid′i va′tion
re cid′i vism
rec″i div′i ty
Recklinghausen, Friedrich D., von
rec″li na′tion
re″com po si′tion
re″com pres′sion
re″con stit′u ent
re″con struc′tion
re co′ver y
rec′re ment
re″cru des′cence
re cruit′ment
rec′tal
rec tal′gi a
rec″ti fi ca′tion
rec″to ab dom′i nal
rec′to cele
rec toc′ly sis
rec″to coc cyg′e al
rec″to coc cyg′e us
rec″to co li′tis
rec″to co lon′ic
rec″to cys tot′o my
rec″to fis′tu la
rec″to gen′i tal
rec″to la′bi al
rec′to pex″y

rec″to rec tos′to my
rec″to ro man′o scope
rec″to scope
rec tos′co py
rec″to sig′moid
rec″to sig″moid ec′to my
rec″to ste no′sis
rec″to u re′thral
rec″to u′ter ine
rec″to vag′i nal
rec″to vag″i no ab dom′i nal
rec″to ves′i cal
rec″to ves i ca′lis
rec′tum
rec′tus
re cum′ben cy
re cum′bent
re cu′per ate
re cu′per a″tive
re cur′rence
re cur′rent
re″cur va′tion
re dresse′ment
re duce′
re duc′tion
re du′pli ca″ted
re du″pli ca′tion
re″ed u ca′tion
re″ev o lu′tion
re″ex ci ta′tion
re fec′tion
re flect′ed
re flec′tor
re′flex
re flex″o gen′ic
re″flex om′e ter
re′flux
re fract″
re frac′ta do′si
re fra′tion
re frac′tion ist
re frac′tive
re″frac tiv′i ty
re frac tom′e ter
re frac′to ry
re frac′ture
re frig′er ant
ref′use
re gen′er ate
reg′i men
re′gion
reg′is ter
reg′is try
reg″le men ta′tion
re gres′sion
re gres′sive
reg″u la′tion
reg″u la″tive
re gur′gi tant
re gur″gi ta′tion
re″ha bil″i ta′tion
re″ha la′tion
re″in fec′tion
re″in force′ment
re″in fu′sion
re″in ner va′tion
re″in oc″u la′tion
re in″te gra′tion
re″in ver′sion
Reiter′s
syn′drome
re ju″ve nes′cence
re lapse′
re la′tion
re lax′
re″lax a′tion
re me′di al
rem″e dy
re″min er al i za′tion
re mis′sion
re mit′tance
re mit′tence

re'nal
ren'i form
re'nin
ren'in ism
ren'net
ren'nin
re pel'lent
re"per co la'tion
re"per cus'sion
re place'ment
re"plan ta'tion
re ple'tion
re"pli ca'tion
re pol"lar i za'tion
re pos'i tor
re pous"soir'
re pres'sion
re"pro duc'tion
re pul'sion
re sect'
re sec'tion
re sec'to scope
re serve'
re sid'u al
res'i due
re sid'u um
re sil'i ence
re sil'i ent
res'in
re sist'ance
res"o lu'tion
re sol'vent
res'o nance
res'o nant
res'o na"tor
re sorb'ent
re sor'cin ol
re sorp'tion
re spir'a ble
res"pi ra'tion
res'pi ra"tor
res pi'ra tory
res"pi rom'e ter
res"pi rom'e try
re sponse'
res'ti form
res"ti tu' ti o ad in'te grum
res"ti tu'tion
res"to ra'tion
re stor'a tive
Res'to ril
re straint'
re sul'tant
re su'pi nate
res"ur rec'tion ist
re sus"ci ta'tion
re sus'ci ta"tor
re su'ture
re tard'er
retch
re'te
re ten'tion
re tic'u la
re tic'u lar
re tic'u la"ted
re tic'u lin
re tic'u lo cyte"
re tic"u lo cy"to pe'ni a
re tic"u lo cy to'sis
re tic"u lo en"do the'li al
re tic"u lo en"do the"li o'ma
re tic"u lo en"do the"li o'sis
re tic"u lo'sis
re tic'u lum
re'ti fism
ret'i na
ret"i nac'u lum
ret'i nal
ret'i nene
ret"i ni'tis
ret"i no blas to'ma
ret"i no cho"roid i"tis
ret"i no cy to'ma
ret"i no pap"il li'tis

ret″i nop″a thy
ret″i nos′co py
re tort′
re tract′
re″trac til′i ty
re trac′tion
re trac′tor
ret″ro ac′tion
ret″ro an′ter o am ne′si a
ret″ro an′ter o grade
ret″ro bul′bar
ret″ro car′di ac
ret″ro ce′cal
ret′ro cele
ret″ro chei′li a
ret″ro col′ic
ret″ro con′dy lism
ret″ro cop″u la′tion
ret″ro de″vi a′tion
ret″ro dis place′ment
ret″ro e soph″a ge′al
ret′ro flex
ret″ro flex′ion
ret″ro gas se′ri an
ret″ro gnath′ism
ret′ro grade′
re trog′ra phy
ret″ro gres′sion
ret″ro jec′tion
ret″ro lab y rin′thine
ret″ro len′tal
ret″ro lin′gual
ret″ro mor′pho sis
ret″ro na′sal
ret″ro per″i to ne′al
ret″ro per″i to ni′tis
ret″ro pha ryn′ge al
ret″ro phar″yn gi′tis
ret″ro phar′ynx
ret″ro pla cen′tal
ret″ro pla′si a
ret′ro posed
ret″ro po si′tion
retro″pul′sion
ret″ro stal′sis
ret″ro tar′sal
ret″ro ton′sil lar
ret″ro tra′che al
ret″ro vac″ci na′tion
ret″ro ver″si oflex′ion
ret″ro ver′sion
ret″ro vert′ed
re trude′
re tru′sion
re″vac ci na′tion
re ver″ber a′tion
rev′er ie
rever′sal
re ver′sion
re″vi taliza′tion
re vive
re viv″i fi ca′tion
rev′o lute
re vul′sant
re vul′sive
Rh
rhab″do my o′ma
rhab″do my″o sar co′ma
rhab″do pho′bi a
rhab″do vi′rus
rha′cous
rhag′a des
rhag′i o crin
rhag′oid
rhan′ter
rhe″bo sce′li a
rheg′ma
rhe′o base
rhe″o car″di og′ra phy
rhe′o cord
rhe ol′o gy
rhe om′e ter

rhe′o nome
rhe′o pex″y
rhe′o phore
rhe′o scope
rhe′o stat
rhe″o ta chyg′ra phy
rhe″o tax′is
rhe′o tome
rhe′o trope
rheu mat′ic
rheu′ma tism
rheu′ma toid
rheu″ma tol′o gy
rheu″mo crin ol′o gy
rhex′is
rhic no′sis
rhi′nal
rhi nal′gi a
rhi″nan tral′gi a
rhi nel′cos
rhi″nen ceph′a lon
rhi″nen chy′sis
rhi″neu ryn′ter
rhin he″ma to′ma
rhin′i on
rhi′nism
rhi ni′tis
rhi″no an tri′tis
rhi″no by′on
rhi″no ceph′a lus
rhi″no ceph′a ly
rhi″no chei′sis
rhi″noc nes′mus
rhi″no dac′ry o lith
rhi″no dym′i a
rhi nog′e nous
rhi″no ky pho′sis
rhi″no la′li a
rhi″no lar″yn gi′tis
rhi″no lar″yn gol′o gy
rhi″no lith
rhi″no li thi′a sis
rhi″nol′o gist
rhi″nol′o gy
rhi″no ma nom′e ter
rhi″no mi o′sis
rhi″nom mec′to my
rhi″no my co′sis
rhi″no ne cro′sis
rhi″nop′a thy
rhi″no pha ryn′ge al
rhi″no phar″yn gi′tis
rhi″no pha ryn′go lith
rhi″no pho′ni a
rhi″no phy′ma
rhi″no plas′tic
rhi′no plas″ty
rhi″no pol′yp
rhi″nop′si a
rhi″nor rha′gi a
rhi″nor′rha phy
rhi″nor rhe′a
rhi nos′chi sis
rhi″no scle ro′ma
rhi″no scope
rhi″no si″nus o path′i a
Rhi″no spo rid′i um
rhi″no ste no′sis
rhi′no thrix
rhi′not′o my
Rhi″pi ceph′a lus
rhi″zo don′tro py
rhi′zoid
rhi′zome
rhi′zo neure
rhi″zo nychi′i a
rhi zot′o my
rho″do gen′e sis
rho″do phy lax′is
rho dop′sin
rhom″ben ceph′a lon
rhom′bo cele

rhom′boid
rhom boi′de us
rhon′chus
Rhus
rhythm
rhyth′mic
rhyth′mi cal
rhyth mic′i ty
rhyt″i do plas′ty
rhyti″i do′sis
rib
ri″bo fla′vin
ri″bo nu′cle ase
ri″bo nu cle′ic
ri″bo nu″cleo pro′tein
ri′bose
rick″ets
Rick ett′si a
rick ett′si al
rick ett′si al pox
Riedel's stru′ma
ri gid′i ty
rig′or
ri′ma
ri′mose
Rinne's test
ri so′ri us
ri′sus sar don′i cus″
rob′o rant
ro′dent
ro den′ti cide
roent′gen
roent″gen i za′tion
roent′gen o gram″
roent′gen o graph″
roent″gen og′ra phy
roent″gen o ky′mo gram
roent′gen o ky mog′ra phy
roent′gen ol″o gist
roent′gen ol′o gy
roent″gen o lu′cent
roent″gen om′e try
roent″gen o paque′
roent″gen os′co py
roent″gen ther′a py
Rikitansky, Carl von
Rolando's a′re a
Romberg's sign
Rorschach test
ro sa ce′a
ro sa′ce i form″
Rosenmuellar, John C.
ro se′ o la
ro se′o lous
ro sette′
ros′trum
ro′ta me″ter
ro ta′tion
ro ta to′res
Roux-en-Y
ru be′do
ru″be fa′cient
ru″be fac′tion
ru bel′la
ru be′o la
ru″be o′sis i′rid is
ru′ber
ru bes′cence
ru′bor
ruc ta′tion
ruc′tus
ru′di ment
ru″di men′ta ry
ru″di men′tum
ru′ga
ru gi′tus
ru′gose
ru gos′i ty
ru′men
ru″men ot′o my
ru′mi nant
ru″mi na′tion

rup′ti o
rup′ture
ru′tin
rye

S

Sabin vac′cine
Sabouraud's me′di a
sab′u lous
sac
sac′cha ride
sac″cha rim′e ter
sac′cha rin'
sac″cha ro ga lac″tor rhe′a
sac″cha ro me tab′o lism
Sac″cha ro my′ces
sac′cha rose
sac″cha ro su′ri a
sac′cu lar
sac′cule
sac″cu lo coch′le ar
sac′cu lus
sac″cus
sa′cral
sa″cral′gi a
sa″cral i za′tion
sa crec′to my
sa″cro an te′ri or
sa″cro coc cyg′e al
sa″cro coc cyg′e us
sa″cro dyn′i a
sa″cro il′i ac
sa″cro lum′bar
sa″cro pos te′ri or
sa″cro sci at′ic
sa″cro spi na′lis
sa″cro u′ter ine
sa′crum
sad′ism
sad′ist
sad″o mas′o chism
sa′fu
sag′it tal
sa′go
sag′u lum
Saint Vitus' dance
sal
sal′i cyl″ate
sal″i cyl″ic ac′id
sal′i cyl ism
sa lim′e ter
sa′line
sa li′va
sal′i vant
sal′i vary
sal″i va′tion
sal′i va″tor
sal″i vo li thi′a sis
Salk vac′cine
Sal″mo nel′la
sal″mo nel lo′sis
sal″pin gec′to my
sal″pin gem phrax′is
sal″pin gi′tis
sal pin″go cath′e ter ism
sal pin′go cele
sal pin″go cy e′sis
sal″pin gol′y sis
sal pin″go-o″o pho rec′to my
sal pin″go-o″o pho ri′tis
sal pin″go-o oph′o ro cele
sal pin″go pal′a tine
sal pin″go per″i to ni′tis
sal pin′go pex″y
sal pin″go pha ryn′ge al
sal pin″go phar″yn ge′us
sal pin′go plas″ty
sal″pin gor′rha phy
sal pin″go sal″pin gos′to my
sal pin′go scope

sal pin″go sten″o cho′ri a
sal″pin gos′to my
sal″pin got′o my
sal″pin gys″ter o cy e′sis
sal′pinx
sal ta′tion
sa lu′bri ty
Sal′var san
salve
sal′vi a
san″a to′ri um
sane
san guic′o lous
san″gui fi ca′tion
san′guine
san guin′e ous
san guin′o lent
san′guis
sa′ni es
san″i ta′ri an
san″i tar′i um
san′i tar″y
san″i ta′tion
san′i tize
san′i ty
san′to nin
Santorini′s
duct
sa phe′na
sa phe′nous
sa′po
sap″o na′ceous
sa pon″i fi ca′tion
sa pon′i form
sap′o nin
sap′phism
sa pre′mi a
sa pre′mic
sap″ro gen′ic
sa proph′a gous
sap″ro phyte
sap″ro zo′ic
sar′a pus
sar ci′tis
sar″co bi′ont
sar′co blast
sar′co cele
sar″co en″do the li o′ma
sar′coid o′sis
sar″co lem′ma
sar co′ma
sar co″ma to′sis
sar co′ma tous
sar′co mere
sar″co mes″ o the li o′ma
sar″co my′ces
sar′co plasm
sar″co poi et′ic
Sar cop′tes
sar″co spo rid″i o′sis
sar′cous
sar″sa pa ril′la
sar to′ri us
sas′sa fras
sat′el lite
sat″el li to′sis
sa ti′e ty
sat′u ra″ted
sat′ur nism
sat″y ri′a sis
sau′cer ize
sau ri′a sis
sau′sar ism
sa′vo ry
scab
scab′bard
sca′bi es
sca″bi o pho′bi a
sca′bi ous
sca bri′ti es
sca′la
sca lene′
sca″le nec′to my
sca″le not′o my

sca le′nus
sca′ler
sca′ling
scape′ goat ing
scalp
scal′pel
scal′ly
scan sor′i us
Scanzoni's
ma neu′ver
sca′pha
scaph″o ceph′a ly
scaph′oid
scap′u la
scap″u lal′gi a
scap′u lar
scap″u lec′to my
scap″u lo cla vic″u la′ris
scap′u lo cos″tal
scap′u lo hu′mer al
scap′u lo pex″y
scar″a bi′a sis
scarf′skin″
scar″i fi ca′tion
scar′i fi ca″tor
scar″la ti′na
scar″la ti nel′la
scar″la ti′ni form
scar″la ti′noid
scar′let fe′ver
Scarpa's fas′ci a
scat″o lo′gi a
sca to′ma
sca toph′a gous
sca tos′co gy
scav′en ger
sche′ma
sche′mo graph
Schick test
Schilders's dis ease′
Schiötz
schis″to ceph′a lus
schis″to cor′mus
schis″to cys′tis
schis′to cyte
schis″to glos′si a
schis tom′e lus
schis tom′e ter
schis″to pro so′pi a
schis tor′rha chis
schis to′sis
Schis″to so′ma
Schis″to so′ma hae″ma to′bi um
Schis″to so′ma ja po′ni cum
Schis″to so′ma man so′ni
schis″to so mi′a sis
schis″to so′mus
schis″to ster′ni a
schis″to tho′rax
schis″to tra′che lus
schiz″o af fec′tive
schiz am′ni on
schiz ax′on
schiz″o ble pha′ri a
schiz″o gen′e sis
schiz″o gnath′ism
schiz og′o ny
schiz″o gy′ri a
schiz′oid
schiz″o ma′ni a
schiz′ont
schiz″o nych′i a
schiz″o pha′si a
schiz″o phre′ni a
schiz″o phren′ic
schiz o phren i form
schiz″o so′ma
schiz″o thy′mic
schiz″o trich′i a
schiz″o type
schiz o ty′pol
Schrimer's dis ease′
schwan no′ma
sci age′

sci ap′o dy
sci at′ic
sci at′i ca
sci″e ro′pi a
scil′lism
scil″lo ceph′a ly
scin′ti gram
scin til′la scope
scin″til la′tion
scin′ti scan′ner
scir′rhoid
scir′rhous
scir′rhus
scis′sion
scis′sors
scis su′ra
scle″ec ta′si a
scle no ther′a py
scle rec″to ir″i dec′to my
scle rec′to my
scler″e de′ma
scle re′ma
scle″ren ce pha′li a
scle ren′chy ma
scle rit′ic
scle ri′tis
scle″ro a troph′ic
scle″ro blas te′ma
scle″ro cat″a rac′ta
scle″ro cho″roid i′tis
scle″ro con″junc ti′val
scle″ro cor′ne a
scle″ro dac tyl′i a
scle″ro der′ma
scle″ro der″ma ti′tis
scle rog′e nous
scle′roid
scle″ro i ri′tis
scle″ro ker″a ti′tis
scle″ro ker″a to i ri′tis
scle ro′ma
scle″ro ma la′ci a
scle rom′e ter
scle″ro nych′i a
scle″ro nyx′is
scle″ro-o″o pho ri′tis
scle′ro plas″ty
scle rose′
scle ros′ing
scle ro′sis
scle″ro ste no′sis
scle ros′to my
scle′ro thrix
scle rot′ic
scle rot″i cec′to my
scle′ro tome
scle rot′o my
scle″ro to nyx′is
scle″ro trich′i a
scle′rous
sco′bi nate
sco lec′i form
sco′lex
sco″li o lor do′sis
sco″li o si om′e try
sco″li o′sis
sco″li o som′e ter
sco′li o tone″
scoop
sco pol′a mine
sco pom′e ter
sco pom′e try
sco″po pho′bi a
scor″a cra′ti a
scor bu′tic
scor′pi on
scot″o din′i a
scot′o gram
sco to′ma
sco to′ma graph
sco tom′e ter
sco″o pho′bi a
scours
scra′per

scrof′u la
scrof″u lo der′ma
scro tec′to my
scro″to plas″ty
scro′tum
scru″pu los′i ty
scu′ba di′ving
scur′vy
scu′tum
scyb′a lum
scy′phi form
scy ti′tis
se ba″ce o fol lic′u lar
se ba′ceous
se bas″to ma′ni a
se bip′a rous
seb′o lith
seb″or rhe′a
se′bum
sec′o dont
Se′co nal
se cre′ta
se cre′ta gogue
se crete′
se cre′tin
se cre′tion
se cre′tor
se cre′to ry
sec′tile
sec′tion
sec to′ri al
se cun″di grav′i da
sec′un dines
sec″un dip′a ra
se da′tion
sed′a tive
sed′en tar″y
sed″i ment
sed′i men ta′tion
seg′ment
seg men′tal
seg″men ta′tion
seg″re ga′tion
seg′re ga″tor
Seitz
  fil′ter
sei′zure
se″la pho bi a
se lec′tion
se lec′tor
se le′ne
se le′nic
se le′ni um
se le′no dont
se le″no gam′i a
sel′la tur′ci ca
se man′tics
se′men
sem″i ca nal′
sem′i car″ti lag′i nous
sem″i co′ma
sem″i com′ a tose
sem″i con′scious
sem″i lu′nar
sem″i lux a′tion
sem″i mem″bra no′sus
sem″i mem′bra nous
sem′i nal
sem″i na′tion
sem″i nif′er ous
sem″i no′ma
sem″i nu′ri a
sem″i pro na′tion
sem″i pto′sis
sem″i so′por
sem″i spi na′lis
sem″i su″pi na′tion
sem″i ten″di no′sus
sem″i ten′di nous
se nec′ti tude
se nes′cence
se′nile

se′nil ism
se′ni um
sen′na
se no′pi a
sen sa′tion
sense
sen′si ble
sen sim′e ter
sen″si tiv′i ty
sen″si ti za′tion
sensi tized
sen″so mo′tor
sen″so pa ral′y sis
sen″so ri mo′tor
sen so′ri um
sen′so ry
sen′su al ism
sen′sus
sen′tient
sen′ti ment
sep′a ra″tor
sep′sis
sep′tal
sep tec′to my
sep′tic
sep″ti ce′mi a
sep″ti co phle bi′tis
sep″ti grav′i da
sep″ti me tri′tis
sep tip′a ra
sep″to der″mo plas′ty
sep″to mar′gi nal
sep tom′e ter
sep′to tome
sep tot′o my
sep′tu lum
sep′tum
sep′tu plet
sep′ul ture
se que′la
se′quence
se ques′ter
se″ques tra′tion
se″ques trec′to my
se ques′trum
se′ries
ser′i flux
se″ro co li′tis
se′ro cul″ture
se″ro der″ma ti′tis
se″ro der″ma to′sis
se″ro di″ag no′sis
se″ro en″ter i′tis
se″ro fi′brin ous
se″ro lem′ma
se″ro li′pase
se″ro log′ic
se rol′o gist
se rol′o gy
se rol′y sin
se ro′ma
se″ro mem′bra nous
se″ro mu′cous
se″ro per″i to ne′um
se″ro prog no′sis
se″ro pu′ru lent
se″ro re ac′tion
se″ro re sis′tance
se ro′sa
se ro″sa mu′cin
se″ro san guin′e ous
se″ro se′rous
se″ro si′tis
se″ro syn″o vi′tis
se″ro ther′a py
ser″o to′nin
se′rous
ser pig′i nous
ser ra′tion
ser ra′tus
Sertoli cells
se′rum

ses′a moid
ses″a moid i′tis
ses′sile
se′ta
se′ton
se′vum
sew′age
sex″i dig′i tal
sex′-in′ter grade″
sex′o-es thet′ic
sex ol′o gy
sex re ver′sal
sex″ti grav′i da
sex tip′a ra
sex′tu plet
sex′u al
sha′king
sheath
shed′ding
shield
Shi gel′la
shi″gel lo′sis
shiv′er
shoul′der
shunt
Shwartzman re ac′tion
si″a go nag′ra
si al′a den
si″al ad″e ni′tis
si al′a gogue
si al′o gram
si″al a po′ri a
si al′ic
si″a li thot′o my
si″a lo ad″e nec′to my
si″a lo ad″e ni′tis
si″a lo ad″e not′o my
si″a lo a″er oph′a gy
si″a lo an gi′tis
si″a lo do chi′tis
si″a lo do′chi um
si″a lo do′cho plas″ty
si″a log′e nous
si al′a gram
si″a log′ra phy
si′a loid
si al′o lith″
si″a lo li thi′a sis
si″a lo li thot′o my
si″al′o mu″cins
si″a lor rhe′a
si″a los′che sis
si″a lo se″mei ol′o gy
si″a lo ste no′sis
si″a lo syr′inx
sib′i lant
sib′ling
sib″i la′tion
sib″i lis′mus
sib′i lus
sib′ship
sic′cant
sic cha′si a
sic′cus
sickle cell
sick le′mi a
sick′ness
sid′er ism
sid″e ro blas′tic
sid″er o dro″mo pho′bi a
sid″er o fi bro′sis
sid″er o pe′ni a
sid′er o phil
sid″er ophi′i lous
sid′er o scope″
sid″er o sil″i co′sis
sid″er o′sis
sigh
sig′ma tism
sig′moid
sig′moid ec′to my
sig″moid i′tis

sig moi′do pex″y
sig moi″do proc tos′to my
sig moi″do rec tos′to my
sig moi′do scope
sig″moid os′co py
sig moi″do sig″moid os′to my
sig″moid os′to my
sig″moid ot′o my
sign
sig′na
sig nif′i cant
sig′num
sil′i ca
sil″i ca to′sis
si li′ ceous
sil′i con
sil″li co si″der o′sis
sil″i co′sis
sil″i co tu ber″cu lo′sis
sil′ver
sim′i an
Simmond′s dis ease′
sim′ple
si′mul
sim″u la′tion
sin′a pis′co py
sin′a pism
sin′ci put
sin′ew
sin gul′tus
sin′is ter
sin′is trad
sin is tral
sin″is tra′tion
sin″is trau′ral
sin″is tro car′di al
sin″is tro cer′e bral
sin″is troc′u lar
sin″is tro gy ra′tion
sin″is tro man′u al
sin″is trop′e dal
sin″is tro′sis
sin″is tro tor′sion
sin′is trous
sin″no a′tri al
si″no bron chi′tis
sin′u ous
si′nus
si″nus i′tis
si′nus oid
si″nus oi′dal
sin″nus oi″dal i za′tion
si″nus ot′o my
si′phon
si′phon age
Sippy di′et
si″re no me′li a
si″ren om′e lus
si ri′a sis
site
sit′fast″
sit″i eir′gi a
si tol′o gy
si″to ma′ni a
si″to pho′bi a
si″to ther′a py
si′tus in ver′sus
skat′ole
ske lal′gi a
skel′e tal
skel″e ti za′tion
skel′e ton
Skene′s gland
ske nei′tis
skene′o scope″
ski′a gram
ski ag′ra phy
ski am′e try
ski′a scope
ski as′co py
skin
skin′ny

Ski′o dan
skull
sli′cer
slough
slum′ber
small′pox″
smear
smeg′ma
smell
Smithwick′s op″er a′tion
smudg′ing
smut
snap
sneeze
snore
soap
so″ci ol′o gy
so″ci o med′i cal
sock′et
so cor′di a
so′di um
sod′om ite
sod′om y
sof′ten ing
sol
sol″lar i za′tion
so′lar plex′us
sole-plate
so′le us
so lid″i fi ca′tion
sol′i ped
sol′ip sism
sol′i tar″y
sol′-lu′nar
sol″u bil′i ty
sol′u ble
so′lum tym′pa ni
sol′ ute
so lu′tion
sol′vate
sol va′tion
sol′vent
so′ma
so″ma tes the′si a
so mat′ic
so mat″i co vis′cer al
so′ma tist
so″ma ti za′tion
so mat′o chrome″
so″ma to did′y mus
so″ma to dym′i a
so ma′to form
so″ma tog′e ny
so″ma tol′o gy
so″ma to mam″mo tro′pin
so′ma tome
so″ma to meg′a ly
so″ma tom′e try
so″ma top′a gus
so′ma to path′ic
so′ma to plasm″
so′ma to pleure″
so″ma to psy′chic
so″ma to splanch″no pleu′ric
so″ma to to′ni a
so″ma to top″ag no′si a
so″ma to top′ic
so″ma to trid″y mus
so″ma to trop′ic
so″ma to tro′pin
so′ma to type″
so″mes the′si a
so″mes thet′ic
so″mes the″tog no′sis
so″mes the″to psy′chic
so′mite
som nam′bu lism
som nam′bu list
som′ni al
som′ni a″tive
som nic′u lous
som″ni fa′cient

som nif′er ous
som nif′ic
som nif′u gous
som nil′o quism
som nil′o quist
som nip′a thist
som nip′a thy
som″no cin″e mat′o graph
som′no lence
som′no lent
som″no len′ti a
som″no les′cent
som′no lism
sone
so no′gra phy
so nom′e ter
so phis″ti ca′tion
soph″o ma′ni a
so′por
sop′o rate
so″po rif′ic
sop′o rose
sor′bi tol
sor′des
sor′did
so ro″ri a′tion
souf′fle
sou′ma
sound
soy′bean
spa
space
span″i o car′di a
spar′a drap
spar ga no′sis
spar go′sis
Spa′rine
spasm
spas mod′ic
spas mol′o gy
spas″mo lyt′ic
spas″mo phe′mi a
spas″mo phil′i a
spas′mus nu′tans
spas′tic
spas tic′i ty
spa′ti um
spat′u la
spav′in
spay
spe′cial ist
spe′cial ty
spe′cies
spe cif′ic
spec″i fic′i ty
spec′ta ces
spec′ta cles
spec″tro col″or im′e ter
spec′tro gram
spec′tro graph
spec trom′e ter
spec″tro pho″te lom′e ter
spec″tro pho tom′e ter
spec″tro po″lar im′e ter
spec′tro scope
spec tros′co py
spec′trum
spec′u lum
speech
sperm
sper″ma cet′i
sperm as′ter
sper″ma ta cra′si a
sper mat′ic
sper′ma tid
sper′ma to cele″
sper″ma to ce lec′to my
sper″ma to ci′dal
sper′ma to cide″
sper″ma to cys ti′tis
sper″ma to cys tot′o my
sper″ma to cyte″

sper″ma to cy to′ma
sper″ma to gen′e sis
sper″ma to gen′ic
sper″ma to go′ni um
sper′ma toid
sper″ma tol′y sin
sper″ma tol′y sis
sper″ma top′a thy
sper′ma to phore″
sper″ma tor rhe′a
sper″ma to zo′i cide
sper″ma to zo′on
sper″ma tu′ri a
sper mec′to my
sper′mi cide
sperm′ism
sper′ mo lith
sper mol′y sin
sphac″e la′tion
sphac′e lism
sphac″e lo der′ma
sphac′e lus
spha″gi as′mus
spha gi′tis
sphe′ni on
sphe″no bas′i lar
sphe″no ceph′a lus
sphe″no ceph′a ly
sphe″no eth′moid
sphe′noid
sphe″noid i′tis
sphe″noid ot′o my
sphe″no man dib′u lar
sphe″no max′il lar″y
sphe″no-oc cip′i tal
sphe″no pal′a tine
sphe″no pa ri′e tal
sphe″no pe tro′sal
sphe no′sis
sphe″no tre′sia
sphe′no tribe
sphe′no trip″sy
sphere
sphe″res the′si a
sphe″ro ceph′a lus
sphe″ro cyl′in der
sphe′ro cyte
sphe″ro cy′tic
sphe″ro cy to′sis
sphe′roid
sphe rom′e ter
spher′ule
sphinc′ter
sphinc″ter al′gi a
sphinc″ter ec′to my
sphinc″ter is′mus
sphinc″ter i′tis
sphinc″ter ol′y sis
sphinc′ter o plas″ty
sphinc″ter ot′o my
sphin″go li pi do′ses
sphin″go my′e lin
sphyg′mic
sphyg″mo bo lom′e ter
sphyg″mo chron′o graph
sphyg″mo chro nog′ra phy
sphyg mod′ic
sphyg″mo dy″na mom′e ter
sphyg′mo gram″
sphyg′mo graph
sphyg mog′ra phy
sphyg′moid
sphyg″mo ma nom′e ter
sphyg″mo-os″cil lom′e ter
sphyg″mo pal pa′tion
sphyg′mo phone
sphyg′mo scope
sphyg′mos′co py
sphyg″mo sys′to le
sphyg′mo tech″ny
sphyg″mo to′no graph
sphyg″mo to nom′e ter

sphyg′mus
spi′ca
spic′ule
spi lo′ma
spi″lo pla′ni a
spi′lus
spi′na bi′fi da
spi′nal
spi na′lis
spin′dle
spine
spi″no cel′lu lar
spi″no gal″va ni za′tion
spi′no graph″
spi″no tec′tal
spin thar′i scope
spin′ther ism
spi′ral
spi′reme
spir″il li ci′dal
spir″il lo′sis
Spi ril′lum
Spi″ro chae′ta
spi″ro chet′al
spi′ro chete
spi″ro che te′mi a
spi″ro che′ti cide
spi″ro che tol′y sis
spi″ro che to′sis
spi′ro gram″
spi′ro graph″
spi rom′e ter
spis′sa ted
spis′si tude
splanch′na
splanch″nec to′pi a
splanch″nem phrax′is
splanch″nes the′si a
splanch″neu rys′ma
splanch′nic
splanch″ni cec′to my
splanch″ni cot′o my
splanch′no cele
splanch″no di as′ta sis
splanch nog′ra phy
splanch′no lith
splanch″no li thi′a sis
splanch nol′o gy
splanch″no meg′a ly
splanch″no mi′cri a
splanch nop′a thy
splanch′no pleure
splanch″not to′sis
splanch″no scle ro′sis
splanch nos′co py
splanch″no skel′e ton
splanch″no so mat′ic
splanch not′o my
splanch′no tribe
spleen
sple nal′gi a
sple nec′to my
splen″ec to′pi a
sple net′ic
splen′ic
splen″i co pan″cre at′ic
splen′i form
sple ni′tis
sple′ni um
sple′ni us
splen″i za′tion
sple′no cele
sple″no clei′sis
sple′no cyte
sple″no dyn′i a
sple″no hep″a to meg′a ly
sple′noid
sple nol′y sis
sple″no ma la′ci a
sple″no meg′a ly
sple nop′a thy
sple′no pex″y

sple″no pneu mo′ni a
sple″no por′tal
sple″no por″to′ graphy
sple″nop to′sis
sple″no re′nal
sple nor′rha phy
sple not′o my
sple″no tox′in
splen′u lus
splice
splint
splint′age
splin′ter
splint′ing
spon″dy lal′gi a
spon″dy lar throc′a ce
spon″dy li′tis
spon″dy lo ar thri′tis
spon″dy lo di dym′i a
spon″dyl od′y mus
spon″dy lo dyn′i a
spon″dy lo lis the′sis
spon″dyl ol′y sis
spon″dyl op′a thy
spon″dy lo py o′sis
spon″dy lo′sis
spon″dy lo syn de′sis
spon″dy lot′o my
sponge
spon′gi o blast″
spon″gi o blas to′ma
spon′gi o cyte″
spon′gi oid
spon′gi o plasm
spon′gi ose
spon″gi o′sis
spon″gi o si′tis
spon′gy
spon ta′ne ous
spo rad′ic
spore
spo′ri cide
spo′ro cyte″
spo″ro gen′e sis
spo′ro phyte
spo″ro tri cho′sis
Spo″ro zo′a
spor′u late
sprain
sprue
spur′gall″
spu′tum
squa′ma
squame
squa″mo-oc cip′i tal
squa mo′sa
squa″mo sphe′noid
squa″mo tym pan′ic
squa′mous
squint
sta′bi li″zer
sta′ble
stac ca′to
stag′gers
stag na′tion
stain
stal″ag mom′e ter
sta′ling
stalk
sta′men
stam′i na
stam′mer ing
stand′ard
stand″ard i za′tion
sta″pe dec′to my
sta′pe des
sta pe′di al
sta pe″di o te not′o my
sta pe″di o ves tib′u lar
sta pe′di us
sta pe″d o plas′ty
sta′pes

Staph cil′lin
staph″y lec′to my
staph″yl e de′ma
staph″y le′us
staph″yl he″ma to′ma
sta phyl′i on
staph″y li′tis
staph″y lo coc′cal
staph″y lo coc ce′mi a
staph″y lo coc′cic
Staph″y lo coc′cus
staph″y lo der″ma ti′tis
staph″y lol′y sin
staph″y lo′ma
staph″y lo phar″yn gor′rha phy
staph′y lo plas″ty
staph″y lop to′sis
staph″y lor′rha phy
staph″y los′chi sis
staph′y lo tome″
staph″y lot′o my
staph″y lo tox′in
starch
star va′tion
stas″i bas″i pho′bi a
stas″i pho′bi a
sta′sis
stat′ic
stat′ics
stat″i den sig′ra phy
stat′im
sta tis′ti cal
sta tis′tics
stat″o ki net′ic
stat′o lith
sta tom′e ter
stat′ure
sta′tus asth ma′ti cus″
sta′tus epi lep′ti cus″
sta′tus thym″i co″lym phat′i cus
sta″tu vo′lence

stau′ri on
steap′sin
stear′ate
ste ar′ic ac′id
stear″o der′mi a
ste″ar rhe′a
ste′a tin
ste″a ti′tis
ste″a to cryp to′sis
ste″a to cys to′ma
ste″a tog′e nous
ste″a tol′y sis
ste″a to′ma
ste″a to py′gi a
ste″a tor rhe′a
steg no′sis
stel′la len′tis hy″a loi′de a
stel′la len′tis i rid′i ca
stel′late
ste nag′mus
ste′ni on
sten″o car′di a
sten″o ceph′a ly
sten″o chas′mus
sten″o cho′ri a
sten″o co ri′a sis
sten″o crot′a phy
sten′o dont
sten″o mer′ic
sten″o pe′ic
ste nosed′
ste no′sis
sten″o sto′mi a
ste nos′to my
sten″o ther′mal
sten″o tho′rax
stent
sten″to roph′o nous
ste pha′ni on
step′page gait
ster″co bi′lin

ster″co bi lin′o gen
ster′co lith
ster″co ra′ceous
ster′co rar″y
ster″co ro′ma
ster′cus
ster″e o an″es the′si a
ster″e o ar throl′y sis
ster″e o cam pim′e ter
ster″e o chem′is try
ster″e o cil′i a
ster″e o en ceph′a lo tome
ster″e o en ceph″a lot′o my
ster″e og no′sis
ster′e o gram″
ster′eo o graph″
ster″e og′ra phy
ster″e o phor′o scope
ster″e op′sis
ster′e op″ter
ster″e o ra′di og′ra phy
ster″e o roent″gen og′ra phy
ster′e o sope
ster‴e o stro′bo scope
ster″e o tax′i a
ster″e o tax′is
ster″e ot′ro pism
ster′e o ty″py
ster″e o vec″tor car′di o graph″
ster′ile
ste ril′i ty
ster″i li za′tion
ster′i lize
ster′i li″zer
ster nal′gi a
ster na′lis
ster″no chon″dro scap″u lar′is
ster″no cla vic′u lar
ster″no cla vic″u lar′is
ster″no clei″do mas′toid
ster″no dyn′i a
ster nod′y mus
ster″no dyn′i a
ster″no hy′oid
ster″no hy oid′e us a zy′gos
ster″no mas′toid
ster″no-om phal″o dym′i a
ster″no per″i car′di al
ster nos′chi sis
ster″no thy′roid
ster not′o my
ster′num
ster″nu ta′tion
ster′nu ta″tor
ster′oid
ster′ol
steth ar″te ri′tis
steth″o pol‴y scope
steth′o scope
steth″o scop′ic
ste thos′co py
sthe′ni a
sthen′ic
sti′fle
stig′ma
stig′ma tism
stil bam′i dine
stil bes′trol
still′birth″
stim′u lant
stim′u late
stim″u la′tion
stim′u li
stim′u lus
stip′pling
stock″i net′
sto′ma
sto mac′a ce
stom′ach
sto mach′ic
sto″ma tal′gi a
sto mat′ic

sto″ma ti′tis
sto″ma toc′a ce
sto″ma to dyn′i a
sto″ma to dy so′di a
sto″ma to gas′tric
sto″ma tol′o gy
sto″ma to ma la′ci a
sto″ma to me′ni a
sto″ma to′mi a
sto mat′o my
sto″ma to no′ma
sto″ma top′a thy
sto′ma to plas″ty
sto″ma tor rha′gi a
sto′ma to scope″
sto″ma to′sis
sto″ma tot′o my
sto men″or rha′gi a
sto″mo de′um
sto mos′chi sis
stool
stop′cock″
stra bis′mus
stra bom′e ter
stra bom′e try
strag′u lum
strait
stra mo′ni um
stran′gle
stran′gles
stran″gu la′tion
stran′gu ry
strat″i fi ca′tion
strat′i fied
stra tig′ra phy
strat′um
streph″o sym bo′li a
strep′i tus
strep″ti ce′mi a
strep″to ba cil′lus
strep″to coc′cal
strep″to coc ce′mi a
strep″to coc′ci
Strep″to coc′cus
strep″to der″ma ti′tis
strep″to dor′nase
strep″to ki′nase
strep″to ly′sin
Strep″to my′ces
strep″to my′cin
strep″to sep″ti ce′mi a
Strep′to thrix
stretch′er
stri′a
stri′ae
stri′a ted
stri a′tum
stric′trure
stri′dor
strid′u lous
strin′gent
string′halt″
strip
strob′ic
stro bi′la
strob″i la′tion
stro′bo scope
stro′ma
Stron″gy loi′des
stron′ti um
stro phan′thin
stroph″o ceph′ a lus
stroph″o ceph′a ly
stroph′u lus
stru′ma
stru‴mi form
stru mi′tis
strych′nine
stupe
stu″pe fa′cient
stu″pe fac′tion
stu″pe ma′ni a

stu pid′i ty
stu′por
Sturge-Weber dis ease′
stut′ter er
stut′ter ing
sty′let
sty″lo glos′sus
sty″lo hy′oid
sty″lo man dib′u lar
sty″lo mas′toid
sty″lo pha ryn′ge us
sty′lus
sty″ma to′sis
styp′tic
sub″ab dom′i nal
sub″a cro′mi al
sub″a cute′
sub al″i men ta′tion
sub an″co ne′us
sub″a or′tic
sub ap′i cal
sub″ap o neu rot′ic
sub a′que ous
sub″a rach′noid
sub″a re′o lar
sub″as trin′gent
sub au′ral
sub″au ric′u lar
sub brach″y ce phal′ic
sub″cal ca′re ous
sub″cal lo′sal
sub cap′su lar
sub chon′dral
sub chron′ic
sub cla‴vi an
sub cla′vi us
sub clin′i cal
sub″col lat′er al
sub″con junc ti′val
sub con′scious
sub con′scious ness
sub″con tin′u ous
sub cor′a coid
sub cor′ti cal
sub cos′tal
sub″cos tal′gi a
sub crep′i tant
sub″crep i ta′tion
sub cul′ture
sub″cu ta′neous
sub″cu tic′u lar
sub cu′tis
sub″de lir′i um
sub del′toid
sub den′tal
sub der′mic
sub″di a phrag mat′ic
sub″di vi′ded
sub dol″i cho ce phal′ic
sub duct′
sub du′ral
sub″e pen‴dy mo′ma
sub″epi the′li al
sub fas′cial
sub ga′le al
sub gle′noid
sub″glos si′tis
sub″grun da′tion
su bic″u lum
sub″in fec′tion
sub″in vo lu′tion
sub ja′cent
sub jec′tive
sub jec′to scope
sub la′tion
sub le′thal
sub′li mate
sub″li ma′tion
sub lime′
sub lim′i nal
sub li′mis
sub lin′gual

sub″lin gui′tis
sub″lux a′tion
sub″mal le′o lar
sub″man dib′u lar
sub′ma rine
sub max″il lar i′tis
sub max′il lar″y
sub men′tal
sub mes′a ti ce phal′ic
sub″mi cro scop′ic
sub mor′phous
sub″mu co′sa
sub nor′mal
sub″nor mal′i ty
sub no″to chor′dal
sub nu′cle us
sub ″nu tri′tion
sub″oc cip′i tal
sub″o per′cu lum
sub or″di na′tion
sub pap′u lar
sub par″a lyt′ic
sub″per i os′te al
sub″per i to ne′al
sub phren′ic
sub″pla cen′ta
sub″pla cen′tal
sub pu′bic
sub″sar to′ri al
sub scap′u lar
sub″scap u la′ris
sub″sen sa′tion
sub se′rous
sub sib′i lant
sub si′dence
sub sig′moid
sub sist′ence
sub spi′nous
sub′stage″
sub′stance
sub ster′nal
sub″sti tu′tion
sub sti tu″tive
sub′strate
sub sul′to ry
sub sul′tus
sub ta′lar
sub″ten to′ri al
sub″te tan′ic
sub thal′a mus
sub thy′roid ism
sub to′tal
sub tro″chan ter′ic
sub trop′i cal
sub u′ber es
sub un′gual
sub vir′ile
sub″vo lu′tion
Su′ca ryl
suc″ce da′ne ous
suc″ce dan′eum
suc cif′er ous
suc′ci nate
suc cin′ic ac′id
suc″cin yl sul″fa thi′a zole
suc″cor rhe′a
suc′cu bus
suc′cu lent
suc cur′sal
suc′cus
suc cus′sion
suck′le
suck′ling
su′crose
suc′tion
suc to′ri al
su da′men
Su dan′
su da′tion
su″da to′ri a
su″da to′ri um
su″do mo′tor

su″do re′sis
su″dor if′er ous
su″dor if′ic
su″dor i ker″a to′sis
su″dor ip′a rous
su′et
suf′fo cate
su″fo ca′tion
suf fu′sion
sug gest″i bil′i ty
sug gest′i ble
sug ges′tion ist
sug″gil la′tion
su′i cide
sul′cus
sul″fa di′a zine
sul″fa guan′i dine
sul″fa mer′a zine
sul″fa meth′a zine
sul″fa mez′a thine
Sul″fa my′lon
sul″fa nil′a mide
sul″fa pyr′a zine
sul″fa pyr′i dine
sulf ars″phen a mine′
Sul″fa sux′i dine
sul′fate
Sul″fa thal′i dine
sul″fa thi′a zole
sulf′he mo glo′bin
sulf he″mo glo″bi ne′
mia
sulf″hy′dryl
sul′fide
sul′fite
sul fon′a mide
sul′fone
sul′fo nyl
sul″fo nyl u re′a
sul′fur
sul fu′ric ac′id
sul′fu rous
Sulkowitch re a′gent
sum ma′tion
su″per ab duc′tion
su″per a cid′i ty
su″per ac tiv′i ty
su″per a cute′
su″per al″i men ta′tion
su″per cer″e bel′lar
su″per cil′i um
su″per di crot′ic
su″per dis ten′tion
su″per e′go
su″per e vac″u a′tion
su″per ex″ci ta′tion
su″per ex ten′sion
su″per fe″cun da′tion
su″per fe ta′tion
su″per fi′cial
su″per im″preg na′tion
su″per in fec′tion
su pe′ri or
su pe″ri or′i ty
su″per lac ta′tion
su″per le′thal
su″per mo′ron
su″per na′tant
su″per nu′mer ar″y
su″per pig″men ta′tion
su″per sat′u rate
su″per se cre′tion
su″per sen′si tive
su″per sen″si ti za′tion
su″per son′ic
su″per spi na′tus
su″per ve nos′i ty
su″per ven′tion
su′pi nate
su″pi na′tion
su′pi na″tor
su pine′
sup″pe da′ne ous
sup″ple men′tal

sup pos′i to″ry
sup pres′sion
sup′pu rant
sup″pu ra′tion
sup′pu ra″tive
su″pra cho′roid
su″pra cla vic′u lar
su″pra con′dy lar
su″pra con′dy lism
su″pra cos ta′lis
su″pra gle′noid
su″pra glot′tic
su″pra hy′oid
su″pra lim′i nal
su″pra mas′toid
su″pra oc clu′sion
su″pra om″pha lo dyn′i a
su″pra or′bit al
su″pra pa tel′lar
su″pra pu′bic
su″pra re′nal
su″pra re″nal ec′to my
su″pra ren′al in
su″pra re″nal op′a thy
su″pra scap′u lar
su″pra scle′ral
su″pra sel′lar
su″pra spi na′tus
su″pra spi′nous
su″pra ster′nal
su″pra ton′sil lar
su″pra troch′le ar
su″pra ver′gence
su″pra vi′tal
su′ra
sur″al i men ta′tion
surd′i ty
sur″ex ci ta′tion
sur′face
sur fac′tants
sur′geon
sur′ger y
sur′gi cal
sur′ro gate
sur″sum duc′tion
sur″sum ver′gence
sur″sum ver′sion
sur vi′vor ship
sus cep″ti bil′i ty
sus cep′ti ble
sus″cep tiv′i ty
sus′ci tate
sus pen′sion
sus pen′soid
sus″pen so′ri um
sus pen′so ry
sus″pi ra′tion
sus″ten tac′u lum
su″sur ra′tion
su sur′rus
su tu′ra
su′tur al
su′ture
sweat
swel′ling
sy co′ma
sy co′sis
Sydenham′s cho re′a
syl lab′ic
syl′la bus
syl lep″si ol′o gy
syl lep′sis
syl vat′ic plague
sym bal′lo phone
sym″bi o′sis
sym″bi ot′ic
sym bleph′a ron
sym bleph″a ro′sis
sym bo′li a
sym′bo lism
sym″bol i za′tion
Syme′s am″pu ta′tion
sy me′li a

sym met′ric
sym′me try
sym″pa ral′y sis
sym″pa thec′to my
sym path″e o neu ri′tis
sym″pa thet′ic
sym″pa thet″i co mi met′ic
sym″pa thet″i co ton′ic
sym″pa thet′o blast
sym path″i co blas to′ma
sym path″i co neu ri′tis
sym path″i cop′a thy
sym path″i co to′ni a
sym path′i co trip″sy
sym path″i co trop′ic
sym path′i cus
sym′pa thism
sym′pa thi″zer
sym path′o blast
sym path″o chro′maf fin
sym path″o go′ni a
sym path″o lyt′ic
sym path″o mi met′ic
sym′pa thy
sym pex′i on
sym phal′an gism
sym″phy o ceph′a lus
sym″phy si ec′to my
sym phys′i on
sym″phy si or′rha phy
sym phys′i o tome″
sym″phy si ot′o my
sym′phy sis
sym″phy so ske′li a
sym′plasm
sym po′di a
symp′tom
symp″to mat′ic
symp″tom a tol′o gy
symp to′sis
sym′pus
syn″ac to′sis
syn″a del′phus
Syn′a lar
syn al′gi a
syn″an as″to mo′sis
sy nan′che
syn an′the ma
syn′apse
syn ap″to lem′ma
syn″ar thro phy′sis
syn″ar thro′sis
syn can′thus
syn ceph′a lus
syn chi′li a
syn″′chon dro′sis
syn″chon drot′o my
syn′chro nism
syn′chy sis
Syn cil′lin
syn′cli tism
syn′clo nus
syn′co pal
syn′co pe
syn cyt′i al
syn cyt′i um
syn dac′tyl ism
syn dac′ty lus
syn dac′ty ly
syn′de sis
syn des″med to′pi a
syn″des mi′tis
syn des″mo cho′ri al
syn des″mo di as′ta sis
syn des′mo pex″y
syn″des mor′rha phy
syn″des mo′sis
syn″des mot′o my
syn′drome
syn ech′i a
syn ech′o tome
syn″ech ot′o my

syn″en ceph′a lo cele
syn er′e sis
syn″er get′ic
syn′der gism
syn′er gy
syn″es the′si a
syn″es the″si al′gi a
syn″gen e′si o plas″ty
Syn′ka min
Syn′ka vite
syn″ki ne′si a
syn oph′rys
syn″oph thal′mi a
syn″oph thal′mus
syn or′chid ism
syn os′che os
syn os′te o phyte″
syn′os tosed
syn″os to′sis
syn o′ti a
syn o′tus
syn″o vec′to my
syn o′vi a
syn o′vi al
syn o″vi o′ma
syn o′vi um
syn″o vi′tis
syn′ta sis
syn tax′is
syn′the sis
syn thet′ic
syn to′ci non
syn ton′ic
syn′tro phus
syn″u lo′sis
syn″u lot′ic
syph″il e′mi a
syph′i lid
syph″il i on′thus
syph′i lis
syph″i lit′ic
syph′i lo derm
syph′i loid
syph″i lol′o gist
syph″i lol′o gy
syph″i lo′ma
syph″i lo ma′ni a
syph″i lo nych′i a
syph″i lop′a thy
syph′i lo phobe″
syph″i lo pho′bia
syph″i lo phy′ma
syph″i lo ther′a py
sy rig″mo pho′ni a
sy rig′mus
syr″ing ad″e no′ma
syr″ing ad″e no′sus
syr′inge
sy rin″go bul′bi a
sy rin″go car″ci no′ma
sy rin′go cele
sy rin″go cyst′ad e no′ma
sy rin″go cys to′ma
syr″in go′ma
sy rin″go my e′li a
sy rin″go my′e lo cele″
sys so′ma
sys so′mus
sys′to le
sys tol′ic
sys trem′ma

T

tab″a co′sis
tab′a gism
Ta ban′i dae
ta bel′la
ta′bes dor sal′is
ta bet′ic

ta bet′i form
ta″bo pa ral′y sis
tab′u lar
tache
ta chet′ic
ta chis′to scope
tach′o gram
ta chog′ra phy
tach″y aux e′sis
tach″y car′di a
tach″y car′di ac
tach′y graph
ta chyg′ra phy
tach″y i a′tri a
tach″y lo′gi a
ta chym′e ter
tach″y pha′gi a
tach″y phy lax′i a
tach″yp ne′a
tach″y rhyth′mi a
tach″y sys′to le
tac′tile
tae′di um vi′tae
Tae′ni a
Tae′ni a
sag i na′ta
Tae′ni a so′li um
tae′ni a cide″
tae′ni a fuge″
tae ni′a sis
tae′ni form
tae″ni o pho′bi a
Tag′ e met
tag′ma
taint
ta lal′gi a
talc
tal′i pes
tal″i pom′a nus
tal′low
ta″lo na vic′u lar
ta′lus
tam′bour
Tam′pax
tam′pon
tam″pon ade′
tam′pon ing
tan′dive dys ki ne′ sia
tan′ gen ti′ al i ty
tan′nic ac′id
tan′nin
tan′ta lum
tan′trum
Tap′a zole
ta pe′tum
tape′worm
tap″i no ceph′a ly
tap″i o′ca
ta′pir oid
ta″pote″ment′
tar′ant ism
ta ran′tu la
ta ras′sis
ta rax′is
tare
tars ad″e ni′tis
tars al′gi a
tars ec′to my
tar si′tis
tar″so chei′lo plas″ty
tar″so ma la′ci a
tar″so met″a tar′sal
tar″so phy′ma
tar′so plas″ty
tar″sop to′si a
tar sor′rha phy
tar sot′o my
tar′sus
tar′tar
taste
tat too′ing
tau′rine
Taussig, Helen B.
tau″to me′ni al

tau tom′er al
tax′is
tax on′o my
tears
tech ni′cian
tech nique′
tec″to ceph′a ly
tec to′ri al
tec″to spi′nal
tec′tum
te′di ous
Teflon
teg′men
teg men′tal
teg men′tum
tei chop′si a
te′la
tel al′gi a
tel an″gi ec′ta sis
tel an″gi ec tat′ic
tel an″gi ec to′des
tel an″gi i′tis
tel an″gi o′ma
tel an′ gi on
tel an″gi o′sis
tel″e car′di o gram″
tel″e car′di o phone″
tel″e cep′tor
tel″e di″as tol′ic
tel″e flu″or os′co py
tel leg′o ny
tel″e ki ne′sis
tel″e lec″tro car′di o gram″
tel″e lec″tro ther″a peu′tics
tel″en ceph′a lon
tel″e ol′o gy
tel″e op′si a
tel″e o roent′gen o gram″
te lep′a thy
tel″e ra″di og′ra phy
tel″e roent″gen og′ra phy
tel″e ster″e o roent″ gen og′ra phy
tel″es the′si a
tel″e systol′ic
tel″e ther′a py
tel′o cele
tel″o den′dron
tel″og nos′sis
tel″o lec′i thal
tel″o lem′ma
tel′o phase
tel″o syn ap′sis
Tem a′ril
tem′per ance
tem′per a ture
tem′po ral
tem′po ral″is su″per fi ci al′is
tem″po ri za′tion
tem″po ro man dib′u lar
tem″po ro-oc cip′i tal
tem″po ro pa ri′e tal
tem″po ro pon′tile
tem′u lence
te na′cious
te nac′i ty
te nac′u lum
ten″di ni′tis
ten′din o plas″ty
ten′di nous
ten dol′y sis
ten″do mu′cin
ten′don
ten″do vag″i ni′tis
te nec′to my
te nes′mus
ten i′o la
ten″o de′sis
ten″o dyn′i a
ten″o fi′bril
ten″o my′o plas″ty
ten″o my ot′o my

ten″o nec′to my
ten″on i′tis
ten″o nom′e ter
te non″to my′o plas″ty
te non″to my ot′o my
ten′o phyte
ten′o pla″sty
ten or′rha phy
ten″os to′sis
ten″o syn″o vec′to my
ten″o syn″o vi′tis
ten′o tome
te not′o my
ten″o vag″i ni′tis
ten′sile
ten″si om′e ter
ten′sion
ten′si ty
ten′sive
ten′sor
ten′sure
ten′ta tive
ten tig′i nous
ten to′ri um
ten′u ate
ten u′i ty
ten′u ous
teph″ro my″e li′tis
tep′id
ter″a mor′phous
te′ras
ter′a tism
ter″a to car″ci no′ma
ter″a tog′e ny
ter′a toid
ter″a tol′a gy
ter″a to′ma
ter″a to pho′bi a
ter″a to′sis
ter″a to zo o sper′mi a
ter″e bra che′sis
te′res
ter′mi nal
ter″mi nol′o gy
ter′na ry
ter′pin hy′drate
Ter″ra my′cin
ter′tian
ter′ti ar ism
ter′ti ar″y
ter tip′a ra
tes′ti cle
tes tic′u lar
tes′tis
tes tos′te rone
tet′a nal
te tan′i form
tet″a nig′e nous
tet″a nil′la
tet′a nism
tet″a ni za′tion
tet′a node
tet′a noid
tet″a no ly′sin
tet″a no ly′sis
tet″a nome′e ter
tet″a no mo′tor
tet″a no pho′bi a
tet″a no spas′min
tet′a nus
tet′a ny
te tar″ta no′pi a
te tar′to cone
te tar″to co′nid
tet″ra bra′chi us
tet″ra chei′rus
tet″ra cy′cline
Te′tra cyn
tet″ra dac′tyl
tet″ra eth′yl
tet″ra gen′ic
te trag′e nous

te′tral o gy of Fallot
tet″ra mas′ti a
tet″ra mas′ti gote
tet″ra ma′zi a
te tram′er ism
tet″ra nop′si a
tet″ra ploid
tet″ra pus
te tras′ce lus
tet″ra so′mic
tet″ra sti chi′a sis
tex′ti form
tex″to blas′tic
tex′ture
tha lam′ic
thal″a mo cor′ti cal
thal″a mo len tic′u lar
thal″a mo mam′mil lar″y
thal″a mo teg men′tal
thal″a mot′o my
thal″a mus
tha las se′ mi a
tha las″so pho′bi a
tha las″so ther′a py
thal′li um
thal″lo tox″i co′sis
tha mu′ri a
than″a to bi″o log′ic
than″a to gno mon′ic
than″a tog′ra phy
than′a toid
than″a tol′o gy
than″a to ma′ni a
than″a to pho′bi a
than′a top sy
than′a tos
thau′ma trope
the′ca
the ci′tis
the′co dont
the co′ma
the″co steg no′sis
the′e lin
the lal′gi a
the lar′che
the las′is
the″la zi′a sis
the′le plas″ty
the li′tis
the′li um
the lon′cus
the″lo phleb″o stem′ma
the″lor rha′gi a
the′lo thism
thel″y ot′o ky
the′nar
the″o ma′ni a
the″ o pho′bi a
the″o phyl′line
the″o ple′gi a
the″o ret′ical
the′o ry
ther″a peu′tic
ther′a pist
ther′a py
ther″en ceph′a lous
The″ri di′i dae
the″ri od′ic
the″ri o′ma
the″ri o mim′ic ry
ther′mal
ther″mal ge′si a
ther″ma tol′o gy
therm″es the′si a
therm″es the″si om′e ter
ther′mic
ther′mite
ther″mo an″al ge′si a
ther″mo an″es the′si a
ther″mo cau′ter y
ther″mo chem′is try
ther″mo chro′ism

ther″mo co ag″u la′tion
ther′mo cou″ple
ther″mo dur′ric
ther″mo dy nam′ics
ther″mo ex ci′to ry
ther″mo gen′ic
ther mog′e nous
ther″mo hy″per al ge′si a
ther″mo hy″per es the′si a
ther″mo hy″pes the′si a
ther″mo in hib′i to″ry
ther″mo la′bile
ther mol′y sis
ther mom′e ter
ther″mo met′ric
ther mom″e try
ther″mo neu ro′sis
ther moph′a gy
ther′mo phile
ther″mo phil′ic
ther″mo pho′bi a
ther′mo phore
ther″mo phyl′ic
ther′mo pile
ther″mo ple′gi a
ther″mo pol″yp ne′a
ther″mo reg″u la′tion
ther′mo scope
ther′mo sta′ble
ther′mo stat
ther″mo ste re′sis
ther″mo sys tal′tic
ther″mo tax′is
ther″mo ther′a py
ther″mo to nom′e ter
ther″mo tox′in
ther″mo tra″che ot′o my
ther mot′ro pism
the′ro morph
the″ro mor′phi a
the sau″ris mo′sis
the′sis
thi′a mine
thigh
thi″o cy′a nate
thi′o nine
thi″o phil′ic
thi″o sul′fate
thi″o u′ra cil
thi″o u re′a
tho″ra cec′to my
tho″ra cen te′sis
tho rac′ic
tho″ra co a ceph′a lus
tho″ra co a cro′mi al
tho″ra co ce los′chi sis
tho″ra co cyl lo′sis
tho″ra co cyr to′sis
tho″ra co dyn′i a
tho″ra co gas″tro did′y mus
tho″ra co gas tros′ chi sis
tho″ra co lap″a rot′o my
tho′ra co lum′bar
tho″ra com′e lus
tho″ra cop′a gus
tho″ra co par″a ceph′a lus
tho′ra co plas″ty
tho″ra cos′chi sis
tho ra′co scope
tho″ra cos′co py
tho″ra cos′to my
tho″ra cot′o my
tho″ra del′phus
tho′rax
Tho′ra zine
tho′ri um
Thornton, M. L.
Tho′ro trast
thre′o nine
threp sol′o gy
thresh′oid
thrill

thrix an″nu la′ta
throm′base
throm″bas the′ni a
throm bec′to my
throm′bin
throm″bo an″gi i′tis
throm″bo ar″te ri′tis
throm′bo blast
throm boc′la sis
throm′bo cyte
throm″bo cy the′mi a
throm″bo cy′to crit
throm″bo cy″to ly′sin
throm″bo cy″to path′i a
throm″bo cy″to pe′ni a
throm″bo cy″to pe′nic
throm″bo cy to′sis
throm″bo em″bo li′sm
throm″bo em″bo li za′tion
throm″bo en″dar ter ec′to my
throm″bo en″do car di′tis
throm″bo gen′ic
throm″bo kin′ase
throm″bo lym″phan gi′tis
throm bol″y sis
throm bop′a thy
throm″bo pe′ni a
throm″bo phil′i a
throm″bo phle bi′tis
throm″bo plas′tic
throm″bo plas′tin
throm″bo plas tin′o gen
throm″bo plas″tin o pe′ni a
throm″bo poi e′sis
throm′bose
throm′bosed
throm bo′sis
throm″bo sta′sis
throm bot′ic
throm′bo zym
throm′bus
thrush
thumb
thyme
thy mec′to my
thy″mer ga′si a
thy′mic
thy′mi on
thy mi′tis
thy′mo cyte
thy″mo ke′sis
thy′mol
thy mo′ma
thy″mo no′ic
thy mop′a thy
thy′mo pex″y
thy″mo priv′ic
thy′mus
thy″re o gen′ic
thy″ro ad″e ni′tis
thy″ro ar″y te′noid
thy″ro car′di ac
thy′ro cele
thy″ro chon drot′o my
thy″ro cri cot′o my
thy″ro ep″i glot′tic
thy rog′en ous
thy″ro glob′u lin
thy″ro glos′sal
thy″ro hy′al
thy′ro hy′oid
thy′roid
thy″roid ec′to my
thy′roid ism
thy″roid i′tis
thy″roid i za′tion
thy″roid ot′o my
thy roid″o tox′in
thy″ro par″a thy″roid ec′to my
thy″ro phar yn ge′us
thy″ro pri′val
thy″ro pri′vus

thy″ro pro′te in
thy″rop to″sis
thy ro′sis
thy″ro ther′a py
thy rot′o my
thy″ro tox′ic
thy″ro tox″i co″sis
thy″ro tox′in
thy″ro tro′pic
thy rot′ro pin
thy rox′in
tib′i a
tib′i al
tib″i al′gi a
tib″i a″lis
tib″i o fib′u lar
tic
tic dou″lou reux′
tick′ling
tic tol′o gy
ti groid
tim′bre
tinc′ture
tine test
tin′e a
tin ni′tus
ti″queur′
tis′sue
ti ta′ni um
ti′ter
tit″il la′tion
titra′tion
tit″u ba′tion
toad′head″
to coph′er ol
to′cus
To′fran il
tok″o dy″na mom′e ter
tok′o graph
to kog′ra phy
tok″o ma′ni a
to kom′e try
tok″o pho′bi a
tol′er ance
tol′er ant
tol′u ene
to lu′i dine
Tome's fi′bers
to′mo gram
to mog′ra phy
to″na pha′si a
tongue
tongue′tie
to nic′i ty
ton″i co clon′ic
ton″i tro pho′bi a
to″no fi′brils
to′no gram
to′no graph
to nom′e ter
to′no plasts
to nos″cil log′ra phy
to no scope
ton′sil
ton′sil lar
ton″sil lec′tome
ton″sil lec′ to my
ton′sil li′tis
ton sil′lo lith
ton sil′lo tome
ton″sil lot′o my
ton sil″lo ty′phoid
ton″sil sec′tor
ton′sure
to′nus
top″ag no′sis
to pal′gi a
to pec′to my
top″es the′si a
to pha′ceous
to′phus
top″o an″es the′si a

top″og nos′tic
to pog′ra phy
top ol′o gy
top″o nar co′sis
top″o neu ro′sis
top″o pho′bi a
top′o phone
Torek's op″er a′tion
tor′mi na
tor′mi nal
tor pes′cence
tor′pid
tor′por
torque
tor″si om′e ter
tor′sion
tor′sive
tor″si ver′sion
tor′so
tor″soc clu′sion
tor″ti col′lar
tor″ti col′lis
tor′tu ous
Tor′u la
tor″u lo′sis
tor′u lus
to′rus
to tip′o tence
tour′ni quet
tox′o phene
tox e′mi a
tox e′mic
tox′ic
tox′i cant
tox′i cide
tox ic′ity
tox″i co den′drol
tox″i co der′ma
tox″i co der″ma ti′tis
tox″i co der″ma to′sis
tox″i co gen′ic
tox′i coid
tox″i col″o gist
tox″i col′o gy
tox″i co ma′ni a
tox″i co path′ic
tox″i co pho′bi a
tox″i co′sis
tox if′er ous
tox″i ge nic′i ty
tox ig′e nous
tox′in
tox″in fec′tion
tox in′i cide
tox″i ther′a py
tox″i tu ber′cu lide
tox′oid
tox′o phil
tox′o phore
Tox″o plas′ma
tox″o plas′min
tox″o plas mo″sis
tra bec′u la
tra′cer
tra′che a
tra″che a ec′ta sy
tra″che al′gi a
tra″che i′tis
trach″e lag′ra
trach″e lec′to my
trach″e le″ma to′ma
trach″e lis′mus
trach″e li′tis
trach″e lo cyl lo′sis
trach″e lo dyn′i a
tra″che lo mas′toid
trach″e lo par″a si′tus
trach″e lo pex′i a
trach″e lo plas′ty
trach″e lor′rha phy
trach″e lor rhec′tes
trach″e los′chi sis

trach″e lo syr″in gor′rha phy
trach″e lot′o my
tra″che o blen″nor rhe′a
tra″che o bron″chi al
tra″che o bron chi′tis
tra″che o bron chos′co py
tra′che o cele
tra″che o e″soph a ge′al
tra″che o fis′sure
tra″che o la ryn′ge al
tra″che or lar″yn got′o my
tra′che oph′o ny
tra′che o plas″ty
tra″che o py o′sis
tra″che or rha′gi a
tra″che or′rha phy
tra″che os′chi sis
tra′che os′co py
tra″che o ste no′sis
tra″che os′to my
tra′che o tome
tra″che ot′o mist
tra″che ot′o mize
tra″che ot′o my
tra″chi el co′sis
tra″ chi el′cus
tra cho′ma
tra″chy o nych′i a
tra″chy pho′ni a
tract
trac′tion
trac tot′o my
trac′tus
tra′gi
tra′gi cus
trag′o mas chal′i a
tra′gus
trait
trance
tran′quil iz″er
trans ac′tion al
trans am i nase
trans au′di ent
trans ca′lent
trans cav′i tar″y
trans″ce den′tal
trans con′dy lar
trans″de am″i na′tion
trans duc′tion
tran sec′tion
trans fer′ence
trans fer′rin
trans fix′ion
trans″fo ra′tion
trans′for a″tor
trans″for ma′tion
trans form″er
trans fuse′
trans fu′sion
tran′sient
trans il′i ac
trans″il lu″mi na′tion
tran sis′tor
tran si′tion al
trans lu′cent
trans lu′cid
trans″mi gra′tion′
trans mis″si bil′i ty
trans mis′sion
trans mit′tance
trans′o nance
trans par′ent
tran spi′ra ble
tran″spi ra′tion
trans′plant
trans″plan ta′tion
trans pose′
trans″po si′tion
trans sa′cral
trans″sub stan″ti a′tion
tran′su date
tran″su da′tion

trans″u re′thral
trans vag′inal
trans″ver sa′lis
trans verse′
trans″ver sec′to my
trans ver′sus
trans ves′ti tism
Tran′xene
tra pe′zi um
tra pe′zi us
trap′e zoid
trau′ma
trau mat′ic
trau′ma tism
trau′ma tize
trau″ma tol′o gy
trau″ma top′a thy
trau″ma top ne′a
trau″ma to′sis
trav′ail
treat
tre′a
Treitz
Trem″a to′da
trem′bles
trem′o gram
trem′o graph
tre″mo la′bile
trem′o lo
tre′mo pho′bi a
trem′or
trem″o sta′ble
trem″u la′tion
trem′u lous
Trendelenburg po sit′ion
trep′a nize
tre pan′ing
tre phine′
tre phin′ing
trep′idant
trep″i da′ti o
trep″i da′tion
Trep″o ne′ma
trep″o ne″ma to′sis
trep″o ne mi′a sis
trep″o ne″mi cid′al
trep op′ne a
tri″acet yl ole an″do my′cin
tri′ad
tri age′
tri″a kai″di ka pho′bi a
tri′an″gle
Tri at′o ma
trib′ade
tri bra′chi us
tri cel′lu lar
tri ceph′a lus
tri′ceps
trich″an gi ec ta′si a
trich″a tro′phi a
trich″es the′si a
trich i′a sis
Tri chi′na
Trich″i nel′la
trich″i no pho′bi a
trich″i no′sis
trich i′tis
tri chlo″ro a ce′tic
tri chlo″ro eth′yl ene
trich″o be′zoar
trich″o car′di a
trich″o clas ma′ni a
trich″o cryp to′sis
trich′o cyst
trich″o ep″i the″li o′ma
trich″o es the′si a
trich″o es the″si om′e ter
trich′o gen
trich″o glos′si a
trich″o hy′a lin
trich′oid
trich′o lith

trich″o lo′gi a
trich ol′o gy
trich o′ma
tri cho″ma de′sis
trich o′ma tose
trich″o ma to′sis
trich′ome
trich″o mo′na cide
trich″o mo′nad
Trich″o mo′nas
Trich″o my ce′tes
trich″o my co′sis
trich″o no′sis
trich″o path″a pho′bi a
trich op′a thy
trich oph′a gy
trich″o pho′bi a
trich″o phy′ta
trich″o phy′tid
trich″o phy′tin
trich″o phy″to be′zoar
Trich″o phy′ton
trich″o phy to′sis
trich″or rhe′a
trich″or rhex′is
trich″or rhex″o ma′ni a
trich o′sis
Trich″o spo′ron
trich″o spo ro′sis
trich″o sta′sis spin″u lo′sa
trich″o stron″gy li′a sis
Trich″o stron′gy lus
trich″o til″lo ma′ni a
tri chot′o my
trich″o zo′a
tri′chro ism
tri′chro mat
tri″chro mat′ic
tri″chro ma top′si a
tri chro′mic
trich″u ri′a sis
Trich u′ris
Trich u′ris trich′i u ra
tri′cro tism
tri′cro tism
tri cus′pid
tri dac′tyl
tri′dent
tri den′tate
tri der′mic
Tri′di one
trid′y mus
tri eth″yl a mine′
tri fa′cial
tri′fid
tri fo″li o′sis
tri″fur ca′tion
tri gas′tric
tri gas′tri cus
tri gem′i nal
tri gem′i nus
tri gem′i ny
tri gen′ic
tri′gone
tri′go nid
tri″go ni′tis
trig″o no ceph′a lus
trig″o no ceph′a ly
tri go′num
Tri lene
tri lo′bate
tri loc′u lar
tri man′u al
tri men′su al
tri mes′ter
tri″oceph′a lus
tri′oph thal′mos
tri″o pod′y mus
tri or′chid
tri or′chis
tri′o tus
trip″a ra

tri″pha lan′gi al
tri phas′ic
tri ple′gi a
trip′let
trip″lo blas′tic
tri ploi′dy
trip″lo ko′ri a
trip lo′ pi a
tri pro′so pus
trip′sis
tri que′trum
tri sac′cha ride
tris′mus
tri so′mus
tri′so my
tris″ti chi′a sis
tris″ti ma′ni a
tris′tis
trit″an o′pi a
trit′u rate
tro′car
tro chan′ter
tro′ che
troch′le a
troch′le ar
troch″le a′ris
troch″o car′di a
troch″o ceph′a lus
troch″o gin′gly mus
tro′choid
Trom bic′u la
trom bic″u lo′sis
trom″o ma′ni a
tro pe′sis
tro″phe de′ma
troph′e sy
troph′ic
tro phic′i ty
troph′ism
tro′pho blast
tro′pho cyte
tro′pho derm
tro″pho dy nam′ics
tro″pho neu ro′sis
tro phop′a thy
tro″pho spon′gi um
tro″pho tax′is
tro″pho ther′a py
tro″pho trop′ic
tro phot′ro pism
tro″pho zo′ite
tro′pism
tro pom′e ter
tro′po sphere
Trousseau′s sign
trun′cat ed
trun′cus
truss
tryp′a nide
Tryp″a no so′ma
try pan′ o some
tryp″a no so mi′a sis
try pan′ o so mide″
tryp ars′ amide
tryp′sin
tryp sin′o gen
tryp′tase
tryp′to phan
tset′se fly
tsu″tsu ga mu′shi fe′ver
tu′bage
tu′bal
tu bec′to my
tu′ber
tu′ber cle
tu ber′cu lar
tuber′cu la″ted
tuber″cu la′tion
tu ber′cu lid
tu ber′cu lin
tu ber″cu lo der′ma
tu ber″cu lo fi′broid

tu ber′cu loid
tu ber″cu lo′ma
tu ber″cu lo pho′bi a
tu ber″cu lo sil″i co′sis
tu ber″cu lo′sis
tu ber′cu lous
tu ber′cu lum
tu″ber os′i tas
tu″ber os′i ty
tu′ber ous
tu″bo ab dom′i nal
tu″bo ad nex′o pex″y
tu″bo cu ra′re
tu″bo lig″a men′tous
tu″bo-o va″ri ot′o my
tu″bo per″i to ne′al
tu″bo plas′ty
tu″bo u′ter ine
tu″bo vag′i nal
tu′bular
tu′bule
tu″bu li za′tion
tu″bu lo al ve′o lar
tu′bu lo cyst″
tu′bu lus
tu′bus
Tu′i nal
tu″la re′mi a
tu″me fa′cient
tu″me fac′tion
tu′me fy
tu men′ti a
tu mes′cence
tu mes′cent
tu′mid
tu mid′i ty
tu′mor
tu″mor i gen′ic
tu′mor ous
tu mul′tus
Tun′ga
tun gi′ a sis
tung′sten
tu′ni ca
tun′nel
tur′bid
tur″bi dim′e ter
tur′bi nate
tur′bi na″ted
tur″bi nec′to my
tur′bi no tome″
tur″bi not′o my
tur ges′cence
tur ges′cent
tur′gid
tur′gor
tur′pen tine
tur″ri ceph′a ly
tus′sal
tus′sis
tus′sive
tweez′ers
twitch′ing
tyl′i on
ty lo′ma
ty lo′sis
ty″lo ste re′sis
tym″pa nec′to my
tym pan′ic
tym′pa nism
tym″pa ni′tes
tym″pa nit′ic
tym″pa ni′tis
tym″pa no mas′toid
tym″pa no mas″toid i′tis
tym″pa no plas′ty
tym″pa no scle ro′sis
tym″pa no′sis
tym″pa no sta pe′di al
tym″pa no sym″pa thec′to my
tym″pa not′o my
tym′pa nous

tym′pa num
tym′pa ny
typh″lec ta′si a
typh lec′to my
typh len″ter i′tis
typh li′tis
typh″lo di″cli di′tis
typh″lo em″py e′ma
typh′loid
typh″lo lex′i a
typh″lo li thi′a sis
typh″lo meg′a ly
typh″lo pto′sis
typh lo′sis
typh″lo spasm
typh″lo ste no′sis
typh los′ to my
ty″pho bac′te rin
ty′phoid
ty″pho ma′ni a
ty″pho pneu mo′ni a
ty′phus
typ′i cal
ty′po scope
tyr′an nism
ty rem′e sis
ty′roid
ty′ro sin ase
ty′ro sine

U

ud′der
u lag″a nac′te sis
u″la tro′phi a
ul′cer
ul′cer ate
ul″cer a′tion
ul′cer a″tive
ul″cer o mem′bra nous
ul′cus
u″le gy′ri a
u ler″y the′ma
u let′ic
u li′tis
ul′na
ul′nar
ul no car′pe us
u loc′a ce
u″lo der″ma ti′tis
u″lo glos si′tis
u′loid
u″lor rha′gi a
u lo′sis
u lot′ic
u lot′o my
ul″ti mo gen′i ture
ul″tra brach″y ce phal′ic
ul″tra cen′tri fuge
ul″tra fil′ter
ul″tra fil tra′tion
ul″tra mi′cro scope
ul″tra phag″o cy to′sis
ul″tra red′
ul″tra son′ic
ul″tra son′o gram
ul″tra son og′ra phy
ul″tra son″o scope
ul″tra struc′ture
ul″tra vi′rus
ul″tra vi′o let
um′ber
um″bi lec′to my
um bil′i cal
um bil′i cate
um bil″i ca′tion
um bil′i cus
um′bo
un′ci form
un′ci nate

un″ci pi″si for′mis
un con′scious
unc′tion
unc′tu ous
un′cus
un dec″y len′ic ac′id
un dine′
un′du lant
un″du la′tion
un′du la to″ry
un guen′tum
un′guis
un′gu la
un′gu late
u″ni ar tic′u lar
u″ni cam′er al
u″ni cel′lu lar
u″ni cen′tral
u″ni cor′nous
u″ni cus′pid
u″ni fa mil′i al
u″ni fi′lar
u″ni grav′ida
u″ni lat′er al
u″ni lo′bar
u″ni loc′u lar
u″ni nu′cle ar
u″ni oc′u lar
u″ni o′val
u″ni ov′u lar
u nip′a ra
u″ni par′i ens
u nip′a rous
u″ni po′lar
u″ni sex′u al
u′ni tar″y
u″ni va′lent
un or′gan ized
un sat′u ra″ted
un sex′
un stri′a ted
un well′
u ra′chal
u ra′chus
u″ra cra′si a
u ra′ni um
u″ra no col″o bo′ma
u′ra no plas″ty
u″ra no ple′gi a
u″ra nor′rha phy
u″ra nos′chi sis
u″ra no staph′y lo plas″ty
u″ra no staph″y lor′rha phy
u″ra ro′ma
u′rate
u″ra tu′ri a
u re′a
u″re am′e ter
u″re am′e try
u″re de′ma
u re′mi a
u re′mic
u re″si es the′si a
u re′ter
u re″ter ec′ta sis
u re″ter ec′to my
u re″ter i′tis
u re′ter o cele
u re″ter o ce lec′to my
u re″ter o co los′to my
u re″ter o cys′tic
u re″ter o cys tos′to my
u re″ter o en ter′ic
u re″ter o en″ter os′to my
u re″ter og′ra phy
u re″ter o hem″i ne phrec′to my
u re″ter o hy″dro ne phro′sis
u re″ter o in tes′ti nal
u re′ter o lith
u re″ter o li thi′a sis
u re″ter o li thot′o my
u re″ter ol′y sis

u re″ter o ne″o cys tos′to my
u re″ter o ne″o py″e los′to my
u re″ter o ne phrec′to my
u re″ter o pel′vic
u re″ter o pel′vi o plas″ty
u re′ter o plas′ty
u re″ter o py″e log′ra phy
u re″ter o py″e lo ne os′to my
u re″ter o py″e lo ne phri′tis
u re″ter o py″e lo ne phros′to my
u re″ter o py″e lo plas′ty
u re″ter o py″e los′to my
u re″ter or rha′gi a
u re″ter or′rha phy
u re″ter o sig″moid os′to my
u re″ter os′to my
u re″ter ot′o my
u re″ter o u re′ter al
u re″ter o u re″ter os′to my
u re″ter o u′ter ine
u re″ter o vag′i nal
u re′ter o ves′ical
u′re thane
u re′thra
u re′thral
u″re threc′to my
u″re thri′tis
u re″thro bulb′ar
u re′thro cele
u re″thro cys ti′tis
u re′thro gram
u re′thro graph
u″re throg′ra phy
u″re throm′e ter
u re″thro phy′ma
u re′thro plas″ty
u re″thro pro stat′ic
u″re thror′rha phy
u re″thror rhe′a
u re′thro scope
u″re thros′co py
u re′thro spasm
u re″thro ste no′sis
u″re thros′to my
u re′thro tome
u″re throt′o my
u re″thro tri″go ni′tis
u re″thro vag′i nal
ur′gen cy
ur″hi dro′sis
u′ric
u′ri nal
u″ri nal′y sis
u″ri na′ry
u′ri nate
u″ri na′tion
u′rine
u″ri nif′er ous
u″ri nif′ic
u″ri nip′a rous
u″ri no cry os′co py
u″ri no gen′i tal
u″ri nog′e nous
u″ri nol′o gy
u″ri no′ma
u″ri nom′e ter
u″ri nom′e try
u″ri no scop′ic
u′ri nose
u″ri sol′vent
u ri′tis
ur′ning
u″ro ac″i dim′e ter
u″ro bi′lin
u″ro bi″li ne′mi a
u″ro bi″lin ic′ter us
u″ro bi lin′o gen
u″ro bi″li nu′ri a
u roch′e ras
u″ro che′si a
u′ro chrome

u″ro chro′mo gen
u″ro clep′si a
u″ro cris′i a
u″ro cy an′o gen
u″ro cy″a no′sis
u″ro gen′i tal
u rog′e nous
u′ro gram
u rog′ra phy
u′ro lith
u″ro li thi′a sis
u″ro li thol′o gy
u″ro lith ot′o my
u rol′o gist
u rol′o gy
u rom′e lus
u″ro nos′co py
u rop′a thy
u″ro por′phy rin
u″ro por″phy rin′o gen
u″ror rha′gi a
u ros′che sis
u ros′co py
u″ro sep′sis
u ro tro′pin
u″ro tox′ic
ur″ti ca′ri a
ur′ti cate
ur″ti ca′tion
u′ter ine
u″ter is′mus
u″ter i′tis
u″ter o ab dom′i nal
u″ter o cer′vi cal
u″ter o col′ic
u″ter o ges ta′tion
u″ter og′ra phy
u″ter o in tes′ti nal
u″ter o ma′ni a
u″ter om′e ter
u″ter o-o va′ri an
u″ter o pa ri′e tal
u″ter o pel′vic
u″ter o pla cen′tal
u′ter o plas″ty
u″ter o rec′tal
u″ter o sa′cral
u″ter o sal″pin gog′ra phy
u′ter o scope″
u″ter o ton′ic
u″ter o trac′tor
u″ter o tu′bal
u″ter o vag′i nal
u″ter o ven′tral
u″ter o ves′i cal
u′ter us
u′tri cle
u tri′ cu lar
u tric″u li′tis
u tric″u lo sac′cu•lar
u′ve a
u″ve i′tis
u″ve o pa rot′id
u′vi o lize″
u″vi o re sist′ant
u′vu la
u′vu lae
u″vu lec′to my
u″vu li′tis
u″vu lop to′sis
u′vu lo tome
u″vu lot′o my

V

vac′ci na ble
vac′ci nal
vac′ci nate
vac″ci na′tion
vac′cine
vac cin′i a

vac cin'i form
vac cin"i o'la
vac'ci noid
vac"ci no pho'bi a
vac'ci no style"
vac"ci no ther'a py
vac'u o lar
vac'u o late
vac'u o la"ted
vac"u o la'tion
vac'u ole
vac'u ome
vac'u um
va'gal
va gi'na
vag'i nal
vag"i nec'to my
vag"i nic'o line
vag"i nif' er ous
vag"i nis'mus
vag"i ni'tis
vag'i no cele
vag"i no dyn'i a
vag"i no fix a'tion
vag"i no my co'sis
vag'i no plas"ty
vag'i no scope
vag"i nos'co py
vag"i not'o my
va gi'tus
va got'o mized
va got'o my
va"go to'ni a
va"go trop'ic
va'gus
va'lence
val"e tu"di na'ri an ism
val'gus
val'ine
Val'i um
val lec'u la
Valsalva's test
valve
val vot'o my
val'vu la
val'vu lar
val"vu li'tis
val' vu lo plas" ty
val'vu lo tome
val"vu lot'o my
vam'pire
vam'pir ism
van"co my'cin
va nil'la
va"po cau"ter i za'tion
va"por i za'tion
va"ri a bil'i ty
va'ri ant
var"i ca'tion
var"i cec'to my
var"i cel'la
var"i cel la'tion
var"i cel'li form
var"i cel'loid
var'i ces
va ric'i form
var"i co bleph'a ron
var'i co cele"
var"i co ce lec'to my
var"i cog'ra phy
var'i coid
var"i co phle bi'tis
var'i cose
var"i co'sis
var"i cos'i ty
var"i cot'o my
va ric'u la
Var'i dase
va'ri form
va ri'o la
va ri'o lar
var'i o late

var″i o′li form
var′i o loid
var′ix
va′rus
vas
vas′cu lar
vas″ cu lar i za′tion
vas″cu li′tis
vas def′e rans
vas ec′to my
vas″i fac′tion
vas i′tis
vas″o con stric′tion
vas″o con stric′tive
vas″o con stric′tor
vas″o de pres′sor
vas″o dil″a ta′tion
vas″o di la′tor
vas″o ep″i did″y mos′to my
vas″o for ma′tion
va″so gen′ic
va sog′ra phy
vas″o in hib′i tor
vas″o li ga′tion
vas″o mo′tion
vas″o mo′tor
vas″o neu ro′sis
vas″o-or″chid os′to my
vas″o pa ral′y sis
vas″o pa re′sis
vas″o pres′sor
va″so pres′sin
vas″o re″lax a′tion
vas or′rha phy
vas″o sec′tion
vas′o spasm
vas″o stim′u lant
vas os′to my
vas ot′o my
vas″o ton′ic
vas″o to′nin
vas″o troph′ic
vas″o va′gal
vas″o vas os′to my
vas″o ve sic″u lec′to my
vas′tus
Vater,
  am pul′la of
vec′tion
vec′tis
vec′tor
vec″tor car′di o gram″
vec″tor car′di o graph
ve′hi cle
vein
ve la′men
vel″a men′tum
vel′li cate
vel″li ca′tion
ve′lum
ve′na ca′va
ve na′tion
ven ec′to my
ven″e nif′er ous
ve ne′re al
ve ne″re ol′o gy
ve ne″re o pho′bi a
ven′er y
ven″e sec′tion
ven″e su′ture
ven″i punc′ture
ve noc′ly sis
ve″no con stric′tion
ve′no gram
ve nog′ra ph
ven og′ra phy
ven′om
ven″o mo sal′i var″y
ve″no mo′tor
ve″no per″i to ne os′to my
ve″no pres′sor
ve″no scle ro′sis
ve nos′i ty
ve″no sta′sis

ve″no throm bot′ic
ve not′o my
ve′nous
ve″no ve nos′to my
vent′er
ven′ti late
ven″ti la′tion
ven″ti lom′e ter
ven′tral
ven′tri cle
ven tric′u lar
ven tric″u li′tis
ven tric″u lo cis″ter nos′to my
ven tric″u lo cor dec′to my
ven tric′u lo gram″
ven tric″u log′ra phy
ven tric″u lo mas″toid os′to my
ven tric″u lom′e try
ven tric″u lo punc′ture
ven tric′u lo scope″
ven tric″u los′co py
ven tric″u los′to my
ven tric″u lo sub″ a rach′noid
ven tric′u lus
ven″tri duc′tion
ven tril′o quism
ven″tri me′sal
ven″tro fix a′tion
ven″tro hys′ter o pex″y
ven″tro lat′er al
ven″tro me′di an
ven tros′co py
ven′trose
ven tros′i ty
ven″tro sus pen′sion
ven″tro ves″i co fix a′tion
ven tu′ri me″ter
ven′ule
ve ra′trum vi′ri de
ver big″er a′tion
ver′gen ces
ver″mi ci′dal
ver′mi cide
ver mic′u lar
ver mic′u late
ver mic″u la′tion
ver mic′u lose
ver′mi form
ver′mi fuge
ver″mi lin′gual
ver′min
ver″mi na′tion
ver′min ous
ver″mi pho′bi a
ver′mis
ver′nal
ver′nix ca″se o′sa
ver ru′ca
ver ru′ci form
ver′ru coid
ver′ru cose
ver′si col″or
ver′sion
ver′te bra
ver″te bro te′ri al
Ver″te bra′ta
ver′te brate
ver″te brec′to my
ver″te bro di dym′i a
ver′tex
ver′ti cal
ver′ti cil
ver tig′i nous
ver′ti go
ver″u mon″ta ni′tis
ver″u mon ta′num
ve sa′ni a
ves′i ca
ves′i cal
ves′i cant
ves″i ca′tion
ves′i ca to″ry

ves′i cle
ves″i co pro stat′ic
ves″i cot′o my
ves″i co u′ter ine
ve sic′u la
ve sic′u lar
ve sic′u lase
ve sic″u la′tion
ve sic″u lec′to my
ve sic″u li′tis
ve sic″u lo bul′lous
ve sic′u lo gram″
ve sic″u log′ra phy
ve sic″u lo pap′u lar
ve sic″u lo pus′tu lar
ve sic″u lot′o my
ves′sel
ves ti′bu lar
ves′ti bule
ves tib″u lot′o my
ves′tige
ves tig′i um
ves″ti men′tum mor′tis
ve′ta
vet″er i na′ri an
vet′er i nar″y
vi′a ble
vi′al
Vi″ bra my′ cin
vi bra′tion
vi′bra to″ry
Vib′ri o
vi bris′sa
vi brom′e ter
vi car′i ous
vid″e og no′sis
vib″il am′bu lism″
vig′i lance
vil li′tis
vil″lo si′tis
vil′lous
vil′lus
vil″lus ec′to my
vin′cu lum
Vi′ne thene
vi′nyl
Vi o′form
vi″o la′tion
vi′per
vir′al
vi re′mi a
vir′gin
vir′gin al
vir gin′i ty
vir′ile
vir″i les′cence
vir′i lism
vi ril′i ty
vi′ri ons
vi rip′o tent
vi rol′o gist
vi rol′o gy
vir′u lence
vir″u lif′er ous
vi′rus
vi′rus cytes″
vis′ce ra
vis′ce ral
vis″cer al′gi a
vis″cer o in hib′i to″ry
vis″cer o meg′a ly
vis″cer op to′sis
vis″cer o sen′so ry
vis′cer o tome
vis″cer ot′o my
vis″cer o to′ni a
vis″cer o troph′ic
vis′cid
vis′co li″zer
vis″co sim′e ter
vis cos′i ty
vis′cous

vis′cus
vis′i ble
vi′sion
vis″u al i za′tion
vis″u o au′di to″ry
vis″u og no′sis
vis″u om′e ter
vis″u o psy′chic
vis″u o sen′so ry
vi′sus
Vis′ ta ril
vi′tal
vi′tal ism
vi tal′i ty
vi′tal ize
Vi tal′li um
vi′tals
vi′ta min
vi′ta zyme″
vit′el lar″y
vi tel′li cle
vi tel′lin
vi tel″lo lu′te in
vi tel″lo mes″en ter′ic
vi tel″lo ru′bin
vi tel′lus
vi″ti a′tion
vit″i lig′i nous
vit″i li′go
vi til′i goid
vit′re in
vit″re o den′tin
vit′re ous
vi tres′cence
vit′re um
vi tri′na
vit′ri ol
vit ri′tis
vit″ro pres′sion
vit′rum
viv″i dif fu′sion
viv″i fi ca′tion
vi vip′a rous
viv″i sec′tion
viv″i sec′tion ist
viv′i sec″tor
vo′cal
vo cal′is
void
vo′la
vol′a tile
vo le′mic
Volkmann′s con trac′ture
Vollmer patch test
vol sel′la
volt
volt′age
volt′a gram″
vol tam′e ter
volt′am″me ter
volt′-am′pere
volt′me″ter
vol′ume
vol″u met′ric
vol′vu lus
vo′mer
vom″er o na′sal
vom′it
vom′i to″ry
vom″i tu ri′tion
vom′i tus
vo ra′cious
Vorhees
vor′tex
vor′ti cose
vox
vo″yeur′
vo″ yeur′ ism
vu″e rom e ter
vul′can ize
vul′ner a ble
vul′ner ar″y

vul′va
vul vec′to my
vul vi′tis
vul″vo vag″i ni′tis

W

wad′ding
wad′dle
waist
wake′ful ness
Wangensteen′s suc′tion
wart
Wassermann test
wa′ter-brax″y
Waterhouse-Friderichsen syn′drome
watt
watt′age
watt′me″ter
Wechsler-Bellevue test
wedge
weep′ing
Weidel re ac′tion
weight
Weil′s dis ease′
wen
Wenckebach′s phe nom′e non
wheal
wheeze
whey
whip′lash″
whip′worm
whit′low
whoop′ing cough
Widal test
Wilms tu′mor
wind′-bro″ken
wind′gall″
wind′lass
wind′stroke″
Wintrobe meth′od
Wirsung′s duct
WISC
with′ers
womb
wound
wrin′kles
wrist
wry′neck″
Wuch″er er′i a

X

Xa′nax
xan″the las′ma
xan′thic
xan′thine
xan″thi nu′ri a
xan″tho chroi′a
xan″tho chro mat′ic
xan″tho chro ma to′sis
xan″tho chro′mi a
xan″tho chro′mic
xan thoch′ro ous
xan′tho cyte
xan″tho der′ma
xan′tho dont
xan″tho gran″u lo″ma to′sis
xan tho′ma
xan tho mat′ic
xan tho″ma to′sis
xan thom′a tous
xan′tho phane
xan′tho phore
xan thop′si a
xan thop′sin
xan thop″sy dra′ci a
xan″thor rhe′a
xan″tho sar co′ma

xan tho′sis
xen o di ag no′sis
xen″o me′ni a
xen″o pho′bi a
xen″oph thal′mi a
xe″no plas′ty
xe ran′tic
xe″ro der′ma
xe″ro me′ni a
xe″ro myc te′ri a
xer on′o sus
xe″ro pha′gi a
xe″roph thal′mi a
xe″ro ra″di og′ra phy
xe″ro si″a log′ra phy
xe ro′sis
xe″ro sto′mi a
xe′ro tes
xe rot′ic
xe″ro trip′sis
xiph″i ster′num
xiph″o cos′tal
xiph od′y mus
xiph″o dyn′i a
xiph′oid
xiph″oid i′tis
xi phop′a gus
X pol y so′my
xy′lene
xy′len ol
xy′lol
xy′ro spasm
xys′ma
xys′ter

Y

yawn
yaws
yeast
Y-plas′ty
yt′tri um

Z

zar an′than
Zeller's test
Zeph′i ran chlo′ride
Ziehl-Neelsen stain
Zika vi′rus
zinc
zo′na
zon″es the′si a
zo nif′u gal
zo nip′e tal
zon′ule
zon″u li′tis
zon″u lot′o my
zo″o er as′ti a
zo og′o ny
zo′o graft
zo″o lag′ni a
zo ol′o gist
zo″o no′sis
zo″o par′a site
zo oph′a gous
zo oph′i lism
zo″o pho′bi a
zo′o plas″ty
zo op′si a
zos′ter
zos ter′i form
zy″ga poph′y sis
zyg′i on
zy″go dac′ty ly
zy go′ma
zy″go mat′ic

zy″go mat″i co fa′cial
zy″go mat″i co tem′po ral
zy″go mat′i cus
zy″go max″il la′re
zy′go spore
zy′gote
Zy′ lo prim
zy mo′sis
zy mot′ic

Section III

LIST OF OFTEN USED WORDS IN MEDICAL SPECIALTIES

- Surgery
- Internal Medicine
- Pediatrics
- Otolaryngology
- Psychiatry

Surgery

ab dom″i no per″i ne′al
ach″a la′si a
ad″e no car″ci no′ma
ad″e no′ma
ad″e no my o′sis
ad he″si o ly′sis
ad he′sion
ad ren″o cor″ti co ster′oids
al dos′ter one
al″i men ta′tion
a mas′ti a
am″e bi′a sis
a nas′to mo′sis
an′eu rysm
an″eu rys mec′to my
an″gi og′ra phy
an″gi o sar co′ma
an″ti chol in er′gic
a or″to il′i ac
a or″to throm bo en″dar te rec′to my
a per″i stal′sis
a pon″eu ro′sis
ap pen″di ci″tis
ar te″ri og′ra phy
ar te″ri ot′o my
ar te″ri o ve″nous
as ci′tes
at″e lec′ta sis
a′tri ot″o my

Balfour
bar′o re cep′tor
Billroth
Blalock
Boeck's sar′coid
bran′chi al
bron″chi ec′ta sis
bron chog′ra phy
bron″cho lith
bron chos′copy
buc′cal
Buerger's dis ease′
bur si′tis

can″nu la′tion
car″ci no em bry on′ic
car″di ot′o my
car″di o pul′mo nary
cath″e ter i za′tion
chem″o pro″phy lax′sis
chol″an″gi o car ci′noma
chol an gi og′ra phy
chol″an gi′tis
chol″e cyst ec′to my
chol′e cys ti′tis
cho led″o chos′ co py
cho led″o chos′to my
cho led″o chot′o my
chon dro′ma
chy″lo tho′rax
cir rho′sis
co lec′to my
co lon′o scope
co los′to my
con″dy lo′ma
cor′ti cos′ter oid
cor″ti co tro′pin
crypt or′ chid ism
cul″do cen te′sis
cyst″ad e no car″ci no′ma
cyst ad e no′ma
cys tos′co py
cys tot″to my

de bride′ment
de cor″ti ca′tion
di al″y sis

di″ver tic″u li′tis
di″ver tic′u lum
du″o de nos′to my
du″o de′num
dys pha′gi a

em″bo lec′to my
em′bo lism
em′bo lus
em″phy se′ma
em″py e′ma
en″dar ter ec′to my
en″do me″tri o′sis
en″ter o ne″ter os′ to my
en″ter os′to my
ep″i did″y mi′tis
ep″i the″li a za′tion
e soph″a ge′al
e soph a gos′co py
e″ven tra′tion
ex″oph thal′mos

fal lo′pi an
fi″bro ad″e no′ma
fi″bro dys plas″tic
fis′sure
fis′tu la
fis″tu lec′to my

gan″gl on ec′to my
gan″gli o neu ro′ma
gas trec′to my
gas″tro en″ter os′ to my
gas″tro je″jun os′to my
gas″tro os′to my
guai′ac
gyn″e co mas′ti a

ham″ar to′ma
he man″gi o′ma
hem′a to cele″
hem″or rhoid ec′to my
hem′or rhoids
hep′a rin i za″tion
Hesselbach″s
Hirschsprungs
Hofmeister
hy′dro cele
hy″dro ne phro′sis
hy″per ka le′mi a
hy″per par″a thy′roid ism
hy″po nat re′mi a
hy″po vo le′mi a
hys″ter ec′to my

ic ter′ic
il″e i′tis
il″e o ce′cal
il″e os″to my
il′e us
incon′ti nence
in nom′i nate
in″tra cel′lu lar
in″tu ba′tion
in″tus sus cep′tion
is che′mi a

je ju′nal
jej″u no jej″u nos′to my
je ju′num
jug′u lar

ka″na my′cin
Kaposi′s
ker″a to′sis
ky pho′sis

lam″i nog′ra phy
lap″a rot′o my
lar yn′ge al
lar″yn gec′to my
lar″yn gos′co py

lo bec′to my
lym phan″gi o′gram
lym″pho ma to′sis

mam mog′ra phy
mam′mo plas ty
mar su″ pi al i za′tion
mas tec′to my
mas ti′tis
Meckel's
me co′ni um
me″di as″ti ni′tis
me″di as ti′num
mes″en ter′ic
me tas′ta sis
my″as the′ni a
my′e lo gram
my ot″o my
myx″e de′ma

na″so phar yn′ge al
na″so phar′ynx
ne cro′sis
ne phrec′to my
ne phros′to my
neu ral′gi a
neu ro′ma
nor ep″i neph′rine

ob″sti pa′tion
Ochsner
Oddi
ol″i gu′ri a
o men′tum
o″o pho rec′to my
or′chi o pex″y
or chi′tis
os″te ot′o my

pal″li a″tive
pan″cre a tec′to my
pap″il lo′ma
par″a cen te′sis
par″a thy′roid
par″a thy″roid ec′to my
par′o nych′i a
per″i to ne′al
per″i to ne′um
per″i to ni′tis
phleb′o gram
phleb″o throm bo′sis
phren′ic
pi″lo ni′dal
pneu″mo nec′to my
pneu″mo tho′rax
pol″py pec′to my
pol″y po′sis
proc″i den′ti a
pros″ta tec′to my
pseu′do cyst″
pseu″do pol′yp
py lor′ic
py lor′o plas ty

rhab″do my″o sar co′ma
Roux-en-Y

sal pin″go-o″o pho rec′to my
sco″li o′sis
sem″i no′ma
sig″moid os′co py
sphinc′ter
sple nec′to my
squa′mous
sym″pa thec′to my

tel an″gi ec′ta sis
tho″ra cen te′sis
tho″ra cot′o my
throm bec′to my
throm″bo em′bo lism″
throm″bo phle bi′tis

thy mec′to my
thy″ro glos′sal
thy″roid ec′to my
tour′ni quet
tra″che o e″soph a ge′al
tra″che os′to my
Treitz

ul′tra son o″graph y
u re″ter os′to my

va got′o my
val′vu lo plas″ty
var′i co cele″
var′i cose
ven og′ra phy
vol′vu lus

xan tho′ma

z-plasty

Internal Medicine

ab″re ac′tion
a can′tho cytes
ac″et a min′o phen
ac′e tyl cho′line
ac′e tyl sal″i cycl′ic
ach″a la′si a
ac″ro meg′a ly
ac″ti no my co′sis
ad″e no car″ci no′ma
ad re″nal ec′to my
ad re″no cor″ti co tro′pic
ad re″no gen′i tal
a gam″ma glob u lin e′mia
a gran″u lo cy to′sis
al dos′ter one
al″o pe′ci a
al″ve o li′tis
am″bly o′pi a
am″e bi′a sis
a men″or rhe′a
a mi″no phyl′line
a mi″tryp′ty lene
A″mox i cil″lin
am″pho ter′i cin
Am″pi cil″lin
am″y loi do′sis
an″ am nes′tic
an″a phy lax′is
an i″so co′ri a
an″ti chol in er′gic
a″pex car″di og′ra phy
a pha′si a
ar rhyth′mic
ar te″ri o ve′nous
ar thral′gi a
ar throp′a thy
as ci′tes
at″e lec′ta sis
ath″er o″scle ro′sis
a″tri o ven tric′u lar
au″to he mol′y sis
au″to im mune′
au″to nom′ic
ag″o te′mi a

Babinski
ba cil′li
bac te″ri u′ri a
bal″a ni′tis
ben′zo di az″e pine
be ryl″li o′sis
bil″i ru′bin
blas″to my co′sis
brad″y car′di a
bron″cho i o al ve′ o lar
bron″chi ec′ta sis
bron′chi ole
bron″cho gen′ic
bron chog′ra phy
bru′it
bul′lous
bur si′tis

Caf′er got
can″di di′as is
can′na bis
car cin′o gen
car″di o e soph″a ge′al
car″di o meg′a ly
cat″e chol′am ines
ceph″a lo spo′rin
chan′cre
che′lat ing
che mo′sis
chlam′y di al
chlor″di az″e pox′ide

chlo′ro quine
chol″an gi og′ra phy
chol″an gi′tis
chol″e cyst ec′to my
chol″e cys ti′tis
chol″e li thi′a sis
chor′dae ten din′e ae
chrys″o ther′a py
chy″lo tho′rax
ci met′i dine
cir rho′sis
col′chi cine
com″mis sur ot′om y
cor″ti co ster′oid
cou′ma din
Cou′ma rin
cre′a tine
cre at′i nine
cre′tin ism
cryp″to coc co′sis
cryp tor′chid
cy″a no′sis
cys″ti nu′ri a

de fib″ril la′tion
de men′ti a
de my′e lin ate
der″ma to my″o si′tis
Des i′pra mine
des ox″y cor″ti cos′te rone
di al′y sis
di′az e pam
di az′ox ide
Di cou′ma rol
di″u re′sis
do′pa mine
dys ar′thri a
dys″di ad″o ko ki ne′si a
dys″ki ne′si a
dys″pa reu′ni a
dys pha′si a
dys u′ri a

e lec″tor pho re′sis
em″phy se′ma
em″py e′ma
en ceph″a lo my″e li′tus
en ceph″a lo′pa thy
en″dar te ri′tis
end or′phrin
en″ter o coc′cus
en″ter o co li″tis
en″ter o vi′rus
er″y sip′e las

fu′run cle

ga lac″tor rhe′a
gas″tro en″ter op′a thy
gas″tro en″ter os′to my
gi″ar di′a sis
glau co′ma
glo mer″u li′tis
glo mer″u lo ne phri′tis
glu″cu ron′i dase
glu tam′ic acid
glu″ta thi′one
gly″co gen′e sis
gly″co ge nol′y sis
gon a″do tro′pin
gran′u lo cyte″
gyn″e co mas′ti a

hem″a to poi e′sis
he″mo chro″ma to′sis
he mol′y sin
He moph′i lus
he mop′ty sis
he″mo sid″er o′sis
hep″a to len tic′lar

ho″mo cys tin u′ria
ho″mo gen tis′ic
hy″drar thro′sis
hy″dro ne phro′sis
hydrox′y lase
hy″per bil″i ru″bi ne′mi a

i at″ro gen′ic
i mip′ra mine
im″mu no de fi′cien cy
im″mu no glob′u lin
in″su lin o′ma
is che′mi a
i″so pro ter′e nol

je ju″no il″e os′to my

Ka″na my′cin
ker″a to con junc″ti vi′tis
ker nic′ter us
Kleb si el′la
ky pho′sis

leu″ko en ceph a lop′athy
leu″ko pe′ni a
leu″ko pla′ki a
lym″phad e ni′tis
lym″pho cy to′sis
lym″pho re tic′u lar

mac′ro phage
me di as″ti nos′co py
meg″a kar′y o cyte
Meniere
me nin″gi o′ma
mes″o the″li o′ma
mon″o nu″cle o′sis
my″as the′ni a
my″lin ol′y sis
myx″e de′ma

nar′co lep″sy
neph″ro li thi′a sis
ne phrop′athy
neu″ras the′ni a
neu″ro fi bro″ma to′sis
neu″ro ni′tis
neu″tro pe′ni a
nys tag′mus

ob′sti pa tion
ol″i ge′mi a
ol″i go den″dro gli o′ma
ol′i gu′ri a
op so′nin
os″mo lar′i ty
os″te o chon dri′tis
os″te o dys′tro phy
os″te o ma la′ci a
os″te o po ro′sis
ox″y to′cin

pan″cre a tec′to my
pan′en ceph a lop″a thy
pa pil″ le de′ma
par″a ple′gi a
par″a thy′roid
par″a thy″roid ec′to my
par″es the′pi a
pel lag′ra
pem′phi gus
per″i neph′ric
pe te′chi a
phen″yl ke″to nu′ri a
phe″o chro″mo cy to′ma
phle bot′o my
pneu″mo co″ni o′sis
pol″y cy the′mi a
pol″y neu rop″a thy
por phy′ri a
pro″pyl thi″o u′ra cil

pro″te in u″ri a
pru ri′tus
pseu″do her maph″ro dit ism
pseu″do hy″per troph′ic
pseu″do hy po par″a thy′roid ism
pto′sis
pur′pu ra
py″e lo ne phri′tis

Raynaud's
re tic″ u lo cy to′sis
re tic u lo en″do the″li al
ret″i no blas to′ma
ri″bo neu cle′ic

sal″mo nel lo′sis
sar″coid o′sis
schis″to so mi′a sis
scle″ro der′ma
shi″gel lo′sis
sig″moid os′co py
so nog′ra phy
sper″ma to gen′e sis
spo″ro tri cho′sis
ste″a tor rhe′a
sym path″o mi met′ic
syn″o vi′tis
sy rin″go my e′li a

tel an″gi ec ta′si a
tha″las se′mi a
tho″ra cen te′sis
throm″bo an″gi i′tis
throm″bo cy″to pe′ni a
throm″bo phle bi′tis
throm″bo plas′tin
thy mec′to my
thy mo′ma
thy″ro tox″i co′sis
to mog′ra phy
tra″che o bron′chi al
tra″che os′to my
tri″cho mon i′a sis
tri bly′ce rides
tri′so my

ul″tra son og′ra phy
ur″ti ca′ri a
u″ve i′tis

Valsalva's test
var″i cel′la
var′i co cele″
var″i cos′i ty
vas′cu li′tis
ver ru′ca
vit′re ous

xan″the las′ma
xan tho′ma

Pediatrics

ac″an thos′sis
ac″e to nu′ri a
ach″a la′si a
a chon″dro gen″e sis
a chon″dro pla′si a
a chy′li a
ac″ro ceph′a ly
ac″ro cy″a no′sis
ac″ti no my co′sis
ad″e nom′a tous
ad″e no vi′rus
ad″ren er′gic
a″er o ti′tis
a fi″brin o gen e′mi a
a gam″ma glob″u lin e′me a
ag″glu tin′o gen
a gran″u lo cy to′sis
al bu″mi nu′ri a
al dos′ter one
al kap″to nu′ri a
al″o pe′ci a
al″ve o li′tis
am″bly o′pi a
am″ni o cen te′sis
am″ni og′ra phy
am′ni ot′ic
a my″o to′ni a
an″a phy lac′toid
an″a phy lax′is
an″gi o car″di og′ra phy
an″gi o e de′ma
an″gi o fi bro′ma
an″gi o ma to′sis
an″gi o neu ro′tic
an i″so co′ri a
an i″so me tro′pi a
an′ky lo′sis
aph tho′sis
aph″thous

a rach′nid ism
a rach″no dac′ty ly
as ci″tes
as per″gil lo′sis
as phyx′i a tion
a stig′ma tism
ath″er om″a tous
au″to im mun″i za′tion
au″to som′al
az″o te′mi a

bac te″ri u′ri a
be′zoar
bil″i ru″bi ne′mi a
bil″i ver′din
Bitot's spots
blas″to my co′sis
bleph″ar it′is
bot′u lism
bron″chi ec′ta sis
bron chi′o lar
bron′chi o li′tis
bron′cho ma la′cia
bul′lous
buph thal′mos

cal″ci no′sis
can″di di′as is
ca′put
car′di o my op″a thy
car″o te ne′mi a
ca″se a′tion
cat′a plex″y
ce″li ac
ceph″al he″ma to′ma
ceph″a lo spo′rin
cer ca′ri a
ce′ru lo plas″min
ce ru′men

cha la′si a
chei lo′sis
che la′tion
chi as′ma
cho′a nal
cho led′o chal
cho″lin er′gic
chon″dro dys′tro phy
cho″re o ath″e to′sis
cho″ri o am″ni on i′tis
cho′ri oid
chro″ma tog′ra phy
chy′lous
cis″tern og′ra phy
cli″no dac″ty ly
co cid″i di oi′dal
coc cid″i oi″do my co′sis
col″o bo′ma
com′e do
con″dy lo′ma
con″san guin′i ty
co″ro na vi′rus
cox al′gi a
cra″ni o fa′cial
cra″ni o pha ryn″gi o′ma
cra″ni o syn″os to′sis
cre′tin ism
cry″o ther′a py
cry pt or′chid ism
cy″clo ple′ gi a
cy″clo tro′pi a
cys″ti cer co′sis
cys″ti no′sis
cys″ti nu′ri a
cy″to me gal′ic
cy″to meg′a ly
cy tox′in

dac″ry o ste no′sis
dac″ty li′tis
de bride′ment
de fib″ril la′tion
de″glu ti′tion
de men′tia
de my′e lin at″ing
der″ma to my″o si′tis
der″mo graph′i a
der′moid
des ox″y cor″ti cos′te rone
dex″tro car′di a
di″a pho re′sis
di aph′y sis
di′en ceph′a lon
di″phen yl hy dan′to in
diph″the ri″tic
di plo′pia
di″zy got′ic
duct′us
du″o de′nal
dys″a cu′sis
dys″au to no′mia
dys co′ria
dys gen′e sis
dys″ger mi no′ma
dys″ker a to′sis
dys″ki ne′si a
dys lex′i a
dys″os to′sis
dys pla′si a
dysp ne′a
dys rhyth′mi a
dys to′ci a
dys to′ni a
dys tro′phi a
dys′tro phy
dys uri a

ec″chy mo′sis
ec″to der′mal
ec′to morph
ec to′pi a
ec′ze ma

ec zem′a toid
a dem′a tous
e las to′sis
e lec″tro en ceph″a log′ ra phy
e lec″tro my og′ra phy
e lec″tro pho re′sis
el lip″to cy to′sis
em′bo lism
em″bry o′ma
em′e sis
em″me tro′pi a
em″phy se′ma
em″py e′ma
en ceph″a lit′i des
en ceph″a li′tis
en ceph′a lo cele″
en ceph″a lo ma la′ci a
en ceph″a lop′a thy
en″co pre′sis
en″do bron″chi o li′tis
en′do bron chi′tis
en′do cri nop′a thy
en′do morph
en″oph thal′mos
en ter′ic
en″ter o co li′tis
ex″ter op′a thy
en″ter o vi′rus
en″u re′sis
en″zy mat′ic
en′zyme
e″o sin′o phil
e″o sin″o phil′i a
ep″i can′thus
ep″i der mol′y sis
ep″i dur′ral
ep″i lep″to gen′ic
e piph′y se al
e piph′y sis
ep″i spa′di as
ep″i stax′is
ep″i troch′le ar
ep u′lis
er″y them′a tous
e ryth″ro blas to′sis
e ryth′ro cyte
e ryth″ro poi e′sis
e″ryth ro poi e″tic
e soph″a gi′tis
es″o tro′pi a
eu sta′chi an
ex an′them
ex″an the′ma tous
ex fo″li a′tion
ex″oph thal′mos
ex″os to′sis
ex″o tro′pi a
ex′stro phy
ex″tra sys′to le

fa′ci es
fe tos′co py
fi brin′o gen
fi″brin ol′y sis
fi″bro e las to′sis
fi bro″ma to′sis
fi′brous
fol lic″u li′tis
fol lic″u lo′sis
fon″ta nel′
fo ra′mi na
fren′u lum
fu run″cu lo′sis

ga lac″tor rhe′a
gal ac″to se′mi a
gan″gli o blas to′ma
gan″gli o neu ro′ma
gar′goyle
gas″ tro en″ter i′tis
gas″tro e soph″a ge′al
gas″tro lith

ges ta′tion al
gi″ar di′a sis
gin″gi vo sto′ma ti′tis
glau co′ma
gli o′ma
glo mer′u lar
glo mer″u lo ne phri′tis
glo mer′u lus
glos″so pha ryn′ge al
glu′co ne″o gen′e sis
glu′co su′ri a
glu″ta thi′one
gly″co ge no′sis
gly″co su′ri a
go na″do trop′in
gon″o coc ce′mi a
gran″u lo cy″to pe′ni a
gran″u lo′ma
gran″u lo″ma to′sis
gran″u lo′ma tous
gyn″e co mas′ti a

Hae moph′i lus
hal lu″ci na′tion
hal lu′ci″no gen
ham″ar to′ma
he″mag glu″ti na′tion
he man″gi o′ma
he″mar thro′sis
he″ma tem′ e sis
hem″a tin′ic
hem″a to′gen ous
he″ma to′ma
hem″a to poi et′ic
hem″i ple′gi a
he″mo chro″ma to′sis
he mol′y sis
he mo lyt′ic
he″mo per″i car′di um
he″mo phil′i a
he mop′ty sis
hem″or rhag′ic
hem′or rhoids
he″mo sid′er in
he″mo sta′sis
he″mo tho′rax
hep″a to′ma
hep″a to meg″a ly
hep″a to sple″no meg′a ly
her maph′ro dism
her pan′gin a
her pet′ic
Herxheimer
het″er o zy′gous
hi a′tal
Hirschsprung
hir′sut ism
his″ti o cy to′sis
his″to plas mo′sis
ho″me o sta′sis
ho″mo sys tin u′ri a
ho″mo zy′gous
hy″a lin i za′tion
hy″a lin o′sis
hy′dro cele
hydro ceph′a lus
hy″dro ne phro′sis
hy″per ad re″no cor′ti cism
by″per bil″i ru″bi ne′mia
hy″per cal ce′mi a
hy″per gam″ma glob u li ne′mi a
hy″per gly ce′mi a
hy″per ka le′mi a
hy″per ki ne′sis
hy″per ki net′ic
hy″per os″mo lar′i ty
hy″per par″a thy′roid ism
hy″per phos pha te′mi a
hy″per pi tu′i ta rism
hy″per pla′si a
hy″per pne′a
hy″per py rex′i a

hy″per tel′or ism
hy″per ther′mi a
hy″per thy′roid ism
hy″per to′ni a
hy″per vol e′mi a
hy phe′ma
hy″po cal ce′mi a
hy″po chon″dro pla′si a
hy″po gly ce′mi a
hy″po kal e′mi a
hy″po nat re′ mi a
hy″po pi tu′i ta rism
hy″po pro″te i ne′mi a
hy″po spa′di as
hy″po ther′mi a
hy″po thy′roid ism
hy″pox e′mi a
hy pox′i a

i at″ro gen′ic
ich″thy o″sis
im″mu no de fi′cien cy
im″mu no glob′u lin
in′fan ti lism
in″ter al ve′o lar
in″ter sti′tial
in″tra u″ter ine
in″tus sus cep′tion
i″so pro te′ren ol

jej″u nos′to my
jux″ta glo mer′u lar

ke′loid
ker″a ti′tis
ker″a to con junc″ti vi′tis
ker nic′ter us
ke″to nu′ri a
ke to′tic
Koplik's
ky′pho sco″li o′sis
ky pho′sis

lab′y rinth
lab′y rin thi′tis
lam″i nec′to my
la nu′go
lar yn″go ma la′ci a
la ryn″go tra″che o bron chi′tis
leish″man i″a sis
lep″to men″in ge′al
leu″ko cy to′sis
leu′ko dys′tro phy
leu′ko pe′ni a
le vo car′di a
lip id o″sis
li po″ma to′sis
lor do′sis
lym phan″gi o′ma
lym″phe de′ ma
lym″pho gran″u lo′ma

mac″ro gen″i to so′mi a
mac″ro glos′si a
man dib″u lo fa′ci al
me″a tot′o my
me co′ni um
med″ul lo blas to′ma
meg″a kar′y o cyte
mel″a no′ sis
men″in git′i des
me nin′go cele
me nin″go en ceph′a lo cele
me nin″go my′e lo cele
mes′en chyme
met″a chro mat′ic
me taph′ y seal
me taph′y sis
met he″mo glo′bin
mi″cren ceph′a ly
mi″cro gna′thi a
mi″croph thal′mi a

mol lus′cum
mon′go lism
mon″o nu″cle o′sis
mu″co vis ci do′sis
mu tism
my al′gia
my″e lo dys pla′si a
myr″in gi′tis
myr″in got′o my
myx″e de′ma

nar′co lep″sy
na″so lac′ri mal
na″so pha″ryn gi′tis
neb″u li″zer
ne′cro tiz″ing
ne″o na′tal
neph″ro blas to′ma
ne phro gen′e sis
ne phrop′athy
ne phro′sis
neu″ro blas′to ma
neu″ro der″ma ti′tis
neu″ro fi bro″ma to′sis
neu″tro pe′ni a
neu″tro phil
ne′vus
nos″o com′i al
nys tag′mus

oc cip″i to front′al
oc″u lo glan′du lar
o don′to blast
ol″i gu′ri a
om″pha li′tis
om′phal o cele″
om″pha lo mes″en ter′ic
oph thal″mo ple′gi a
op″is thot′o nos
or″chi ec′to my
or′chi o pex″y

o″ro phar yn′ge al
os″mo lar′ity
os″te o ar throp′a thy
os″te o chon dri′tis
os″te o chon dro′sis
os″te o ma la′ci a
os″te o po ro′sis
os″ti um
o″tor rhe′a
o″to scle ro′sis
ox y to′cin

pal′pe bral
pan cre a ti′tis
pan hy″po pi tu′i ta rism
pan nic′u li tis
pan″oph thal mi′tis
pap″il li′tis
par′a cen te′sis
par″a per tus′sis
pa ren′chy ma
par″o ti′tis
pe dic″u lo′sis
pen to su′ri a
per″i bron chi′tis
per″i ne phri′tis
per″i o don′tal
per″i or′bi tal
per″i os′te al
per″i os′te um
per leche′
per tus′sis
pe te′chi a
pe tit′mal
phen″yl ke″to nu′ri a
phe″o chro′mo cy to′ma
phi mo′sis
phlyc ten′u lar
phos″pha tu ri a
pit′y ri′a sis
pleu′ro dyn′i a

pneu′ma to cele″
penu″mo en ceph″a log′ra phy
pneu″mo tho′rax
pol″y ar thral′gi a
pol″y chro″ma to phil′i a
pol′y cy the′me a
pol′y dac′ty ly
pol′y dip′si a
po ren ce phal′ic
por′phy rin
por″phyr u′ri a
pre′puce
pri mor′di al
prop to′sis
pseu″do ar″thro′sis
pseu″do her maph′ro dit ism
pseu″do hy″per troph′ic
pseu″do mem″bran ous
pso ri′a sis
pu″er pe′ri um
pur′pu ra
py″e lo ne phri′tis
py″lor o my ot′o my
py lor′ o spasm″

ra chit′ic
ra dic″u li′tis
ran′u la
re tic″u lo cy to′sis
re tic″u lo en″do the′li al
ret″i no blas to′ma
ret″i nop′a thy
ret″ro len′tal
rhi″nor rhe′a
ru be′o la

sag′it tal
sal′i cyl ism
sal′mo nel lo′sis
scap″u lo hu′mer al
schis″to so mi′a sis
scle″ro der′ma
sco″li o′sis
seb″or rhe′ic
shi″gel lo′sis
sphe′ro cyte
sphe″ro cy to′sis
sphinc″ter ot′o my
sphin″go my′e lin
spi na bi′fi da
spon″dy li′tis
spon″dyl ol′y sis
staph″y lo coc′cal
ste″a tor rhe′a
ster″co bi′lin
strep″to dor′nase
strep″to ki′nase
stri′dor
sub″a rach′noid
sub un′gu lal
sym″pa thet″i co mi met′ic
syn′co pe
syn dac′ty ly
syn″os to′sis
syn″o vi′tis

tel an″gi ec′ta sis
te nes′mus
ter″a to′ma
tha las se′mi a
tho″ra cen te′sis
throm″bo cy″to pe′ni a
throm″bo cy to′sis
thy mec′to my
thy″ro glos′sal
tin′e a
tor″ti col′lis
tox″o plas mo′sis
tra″che o bron′chi al
tra″che o e soph″a ge′al
tra″che os′to my
tra″che ot′o my

trich″u ri′a sis
tri gly′cer ide″
tris′mus
tri′so my
tryp sin′o gen
tryp′to phan″
tym pan′ic
tym″pa no cen te′sis
ty′ro sinase

u re′ter o cele
u″reth rot′o my
u″ro bi lin′o gen
u″ro li thi′a sis
ur″ti ca′ri a
u″ve i′tis

vac cin′i a

var″i cel′la
va ri′o la
var′i o loid
ver′nix
ver ru′ca
ves ti′bu lar
vi re′mi a
vit″i li′go
vol′vu lus
vul″vo vag″i ni′tis

wry′neck

xan″thi nu′ri a
xan″tho chro′mic
xan tho′ma
xan tho″ma to′sis
xe ro′sis

Otolaryngology

ac″an tho′ma
ac″an tho′ sis
ach″a la′si a
a chon″dro pla′ si a
ac″ti no my co′sis
ad′a man ti no′ma
am pho ter′i cin
am″y loi do′sis
an″gi o fi bro′ma
an″ gi o neu ro′ tic
an os′mia
an″ti he′lix
an″ti tra′gus
a tre′si a

blas″to my co′sis
bron″chi o li′tis
bul la
bull′ae(pl)

can″di di′as is
ce ru″mi no′ma
chlo′ro cy″cli zine
cho a′nal
cho les″te a to′ma
chon dro′ma
Chvosteck's sign
cis ter′no gram
coch″le ar′i form
con′cha
cra″ni o pha ryn″gi o′ma
crib′ri form
cri″co thy rot′o my
cyl″in dro′ma

dec′i bel
den″ti no′ma
dip″la cu′sis
di plo′pi a

dys″a cu′sis
dys pha′gi a

en″do tra′che al
ep″i glot′tis
ep″i stax′is
ep″i the″li o′ ma
ep″i tym′pa num
eth′ moid
eu sta′chi an
ex″oph thal′mos
ex″os to′sis

fa rad′ic
fen″es tra′tion
fo ra′men
fo ra′mi na
fren′u lum

glo′mus
glos′so pal′a tine
glot′tic
goi′tre

ham″ar to′ma
he′lix
hem″i lar″yn gec′to my
her″pan gi′na
hi a′tus

in″fun dib′u lum
I′su prel

jug′u lar og″ra phy

Kiesselbach's plex′us
Kleb si el′la

lab″y rin′thine

lab″y rin thi′tis
lam′i na
la ryn′go cele
lar″yn go ma la′ci a
la ryn″go tra″che o bron chi′tis
len tic′u lar
leu″ko pla′ ki a
lym″phan gi′na

mac″ro glos′si a
mas″toid ec to my
me nin″gi o′ma
Mikulicz's cells
mo″ni li a sis
mu″co cu ta′ ne ous
mu″co vis ci do′sis
my″co bac te′ri um
my rin′go plas″ty
my rin′go scle′ro sis
myx o′ma

na″so pal′a tine
na″so pha ryn′go gram
neu″ro blas to′ma
nys tag′mus

o″don to′ma
oph thal″mo ple′gi a
or′bi to gram
o″ro phar′ ynx
os sic′u lar
os″te i′tis
os″te o gen′ic
os″te o ma la′ci a
os″te o my″e li′tis
os′ti a
o″tor rhe a
o″to scle ro′sis

pal″a to pha ryn′ge us
par″a na′sal
par″a phar″yn ge′al
per″i lab″y rin thi′tis
per′i lymph
pet″ro si′tis
pet′rous
pneu″ma ti za′tion
pneu′ma to cele″
pres″ by a cu′sis
prop to′sis
pter″y go man dib′u lar
pty′ a lism

ra″di o si a log′ra phy
ran′u la
ret″ro lab y rin′thine
ret″ro pha ryn′ge al
rhi′no lith
rhi″no phy′ma
rhi″no scle ro′ma
rhom″ben ceph′a lon

sac′cus
sca′la
sca le′nus
sep″to derm o plas′ty
si al″o gram
sphe″no eth′moid al
sta″pe dec′to my
sta pe′di us
sta′pes

teg′men
thy″ro ep″i glot′tic
thy″ro hy′oid
ton sil′lo lith
Trousseau's sign
tym pan′o gram
tym″pa nom′e try
tym″pa no plas′ty
tym″pa no scle′ro sis

un′ci nate
u tri′cu lar
u″ve o pa′rot id

Valsalva test
ver tig′i nous
ver′ti go

Waldeyer's ring

xe′ro ra″di og′ra phy
xe′ro si″a log′ra phy

zy go′ma

Psychiatry

a ba′si a
a bu′li a
a can″thes the′si a
ac″a ro pho′bi a
ac a thex′is
ac cre′tion
ac″ro cy″a no′sis
ac″ro dyn′i a
a″di ad″o cho ki ne′sis
a″er o pha′gi a
a″er o pho′bi a
ag no′si a
ag″o ra pho′bi a
a graph′i a
ak″i ne′si a
a la′li a
Alz′hei mer's dis ease′
am″bly o′pi a
a men′ti a
am ne′si a
am phet′a mine
a na clit′ ic
a nal′i ty
an″a phy lax′is
an″o rex′ia ner vo′sa
an″ta buse
a pha′si a
a prax′i a
ar′che type″
a tax′i a
ath″e to′sis
au′tism

Babinski's reflex
bi″o feed′back
bi sex′u al
brux′ism
bu lim′i a

ca chex′i a
can′na bis
cas tra′tion
ca tab′o lism
cat′a lep″sy
cat′a plex″y
cat″a to′ni a
cat′e chol″am′ine
ca thar′sis
ca thex′is
ceph″a lal′gi a
ce′re lo″plas min
Charcot-Marie-Tooth's dis ease′
che la′tion
cho″lin er′gic
cho″lin es′ter ase
cho re′a
cho re′i form
cho″re o ath″e to′sis
chro′ma tin
cir ca′di an
clau″di ca′tion
claus″tro pho′bi a
cli mac′ter ic
co cain′ism
coc″cy go dyn′ i a
co′i tus
con′scious ness
cop″ro phil′i a
cun″ni lin′gus
cy′cloid
cy″clo thy′mic
cy″to me gal′ic

de ja vu′
de lin′quen cy
de lir′i ous

de lir′i um
de lu′sion
de men′ti a
de my″e lin a′tion
de per″son al i za′tion
de″ter i or a′tion
di ath′e sis
di″en ceph′a lon
de ple′gi a
di plo′pi a
dip″so ma′ni a
dis so″ci a′tion
di ur′nal
dys ar′thri a
dys″au to no′mia
dys ba′si a
dys bu′li a
dys gen′e sis
dys″ki ne′si a
dys″pa reu′ni a
dys pha′gi a
dys pho′ri a
dys pla′si a
dys prax′i a
dys to′ni a

e″cho en ceph″a log′ra phy
ech″o la′li a
e′go-syn ton′ic
e″go cen′trism
e′go tism
e′jac u la″tio prae′cox
e lec″tro en ceph′a lo gram″
em′pa thize
en ceph″a lo my″e li′tis
en ceph″a lop′a thy
en dor′phins
en″u re′sis
ep′i lep″sy
er′got ism
e rot′i cism

eu′nuch
eu′nuch oid
eu pho′ri a
ex is ten′tial
ex pi a′tion

fac ti′tious
fa nat′i cism
fan′ta sy
fel la′ti o
fe′tish
fe′tish ism
flag″el la′tion
fo lie′a deux
fu′gue

Gaucher′s dis ease′
gen′e al′o gy
gen′i tal ize
gib′ber ish
glos″so la′li a
gnos′tic
gran′deur
Guillain-Barrè syn′drome
gy′rus

ha bit″u a′tion
hal lu″ci na′tion
hal lu′ci″no gen
he″be phre′ni a
he′don ism
ho lis′tic
ho″me o sta′sis
ho mo′gamy
ho mol′o gous
ho″mo sex′u al
ho″mo zy′gous
hy″brid i za′tion
hy″per ki ne′sis
hy″per tel′or ism
hy″po chon dri′a sis

hy″po pla′si a
hy″po som′ni a
hy″po thal′a mus
hy″po to′ni a
hys te′ri a

im′po tence
im″pul siv′ i ty
in″con gru′i ty
in″tro jec′tion
in″tro ver′ sion

kin″es the′si a
klep″to ma′ni a
Klinefelter's syn′drome
Klippel-Feil syn′drome
Korsakoff psy cho′sis

lal la′tion
li bid′i nal
li bi′do
lin guis′tics
lo″go ther′ a py

mas′ o chism″
mel″an cho′li a
mel′an choly
meth′a done
meth″od ol′ogy
mi″cro ma′ni a

nar cis′sism
nec″ro phil′i a
neg′a tiv ism
ne ol′ o gism
neu″ras the′ni a
neu″ro fi bro″ma to′sis
neu″ro lep′tic
neu rop′a thy
neu ro′sis
nor ep″i neph′rine

nym″pho ma′ni a
nys tag′mus

ob ses′sion
oed′i pal com′plex
ol″i go phre′ni a
om ni′po tence
or′gasm
or″tho psy chi′a try

pan sex′u al ism
pa pil″le de′ma
par′a dox
par″a hyp no′sis
par″a noi′a
pa re′sis
Par′kin son ism
path″o psy chol′o gy
Pavlov's theory
pa′vor noc tur′nus
pe″do phil′i a
per sev″er a′tion
per va′sive
phal′lic
phal′lus
phan′ta sy
phen cy′cli dine
phe nom″e nol′ogy
phe″no thi′a zine
phen″yl ke″to nu′ri a
phen″yl py ru′vic oligophrenia
pho′bi a
pho″to pho′bi a
phre nol′o gy
phy″lo ge ne′tic
pi′ca
pla ce′bo
plat″y ba′si a
plu′ral ism
pneu″mo en ceph′a lo gram″
prae′cox

pre coc′i ty
pre cons′cious
pre″dis po si′tion
pri′a pism
pri″mi ti va′tion
proc tal′gi a
prom″is cu′i ty
pro″phy lax′is
pseu″do ag gres′sion
psy″chas the′ni a
psy′che
psy″cho mo′tor
psy″cho neu ro′sis
psy″cho pa thol′o gy
psy″cho′sis
psy″cho so mat′ic
psy″cho ther′a py
psy″cho tro′pic
py″ro ma′ni a

ra dic″u li′tis
rap port′
re″ca pit″u la′tion
re juv″e na′tion
re nun″ci a′tion
ret″ro gres′sion
rhi″nen ceph′a lon
Romberg sign
Rorschach test
ru″mi na′tion

sad′ism
sad″o mas′o chism
scape′goat ing
schiz″o af fec′tive
schiz′oid
schiz″o phre′ni a
ser″o to′ nin
sex″u al′i ty
so″ma ti za′tion
so ma′to form
som nam′bu lism
som′no lent″
so″po rif′ic
sta′tus epi lep′ti cus″
ster′e o ty″py
sthen′ic
stra bis′mus
streph″o sym bo′li a
sub″li ma′tion
sug gest″i bil′i ty
su″per e′go
sur′ro gate
sym′bo lism
syn′er gism
sy rin″go my e′li a

ta′ bes
tan″ gen ti al′ ity
tel″ en ceph′ a lon
tel″e ol′o gy
throm″bo an″gi i′tis ob lit′er ans
thy″ro tox″i co′sis
tic dou″lou reux′
to′mo graph
tran′quil iz″er
trans act′ion al
trans″ce den′tal
trans ves′ti tism
tri′ad
tu mes′cence

un con′scious
u″ni po′lar

vag″i nis′mus
vam′pir ism
vas″o va′gal
ven tric″u log′ra phy
vo″yeur′ism

Section IV

PHONETICALLY SPELLED WORD LIST

- Selected Medical Words

AS PHONETICALLY SPELLED	*AS CORRECTLY SPELLED*
ack′nee	acne
ack″row me gal′ic	acromegalic
ack row my′sin	Achromycin
ack′tar	Acthar
ack″ti no mye ko′sis	actinomycosis
a cue′i ty	acuity
a fan′i sis	aphanisis
a fay′je ah	aphagia
a fay′ke ah	aphakia
a fay′zhuh	aphasia
a fee′me ah	aphemia
a fo′nee uh	aphonia
a fon′ic	aphonic
a′fose	aphose
a fray′zhuh	aphrasia
af″ro diz′ee ack	aphrodisiac
af″ro diz′ee uh	aphrodisia
af′tha	aphtha
af tho′sis	aphthosis
af′thus	aphthous
ah′foze	aphose
ah koosh′munt	accouchement
ahr jirr′ee uh	argyria
ahr kay′ick	archaic
ahrs fen′uh meen	arsphenamine
air″en tur eck tay zhuh	aerenterectasia
air o′bik	aerobic
air′o fil″	aerophil
air′o form″	aeriform
air′o lin	Aerolin
air′o seel″	aerocele
air′o sol″	aerosol
a kay′shuh	acacia
a kye′lee uh	achylia
A kil′eez	Achilles
ak″ro meg′a ly	acromegaly
al″i fat′ick	aliphatic
al″kuh lee′mee uh	alkalemia
al″o pee′shee uh	alopecia
a men′shee uh	amentia

AS PHONETICALLY SPELLED	*AS CORRECTLY SPELLED*
am fet′uh meen	amphetamine
am″fe the′a ter	amphitheater
am″fi blas′tic	amphiblastic
am″fo gel′	Amphojel
am for′ick	amphoric
am″fo sill′in	amphocillin
am″fo ter′ick	amphoteric
am′i lace	amylase
am′i loyd	amyloid
am′i tol	Amytal
a mor′fick	amorphic
a mor′fus	amorphous
an″gee or′uh fee	angiorrhaphy
ang″kil ozh′is	ankylosis
an″jee o ko lye′tis	angicholitis
an″o for′ee uh	anophoria
an″o nick′ee uh	anonychia
an″te hee″mo fil′ick	antihemophilic
an″ti fag o sit′ick	antiphagocytic
an″ti hem″o roy′dal	antihemorrhoidal
an″ti lit′ick	antilytic
an″ti pye ret′ick	antipyretic
an″ti ra kit′ick	antirachitic
an″ tispy″ro kee′tic	antispirochetic
an″ti tye′foyd	antityphoid
an′uh fayz	anaphase
an″uh fuh lax′is	anaphylaxis
an′yoo rizm	aneurysm
a pof′i seal	apophyseal
a pof′i sis	apophysis
ap″o mor′feen	apomorphine
ap tye′uh liz um	aptyalism
a rack″nye′tis	arachnitis
a rack′noyd	arachnoid
Argile Robertson	Argyll Robertson
ar″i epi″glot′ick	aryepiglottic
a reno″blast toe′muh	arrhenoblastoma
a ri″no′ma	arrhenoma
ar′i tee″noyd	arytenoid
a rith′me ah	arrhythmia

AS PHONETICALLY SPELLED	*AS CORRECTLY SPELLED*
ar'ke type	archetype
ar'kus	arcus
a sef'uh ly	acephaly
as fik'se ah	asphyxia
as fik'se ant	asphyxiate
a sigh'lum	asylum
a sigh'teez	ascites
ass"i do'sis	acidosis
ass'i nye	acini
ass"i tab'yoo lum	acetabulum
ass'i tate	acetate
ass"i til sal i sil'ick	acetylsalicylic
ass"i tone	acetone
a'tro fe	atrophy
aus kul'tah tor"y	auscultatory
aw"toe fo'bi a	autophobia
aw"toe lil'tick	autolytic
aw tol'i sis	autolysis
Ay ee'deez	Aëdes
ay jy'ree uh	agyria
ay ko"lee uh	acholia
ay sigh"uh not'ick	acyanotic
ay sim'i tree	asymmetry
ay thi"re o'sis	athyreosis
ay thy'mick	athymic
az'muh	asthma
az mat'ic	asthmatic
bay'so fil	basophil
Beck's sar'coyd	Boeck's sarcoid
bew'bon ick	bubonic
blef"a ror'ah fe	blepharorrhaphy
blef'a ron	blephoron
blef'a ro pla sty	blepharoplasty
blef"a ro plee'gee a	blepharoplegia
blef"a rop'toe sis	blepharoptosis
blef"a ro spa'zm	blepharospasm
blef"a rot'o me	blepharotomy
blen"o re'ah	blenorrhea
brang'kee ul	branchial

AS PHONETICALLY SPELLED	*AS CORRECTLY SPELLED*
bray″kee al	brachial
bray″kee ce fal′ic	brachycephalic
bray″kee ot′o me	brachiotomy
bray′kee um	brachium
brong′kee ol	bronchiole
brong′kye	bronchi
brong″ko gen′ick	bronchogenic
brong kog′gra fe	bronchography
brong″ko nu mo′ne ah	bronchopneumonia
brong″ko ploor′ul	bronchopleural
brong″ko seel′	bronchocele
brong′kus	bronchus
bron kye′tis	bronchitis
broo ee′	bruit
brooz′	bruise
buck″o fa rin′jul	buccopharyngeal
buck′o lay′bi al	buccolabial
by rine′ee uh	birhinia
ca kec′tic	cachectic
care″ee ol′e sis	karyolysis
care″ee o rek′sis	karyorrhexis
care′ee o type″	karyotype
care′ee o fayj″	karyophage
caw′duh	cauda
cawl	caul
caw′ter ize	cauterize
Chain Stokes	Cheyne Stokes
clam′i do spore″	chlamydospore
clam y′di al	chlamydial
cly″do mass′toyd	cleidomastoid
cly″do stur′nal	cleidosternal
co′cane	cocaine
cock′lee uh	cochlea
cock′sicks	coccyx
Coksacki vi′rus	Coxsackie virus
co″le cys′tic	cholecystic
co′lic	cholic
Con test	Kahn test
coo′ma din	coumadin

AS PHONETICALLY SPELLED	*AS CORRECTLY SPELLED*
Coplik's spots	Koplik's spots
craw ro′sis	kraurosis
crip tor′kid ism	cryptorchidism
crow′mo some	chromosome
crow″mo so′mal	chromosomal
deh bree′	debris
deng′ghee	dengue
de send′enz	descendens
de sid′u ah	decidua
de sid′u us	deciduous
dess′i bel	decibel
di af″y seal′	diaphyseal
die′uh foe re′sis	diaphoresis
di fo′ne uh	diphonia
dif the′re ah	diphtheria
dif′the royd	diphtheroid
dine	dyne
dis ar′thre ah	dysarthria
dis″ar thro′sis	dysarthrosis
dis′en ter″e	dysentery
dis fay′je ah	dysphagia
dis fay′zhuh	dysphasia
dis funk′shun	dysfunction
dis′ki nee′ze ah	dyskinesia
dis kon″dro pla′zhuh	dyschondroplasia
dis ko′ree ah	dyscoria
dis play′zhuh	dysplasia
disp nee′ah	dyspnea
dis rith′mee uh	dysrythmia
dis toe′ne ah	dystonia
dis toe′se ah	dystocia
dis′tro fe	dystrophy
dis″uh koo′zhuh	dysacousia
dis u′re ah	dysuria
doosh	douche
dur′mis	dermis
dur′moyd	dermoid
dur″muh toe′sis	dermatosis
dur″muh ti′tis	dermatitis

AS PHONETICALLY SPELLED	*AS CORRECTLY SPELLED*
dye nam′ick	dynamic
dye′uh fram	diaphragm
dye″uh ree′a	diarrhea
eck″o la′le ah	echolalia
eck′zi muh	eczema
ed′i pal	oedipal
ee″lew rop′sis	aeluropsis
ee kol′o je	ecology
eh fed′rin	ephedrine
eh rith′ro cite	erythrocyte
eh rith″ro po ee′sis	erythropoiesis
eh rith″ro sigh toe′sis	erythrocytosis
ek lamp′se ah	eclampsia
ek tah′pic	ectopic
ek′to derm	ectoderm
ek tro′pe on	ectropion
E kye″no kok′us	Echinococcus
el″e fan tye′ah sis	elephantiasis
em″fi see′muh	emphysema
em″pye ee′muh	empyema
en″kon dro′muh	enchondroma
en′sef a li″tic	encephalytic
en sef″ah log′rah fe	encephalography
en sef′ah lo gram	encephalogram
en sef″ah lop′ah the	encephalopathy
en″sef ah lye′tis	encephalitis
en sist′ed	encysted
en′zime	enzyme
e pif′i sis	epiphysis
e pif′o rah	epiphora
er″i thee′mah	erythema
er″i them′ah tus	erythematous
er ith′royd	erythroid
Esh″ur eek′ee uh	Escherichia
e sof′ah gus	esophagus
e sof″ah je′al	esophageal
e sof″ah jye′tis	esophagitis
es″o fo′re ah	esophoria
ess″car	eschar

AS PHONETICALLY SPELLED	*AS CORRECTLY SPELLED*
ess′truss	oestrus
eth′il	ethyl
eth′i leen″	ethylene
eye′kon	icon
eye′kor	ichor
eye′let	islet
eye o″do fil′e yuh	iodophilia
eye″so fo′ri a	isophoria
eye″so ko′ri a	isocoria
eye″so kro mat′ick	isochromatic
fag o sigh′toe blast	phagocytoblast
fag″o sigh toe′sis	phagocytosis
fag′o site	phagocyte
fahr′mi sist	pharmacist
fahr″muh ko pee′uh	pharmacopeia
fahr″muh sue′tick	pharmaceutic
fair′inks	pharynx
fal′ic	phallic
fal′lus	phallus
Falow	Fallot
Fanensteel's in ci′sion	Pfannenstiel's incision
fan′tum	phantom
Fa′ren hite	Fahrenheit
fa ring′go scope	pharyngoscope
fa ring′go spaz″um	pharyngospasm
far ing jiz′mus	pharyngismus
fa rin″go nay′sal	pharyngonasal
fa ring″o pal′a teen	pharyngopalatine
far″in got′o me	pharyngotomy
far″in jeck′to me	pharyngectomy
far″in jye′tis	pharyngitis
fash′ee uh	fascia
fa sigh′tis	phacitis
fat no re′ah	phatnorrhea
fay kol′e sis	phacolysis
fay″ko muh toe′sis	phacomatosis
fay′ko scope	phacoscope
fay′ko sist	phacocyst
fay′koyd	phacoid

AS PHONETICALLY SPELLED	*AS CORRECTLY SPELLED*
fay′langks	phalanx
fay lan′jeez	phalanges
fay″lan jye′tis	phalangitis
Fayling's re a′gent	Fehling's reagent
faze	phase
fee″no bahr′bi tol	phenobarbital
fee′nol	phenol
fee′no lat ed	phenolated
fee′no type	phenotype
fe nas′i tin	phenacetin
fen′il kee″to nu′ri a	phenylketonuria
fen″yl bu′ta zone	phenylbutazone
fen y′toin	phenytoin
Fye″ko my see′teez	Phycomycetes
fye ma toe′sis	phymatosis
fye mo′sis	phimosis
figh′tase	phytase
figh′tin	phytin
figh″to bee′zor	phytobezoar
fish′er	fissure
fiz″i a′tricks	physiatrics
fizz″ee o lodj′ick	physiologic
fizz″ee ol′o jee	physiology
fleb eck′to me	phlebectomy
fleb′o gram	phlebogram
fle′bo lith	phlebolith
fleb′o plas″te	phleboplasty
fleb os′tas sis	phlebostasis
fleb′o tome	phlebotome
Fleb ot′o mus	Phlebotomus
fleb bot′o me	phlebotomy
fle bye′tis	phlebitis
flee″bo throm bo′sis	phlebothrombosis
fleg ma′tick	phlegmatic
flem	phlegm
flik ten′yool	phlyctenule
flik ten′yool ur	phlyctenular
fo′bi a	phobia
fo″ko mee′li uh	phocomelia
fo nay′shun	phonation

AS PHONETICALLY SPELLED	*AS CORRECTLY SPELLED*
fo net′ick	phonetic
fo′niks	phonics
fo nop′si uh	phonopsia
fos′fate	phosphate
fos for′ick	phosphoric
fo′tizm	photism
fo″to fo′bi uh	photophobia
fo tom′e ter	photometer
fo″to mye′kro graf	photomicrograph
fren″eh cot′o mee	phrenicotomy
fren′ick	phrenic
fren o kol′ick	phrenocolic
fren ol′o je	phrenology
Froid, S.	Freud, S.
Fry test	Frei test
fye′brus	fibrous
Gheem′suh	Giemsa
gin″e co mas′tia	gynecomastia
ghil′o teen	guillotine
gin′i koyd	gynecoid
glaw ko′mah	glaucoma
gliss′ur ide	glyceride
gliss′ur il	glyceryl
gliss′ur in	glycerin
glye′ko jen	glycogen
glye″ko jen′e sis	glycogenesis
glye″ko jen′ick	glycogenic
glye kol′i sis	glycolysis
glye′ko side	glycoside
glye″ko su′re ah	glycosuria
glye see′mee uh″	glycemia
glye′seen	glycine
Goan	Ghon
goo″bur nack′u lum	gubernaculum
grye po′sis	gryposis
guy″ni kol′o jee	gynecology
guy″ni kol′o jist	gynecologist
Guy so′muh	Geisoma
gwy′ack	guaiac

AS PHONETICALLY SPELLED	*AS CORRECTLY SPELLED*
heem	heme
hee″mo fill′e ack	hemophiliac
hee″mo fill′ee uh	hemophilia
hee′mo lize	hemolyze
hee″mo new″mo thor′acks	hemopneumothorax
He mof′i lus	Hemophilus
he mop′ti sis	hemoptysis
hem′o ridj	hemorrhage
hem′o royd	hemorrhoid
het′er fo ne ah	heterophonia
het′er o fil	heterophil
hi′ah lin	hyalin
hi′ah loyd	hyaloid
hi″al u ron′i dase	hyaluronidase
hi′brid	hybrid
hi dan′toin	hydantoin
hi dat′id	hydatid
hi′dra gog	hydragogue
hi′drate	hydrate
hi dro fil	hydrophil
hi″dro fo′bi a	hydrophobia
hi″dro noo″mo tho′racks	hydropneumothorax
hi′drops	hydrops
hi′dro seel	hydrocele
hi″dro se fal′ick	hydrocephalic
hi″dro sef′uh lus	hydrocephalus
hi′druh zeen	hydrazine
hi′fa	hypha
hi fee′mee uh	hyphemia
hi gro′mah	hygroma
hi′jeen	hygiene
hi′men	hymen
hi′oid	hyoid
hi″pah ku′ze ah	hypacusia
hip no′sis	hypnosis
hip′no tize	hypnotize
hi″per ee′mi a	hyperemia
hi″po cal ee′mee uh	hypokaliemia
hi″po far′inx	hypopharynx
hi″pof′i sis	hypophysis

AS PHONETICALLY SPELLED	*AS CORRECTLY SPELLED*
hi″po fon′ia	hypophonia
hi″po for′ia	hypophoria
hi″po gly see′mee uh	hypoglycemia
hi″po klor high′dree uh	hypochlorhydria
hi″po kon′dree ack	hypochondriac
hi″po kon′dree uh	hypochondria
hi″po kon′dree um	hypochondrium
hi″po nath′us	hypognathous
hi″pur cal ee′mee uh	hyperkalemia
hi pur faj′ee uh	hyperphagia
hi″pur gly see′mee uh	hyperglycemia
hi″pur kye′lee uh	hyperchylia
hi″pur koe′lee uh	hypercholia
hi″pur o nick′ee uh	hyperonychia
hi″pur pye ee′zhuh	hyperpiesia
hi″pur pye reck′see uh	hyperpyrexia
hi″pur tri ko′sis	hypertrichosis
hi pur′tro fe	hypertrophy
hiss tear′ia	hysteria
hiss″tur ec′to me	hysterectomy
hiss″tur or′rafy	hysterorrhapy
hoop′ing cough	whooping cough
Hoosay	Houssay
ick ter′ick	icteric
ick′ter us	icterus
ick′thee o′sis	ichthyosis
ick′thee oyd	ichthyoid
ick′tul	ictal
ick′tus	ictus
il″e or′ah fe	ileorrhaphy
ill′eh um	ileum
ill′eh um	ilium (bone)
in″o kon dry′tis	inochondritis
in′sest	incest
in sigh′zor	incisor
in size′d	incised
in″tur ass′i nus	interacinous
in″tur kon′drul	interchondral
in″tur kon′du lur	intercondylar

AS PHONETICALLY SPELLED	*AS CORRECTLY SPELLED*
ip'i kack	ipecac
irr"i do ko"royd i'tis	iridochoroiditis
irr"i do recks'is	iridorhexis
irr"i do sigh klye'tis	iridocyclitis
irr"i do sigh kleck'to mee	iridocyclectomy
ir"uh sip'e las	erysipelas
is ku're ah	ischuria
iss kee' mee ah	ischemia
iss"kee o bul bo'sus	ischiobulbosus
iss"kee o pew'bis	ischiopubis
iss"kee o reck'tul	ischiorectal
iss'kee um	ischium
iss'mus	isthmus
jawn'dis	jaundice
jin"i kol'o jee	gynecology
jin"i kol'o jist	gynecologist
jin'i koyd	gynecoid
jin'ji vah	gingiva
jin"ji vek'to me	gingivectomy
jin"ji vye'tis	gingivitis
jin'o plas"te	gynoplasty
juck"sta po zish'un	juxtaposition
jye'rus	gyrus
ka cof'o ny	cacophony
kahl'ick	colic
kahr"dee o new mat'ick	cardiopneumatic
kahr"po fa lan'je al	carpophalangeal
kah tahr'	catarrh
kah tahr'ul	catarrhal
ka keck'see uh	cachexia
ka'se us	caseous
kar"si no'mah	carcinoma
kay'licks	calyx
kay'seck	Casek
Keeahri's net'work	Chiari's network
kee'late	chelate
kee'loyd	keloid
kee'lo plas"ty	cheiloplasty

AS PHONETICALLY SPELLED	AS CORRECTLY SPELLED
kee mo′sis	chemosis
kee″mo tak′sis	chemotaxis
kye az′muh	chiasma
kye fo′sis	kyphosis
kye ligh′tis	cheilitis
kye lo′sis	cheilosis
kye″lo tho′racks	chylothorax
kye′mo graf	kymograph
kye″mo trip′sin	chymotrypsin
kile	chyle
klav′i kul	clavicle
klo az′muh	chloasma
klo″ro my see′tin	Chloromycetin
kly″do mas′toyd	cleidomastoid
kly′noyd	clinoid
ko ag′yoo late	coagulate
Koksacki vi′rus	Coxsackie virus
kol″an gi′tis	cholangitis
ko led′o kus	choledochus
ko′leen	choline
Kolee's frac′ture	Colles's fracture
ko les′ter ol	cholesterol
ko″le li thigh′ah sis	cholelithiasis
kol″i sis tek′to me	cholecystectomy
kol″i sis ti′tis	cholecystitis
kol″i sis′to gram	cholecystogram
ko′lon	colon
ko los′to me	colostomy
ko los′trum	colostrum
kom′uh	coma
kom′uh toce	comatose
kon″di lo′mah	condyloma
kon″dro kos′tal	chondrocostal
kon dro′mah	chondroma
kon′droyd	chondroid
kon′drul	chondral
kon dry′tis	chondritis
koo′muh rin	coumarin
Koos mahl's res″pi ra′tion	Kussmaul's respiration
kor′duh	chorda

AS PHONETICALLY SPELLED	*AS CORRECTLY SPELLED*
ko ree′i form	choreiform
ko ree′′uh	chorea
kor′ne ah	cornea
ko′roid	choroid
koo′ma din	coumadin
kor′pus ul	corpuscle
korr′o nerr″ee	coronary
kouch′ing	couching
krep′i tant	crepitant
kript	crypt
kro′mo fobe	chromophobe
kro′mate	chromate
krome	chrome
kron′ick	chronic
kroop	croup
kro nis′i te	chronicity
kur nick′tuh rus	kernicterus
Kweckenstedt's sign	Queckenstedt's sign
kwin′i deen	quinidine
kwin′zee	quinsey
kwod″ri plee′juh	quadriplegia
kwod′ri seps	quadriceps
kwor′en teen	quarantine
kwor′tan	quartan
kwye′nine	quinine
ky″lo tho′rax	chylothorax
ky′lous	chylous
lab′i rinth	labyrinth
lack′ri mul	lacrimal
lack′tate	lactate
lack′tick	lactic
lack′tos	lactose
lar″ing go far′iinks	laryngopharynx
lar″ing gol′o gy	laryngology
lar″ing go scope′	laryngoscope
lar″in jeck′to mee	laryngectomy
lar″in ji′tis	laryngitis
lar″in jiz′mus	laryngismus
lar′inks	larynx

AS PHONETICALLY SPELLED	*AS CORRECTLY SPELLED*
lass′uh rate	lacerate
Layehneck′cir rho′sis	Laennec's cirrhosis
Leesh may′nee uh	Leishmania
leesh″mun eye′uh sis	leishmaniasis
Leffler's syn′drome	Loeffler's syndrome
lew′eez	lues
lew kee′mee ah	leukemia
lew kee′moyd	leukemoid
lew″ko durma′	leukoderma
lew ko′muh	leukoma
lew″ko pee′ne ah	leukopenia
lew″ko pee′nic	leukopenic
lew″ko ree′ah	leukorrhea
lew′ko site	leukocyte
lew″ko si toe′sis	leukocytosis
lew′pus	lupus
lew′te al	luteal
limf	lymph
lim fad″eh nop′ah the	lymphadenopathy
lim fad″en ni′tis	lymphadenitis
lim fan″je o′mah	lymphangioma
lim″fan ji′tis	lymphangitis
lim foj′en us	lymphogenous
lim fo′mah	lymphoma
lim″fo sar ko′mah	lymphosarcoma
lim′fo site	lymphocyte
li′sis	lysis
lo″kee o ree′uh	lochiorrhea
lo′kee uh	lochia
lo′shee o	lotio
lo′sigh	loci
lye′kin	lichen
lye kun″if i kay′shun	lichenification
lye″o my o′ma	leiomyoma
ma lay′shee uh	malacia
Mantoo test	Mantoux test
mass′er rate″	macerate
mame	maim
meel′yoo	milieu

AS PHONETICALLY SPELLED	*AS CORRECTLY SPELLED*
me nar'kee	menarche
me seng'kye muh	mesenchyma
mess'eng kima	mesenchyme
mew'koyd	mucoid
mew ko'zuh	mucosa
mew'kus	mucous
micks'oyd	myxoid
micks o'muh	myxoma
mid ri'a sis	midriasis
migh at'ro fe	myatrophy
migh cot'ick	mycotic
migh"eh ligh'tis	myelitis
migh'eh lin	myelin
migh'eh lin ayt"ed	myelinated
migh"ek'to me	myectomy
migh"e lo po ee'sis	myelopoiesis
migh'koyd	mycoid
migh kol'o je	mycology
migh ko'sis	mycosis
migh o clo'ne ah	myoclonia
migh'oyd	myoid
migh o'ma	myoma
migh o'ma tus	myomatous
migh"o meck'to me	myomectomy
migh"o me try'tis	myometritis
migh'ope	myope
migh o'pee uh	myopia
migh o'pick	myopic
migh orr'uh fee	myorrhaphy
migh"o si'tis	myositis
migh ot'o me	myotomy
migh o ton'ick	myotonic
migh se toe'ma	mycetoma
mi"ring got'to me	myringotomy
mi ring'o plast te	myringoplasty
mirr"in jy'tis	myringitis
mix"e de'ma	myxedema
mix'oyd	myxoid
mix o'ma	myxoma
mon o rine'ick	monorhinic

AS PHONETICALLY SPELLED	*AS CORRECTLY SPELLED*
mon o ti'ke al	monotychial
moo'lahjh	moulage
mor fe'ah	morphea
mor'feen	morphine
mor"fo jen'eh sis	morphogenesis
mor fol'o je	morphology
mor'guh	morgue
my'krobe	microbe
naf'thuh	naphtha
naf'thu leen	naphthalene
Nah thos'to mah	Gnathostoma
nat	gnat
nath'ik	gnathic
na'tho plas"te	gnathoplasty
naw'zee uh	nausea
nayth'ee on	gnathion
nee fral'juh	nephralgia
nee frek'to me	nephrectomy
nee fro'muh	nephroma
nee fro'sis	nephrosis
nee frot'o me	nephrotomy
nee"mass thee'ne uh	mnemasthenia
nee"mo dur'me uh	mnemodermia
nee mon'icks	mnemonics
neh'frick	nephric
neh fry'tis	nephritis
new'klee ate"ed	nucleated
new'klee eye	nuclei
new klee'o lus"	nucleolus
new'klee ur	nuclear
new'kle us	nucleus
new mat'ick	pneumatic
new"mat o seal'	pneumatocele
new"ma ti za'tion	pneumatization
new"mo cock'al	pneumococcal
new"mo cock see'mee uh	pneumococcemia
new"mo cock'us	pneumococcus
new"mo en sef'a lo gram	pneumoencephalogram
new'mo graf	pneumograph

AS PHONETICALLY SPELLED	*AS CORRECTLY SPELLED*
new″mo hee″mo thor′acks	pneumohemothorax
new″mo mee dee uhs tine′um	pneumomediastinum
new″mo neck′to mee	pneumonectomy
new mon′ick	pneumonic
new″mo nigh′tis	pneumonitis
new mo′ni uh	pneumonia
new″mo per″i card′i um	pneumopericardium
new″mo per′i to ne um	pneumoperitoneum
new″mo tho′racks	pneumothorax
new″muh toe′sis	pneumatosis
new rite′is	neuritis
new″ro jen′ick	neurogenic
new ro′ma	neuroma
new′ron	neuron
new ro′sis	neurosis
new′ral	neural
new′tron	neutron
nick tal′je uh	nyctalgia
nigh seer′ee uh	neisseria
nigh stag′mus	nystagmus
nimf	nymph
nim″foe may′ne ack	nymphomaniac
nos′tick	gnostic
o ee″de o migh ko′sis	oidiomycosis
Oee′de um	Oidium
off thal′mee uh	ophthalmia
off thal′mick	ophthalmic
off′thal mo din′e ah	ophthalmodynia
off″thal mol′o jist	ophthalmologist
off thal′mo scope	ophthalmoscope
off thal mos′co pe	ophthalmoscopy
o fi′as is	ophiasis
ok′u lar	ocular
ok″u lo mo′tur	oculomotor
ome	ohm
om fal′ick	omphalic
om″fal i′tis	omphalitis
om″fal o mez″en ter′ick	omphalomesenteric
om″fa lot′me	omphalotomy

AS PHONETICALLY SPELLED	*AS CORRECTLY SPELLED*
om fal'o seel	omphalocele
Ong"ko sur'ca	Onchocerca
o nick'ee uh"	onychia
o nik i'tis	onychitis
o nik"ko din'e ah	onychodynia
o nik o'mah	onychoma
on"i ko migh ko'sis	onychomycosis
on ik o'sis	onychosis
on ik'sis	onyxis
on kol'o gy	oncology
o"off or'af ee	oophorrhaphy
o"o foe reck'to me	oophorectomy
o"o foe ro hiss"tyr eck'to me	oophorohystercetomy
o"o foe ro pex se	oophoropexy
or"kee eck'to me	orchiectomy
or"kee o peck'see	orchiopexy
or kye'tis	orchitis
o"to rea'ah	otorrhea
Oxner, Alton	Ochsner, Alton
pack"e durm'a tus	pachydermatous
pack e ji're ah	pachygyria
pack"e kro mat'ick	pachychromatic
pack"i men"in jy'tis	pachymeningitis
pack"i men'inks	pachymenix
pan"flee bi'tis	panphlebitis
pan"his tur eck'to me	panhysterectomy
par"o nick'ee uh	paranychia
pew'bur ty	puberty
pew'biz	pubis
pick'no lep"se	pyknolepsy
Pirkay test	Pirquet test
ploo'rah	pleura
ploo'ri se	pleurisy
ploo"ro din'ee yuh	pleurodynia
pre'cox	praecox
pro"fi lack'tick	prophylactic
pro'fayz	prophase
pro"fi lacks'is	prophylaxis
pur"pe'ri um	puerperium

AS PHONETICALLY SPELLED	AS CORRECTLY SPELLED
pur′pur uh	puerpera
pur′pur al	puerperal
rab″do migh o′muh	rhabdomyoma
rab″do migh″o sar co′muh	rhabdomyosarcoma
raf a′ne ah	raphania
rag′uh deez	rhagades
ra kit′ick	rachitic
ray′fee	raphe
ra″kee o din′ee ah	rachiodynia
ra″kee op′a the	rachiopathy
ra″kee o ple′je ah	rachioplegia
ray′cus	rhacous
ray′ki om′e ter	rachiometer
ray′ki o tome″	rachiotome
ray″ko ot′o me	rachiotomy
ray′kis	rachis
Re′delz stru′ma	Riedel's struma
ree′o base	rheobase
ree″o card″i og′ra fe	rheocardiography
ree′o cord	rheochord
ree ol′o ge	rheology
ree om′e ter	rheometer
ree′o stat	rheostat
ree″o tack′sis	rheotaxis
ree′o tome	rheotome
ree′o trope	rheotrope
reg′mah	rhegma
rent′ghin	roentgen
rent″ghin og′ra fe	roentgenography
rent′ghin o gram″	roentgenogram
rent′ghin ol′o je	roentgenology
rent″ghin ol′o jist	roentgenologist
reo′stat	rheostat
rew ma tal′je ah	rheumatalgia
rew ma′tick	rheumatic
rew′ma tizm	rheumatism
rew′ma toyd	rheumatoid
rex′is	rhexis
rye′neck	wryneck

AS PHONETICALLY SPELLED	*AS CORRECTLY SPELLED*
rye nigh'tis	rhinitis
Ri'terz syn'drome	Reiter's syndrome
ri'thum	rhythm
rit"i doe plas'te	rhytidoplasty
rit i doe'sis	rhytidosis
ro dop'sin	rhodopsin
rom'boyd	rhomboid
rong'cus	rhonchus
roo-en-y	roux-en-y
Roos	Rhus
rowl	rale
rye'nal	rhinal
rye nal'jee ah	rhinalgia
rye"no an try'tis	rhinoantritis
rye"no fye'muh	rhinophyma
rye"no foe'ne ah	rhinophonia
rye'no lith	rhinolith
rye nol'o jist	rhinologist
rye"no plas'te	rhinoplasty
rye nop'uth ee	rhinopathy
rye"nor ray'je ah	rhinorrhagia
rye no ree'uh	rhinorrhea
rye nor'uh fee	rhinorrhaphy
rye'ne scope	rhinoscope
rye"no sef'a le	rhinocephaly
rye"no sef'a lus	rhinocephalus
Rye"no spor rid'i um	Rhinosporidium
rye not'o me	rhinotomy
rye'zome	rhizome
rye zot'o me	rhizotomy
sack'uh rin	saccharin
sac'uh ryde	saccharide
sack'yoo lar	saccular
saf'eh nus	saphenous
sam o'muh	psammoma
see'kum	cecum
see'lee ack	celiac
sef'ah lad	cephalad
se fal'gic	cephalgic

AS PHONETICALLY SPELLED	*AS CORRECTLY SPELLED*
sef′al hee″muh toe′muh	cephalhematoma
sef′al in	cephalin
se fal′ick	cephalic
sef″a lo′ma	cephaloma
sel	cell
sel″u li′tis	cellulitis
ser″e bel′ar	cerebellar
ser″e bel′lum	cerebellum
ser′e bral	cerebral
se roo′men	cerumen
ser′vicks	cervix
ser″vi sy′tis	cervicitis
sfee′ne on	sphenion
sfee″no eth′moyd	sphenoethmoid
sfee″no max′i lar ee	sphenomaxillary
sfee″no pal′uh teen	sphenopalatine
sfee″ne pe tro′sal	sphenopetrosal
sfee″no tree′ze ah	sphenotresia
sfee no′tribe	sphenotribe
sfee′noyd	sphenoid
sfee″noyd i′tis	sphenoiditis
sfeer′o site	spherocyte
sfeer′oyd	spheroid
sfeer′ule	spherule
sfig mo′graf	sphygmograph
sfig′moyd	sphygmoid
sfig″mo ma nom′e ter	sphygmomanometer
sfing′go my′eh lin	sphyngomyelin
sfink″ter al′je ah	sphincteralgia
sfink″ter i′tis	sphincteritis
sfink″ter ot′o me	sphincterotomy
sfink′tur	sphincter
shang′ker	chancre
Shick test	Schick test
Shil′derz dis ease′	Schilder's disease
shis″to so mye′a sis	schistosomiasis
shwon o′muh	schwanoma
sib′a lum	scybalum
Sidinham's cho re′a	Sydenham's chorea
sif′i lid	syphilid

AS PHONETICALLY SPELLED	*AS CORRECTLY SPELLED*
sif″i lit′ick	syphilitic
sif il o′mah	syphiloma
sif′i loyd	syphiloid
sif″i lo ther′a pe	syphilotherapy
sif′i lus	syphilis
sigh at′ick	sciatic
sigh at′i kuh	sciatica
sigh″kass thee′ne uh	psychasthenia
sigh′kee	psyche
sigh″kee at′rick	psychiatric
sigh′kick	psychic
sigh″ko an al′i sis	psychoanalysis
sigh″ko dye nam′icks	psychodynamics
sigh kol′o gee	psychology
sigh kol′o jist	psychologist
sigh″ko me′trics	psychometrics
sigh″ko mo′tor	psychomotor
sigh″ko new ro′sis	psychoneurosis
sigh″ko new rot′ick	psychoneurotic
sigh′ko path	psychopath
sigh ko′sis	psychosis
sigh″ko so ma′tick	psychosomatic
sigh′nate	cynate
sigh tite′is	scytitis
sigh tol′ogy	cytology
sik′ah triks	cicatrix
si kye′uh tree	psychiatry
si kye′uh trist	psychiatrist
sil′a bus	syllabus
sil′e air″ee	ciliary
sil′e ate″ed	ciliated
sil′ee ah	cilia
sim blef′uh ron	symblepharon
sim″bi o′sis	symbiosis
sim e′le ah	symelia
Sime′s am″pu ta′tion	Syme′s amputation
sim′fi sis	symphysis
sim fiz′ee o tome″	symphisiatome
sim′i try	symmetry
sim″pa theh′tick	sympathetic

AS PHONETICALLY SPELLED	*AS CORRECTLY SPELLED*
sim″pa thek′to me	symphathectomy
sim path″e kop′a the	sympathicopathy
sim path″e o nu ri′tis	sympathoneuritis
sim″pa thet″i ko mi met′ick	sympatheticomimetic
sim path″o lit′ick	sympatholytic
sim path″o mi met′ick	sympathomimetic
simp′tom	symptom
sin′aps	synapse
sin″ar thro′sis	synarthrosis
sin dack′til ee	syndactyly
sin′drome	syndrome
sing′ko pee	syncope
sing″kon dro′sis	synchondrosis
sink′a men	Synkamin
sin′ka vite	Synkavite
sin′ko py	syncopy
sin″os toe′sis	synostosis
si no″vee o′muh	synovioma
si no′vee ah	synovia
sin″o vy′tis	synovitis
sin sill′in	Synicillin
sin thet′ick	synthetic
sint′ti gram	scintigram
sin′ur jiz um	synergism
si″ring go′ma	syringoma
si ring″go migh ee′lee ah	syringomyelia
si ring″go seel′	syringocele
si ring″o sist toe′mah	syringocystoma
si′rinj	syringe
si row′sis	cirrhosis
sist	cyst
sis′tick	cystic
sis′to lee	systole
sis tol′ick	systolic
sis′to seel	cystocele
sis′to scope	cystoscope
sis tos′ko pe	cystoscopy
sis′turn	cistern
sis tur′nah	cisterna
sit″a ko′sis	psittacosis

AS PHONETICALLY SPELLED	*AS CORRECTLY SPELLED*
Skanzoni's ma neu′ver	Scanzoni's maneuver
skee′mo graf	schemograph
skil′izm	scillism
skirr′oyd	scirrhoid
skirr′us	scirrhous or scirrhus
skiz″o fren′ick	schizophrenic
skiz″o fren′i ah	schizophrenia
skiz og′o ne	schizogony
skiz″o may′ni ah	schizomania
skiz′oyd	schizoid
skle″ro ma la′she ah	scleromalacia
skle ro nik′e ah	scleronychia
skle ro′sis	sclerosis
sklerr eck′to me	sclerectomy
sklerr ee′muh	sclerema
sklerr eye′tis	scleritis
sklerr o′muh	scleroma
sklerr″ro durm′ah	scleroderma
skle′ruh	sclera
skli rot′ick	sclerotic
skli roze′	sclerose
sko″lee o′sis	scoliosis
sko′lex	scolex
sko toe′muh	scotoma
skra′fu luh	scrofula
sku′ba di′ving	scuba diving
skur′vee	scurvy
soo′do cyst′	pseudocyst
sor″ee at′ick	psoriatic
so″rye ass′i form	psoriasiform
so rye′uh sis	psoriasis
so′us	psoas
spy′ro keet	spirochete
staf″i lo cock′al	staphylococcal
staf′i lo cock see′me uh	staphylococcemia
staf″i lo cock′us	staphylococcus
staf′i loma	staphyloma
stip′tick	styptic
strick′nin	strychnine
sty′lit	stylet

AS PHONETICALLY SPELLED	*AS CORRECTLY SPELLED*
sty″lo high′oyd	stylohyoid
sty′lus	stylus
sue″dar thro′sis	pseudarthrosis
sue″do an jye′angina	pseudoangina
sue″du bul′bar	pseudobulbar
sue″do hee″mo fill′ee ah	pseudohemophilia
sue″do high pur′tro fee	pseudohypertrophy
sue″do hur maf′ro dite	pseudohermaphrodite
sue″do mem′brane	pseudomembrane
sue″do mo′nus	pseudomonas
sue″do mew′sin	pseudomucin
sue″do pa ree′sis	pseudoparesis
sue″do par ral′e sis	pseudoparalysis
sue″do po′dee um	pseudopodium
sue″do sigh ee′sis	pseudocyesis
sue″do sist′	pseudocyst
sue″do tay′beez	pseudotabes
sue″do tie′foyd	pseudotyphoid
sub fren′ick	subphrenic
su′krose	sucrose
sul′fur	sulphur
supra high′oyd	suprahyoid
sur″kum sizh′un	circumcision
tack′ee card′i uh	tachycardia
tack″ip nee′uh	tachypnea
tahr′mick	ptarmic
taw′reen	taurine
tee′nee uh	taenia
tee′nee uh fuj″	taenifuge
Teet′see fly	tsetse fly
teh ridj′ee um	pterygium
tel′o faze	telophase
terr′ee on	pterion
terr′i goyd	pterygoid
thigh′mawl	thymol
thigh meck′to mee	thymectomy
thigh′mick	thymic
thigh mo′muh	thymoma
thigh′mus	thymus

AS PHONETICALLY SPELLED	*AS CORRECTLY SPELLED*
thigh my'tis	thymitis
thigh rock'sin	thyroxin
thigh"ro gen'ick	thyrogenic
thigh"ro gloss'ul	thyroglossal
thigh"ro high'oyd	thyrohyoid
thigh ro'sis	thyrosis
thigh"ro trope'in	thyrotropin
thigh'royd	thyroid
thigh"royd eck'to mee	thyroidectomy
thigh"royd i'tis	thyroiditis
tie lo'sis	ptilosis
tif leck'to mee	typhlectomy
tif lye'tis	typhlitis
ti flos'to mee	tiphlostomy
ti'foyd	typhoid
ti'fus	typhus
tim'pa nee	tympany
tim pan'ick	tympanic
tim"pan it'ick	tympanitic
tim'pan um	tympanum
ti'ro seen	tyrosine
toe'sis	ptosis
track'i lor'ud fee	trachelorrhaphy
track"i lot'o mee	trachelotomy
track"i lye'tis	trachelitis
tra ko'muh	trachoma
traw mat'ick	traumatic
traw'muh	trauma
traw'muh tize	traumatize
tray"kee i'tis	tracheitis
tray'kee o brong'kee ul	tracheobronchial
tray"kee o brong kigh'tis	tracheobronchitis
tray"kee o lar in'jul	tracheolaryngeal
tray"kee o ste no'sis	tracheostenosis
tray"kee os'tomy	tracheostomy
tray"kee ot'o mee	tracheotomy
tray'kee uh	trachea
tree ahj'	triage
tre fine'	trephine
Trick"i nel'uh	Trichinella

AS PHONETICALLY SPELLED	AS CORRECTLY SPELLED
trick″i no′sis	trichinosis
trick″ko bee′zoar	trichobezoar
tric′ko lith	tricholith
Trick″o migh ko′sis	Trichomycosis
Trick″o mo′nas	Trichomonas
Trick yoo′ris	Trichuris
tri kye′nuh	trichina
Tri kof′e tin	Tricophyton
trip′sin	trypsin
tro can′tur	trochanter
trock′lee uh	trochlea
trock′lee ur	trochlear
tro′fick	trophic
tro′fizm	trophism
tro′fo blast	trophoblast
tro″fo zo′ite	trophozoite
tro′kee	troche
try cot′o mee	trichotomy
try fay′zick	triphasic
turn′eh kit	tourniquet
tye′al in	ptyalin
ty′a lism	ptyalism
tye al′o gog	ptyalogogue
tye′sis	ptysis
u′fo ni a	euphonia
u′fo ri a	euphoria
u jen′ics	eugenics
u ko′le ah	eucholia
u mor′fic	eumorphic
u′nuch oild	eunuchoid
u′nuck	eunuch
u ray′cus	urachus
u sta′shi an	eustachian
u″thah nay′ze ah	euthanasia
vack′seen	vaccine
vack sin′ee uh	vaccinia
vack′sin oyd	vaccinoid
vair′icks	varix

AS PHONETICALLY SPELLED	*AS CORRECTLY SPELLED*
vane	vein
veck′tor	vector
vur′gin	virgin
waw bain	ouabain
zan′theen	xanthine
zan″thi laz′muh	xanthelasma
zan″tho crow′mee uh	xanthochromia
zan tho″ma toe′sis	xanthomatosis
zan tho′ma tus	xanthomatous
zan tho′muh	xanthoma
zan tho′sis	xanthosis
zeer″o dur′muh	xeroderma
zeer″of thal′mee uh	xerophthalmia
zef′e ran	Zephiran
zer an′tic	zerantic
ae ro′sis	xerosis
ze rot′ick	xerotic
zi′goma	zygoma
zif′oyd	xiphoid
zi′gee on	zygion
zi′goat	zygote
zi go mat′ick	zygomatic
zi′leen	xylene
zi′lol	xylol

Section V

ALPHABETICAL LIST OF:

- Arteries
- Veins
- Muscles
- Diseases
- Syndromes
- Commonly Performed Tests
- Surgical Incisions
- Dental Surfaces
- Descriptive Positions, i.e., Anatomical

Arteries

aberrant
acetabular
acromial
acromiothoracic
alveolar
angular
antral
aorta
appendicular
arciform
arcuate (foot, kidney)
auditory
aruicular
axillary
azygos (of vagina)

basilar
brachial
bronchial
buccal
buccinator

calcaneal
calcarine
caroticotympanic
carotid
carpal
cavernous
celiac
central (of retina)
cerebellar
cerebral
cervical
choroid
ciliary
circumflex
clitoral
colic
collateral
communicating
conjunctival
coronary
costocervical
cremasteric
cricothyroid
crural
cystic

deferential
dental
digital (fingers, toes)
diploic
dorsalis pedis

epigastric
episcleral
esophageal
ethmoidal

facial
femoral
frontal

gastric
gastroduodenal
gastroepiploic
genicular
gluteal

hallucis
helicine
hemorrhoidal
hepatic
humeral
hypogastric
hypophyseal

ileal

ileocolic
iliac
iliolumbar
infraorbital
innominate
intercostal
interlobar (of kidney)
interosseous
intestinal

jejunal

labial
lacrimal
laryngeal
lenticulostriate
lienal
lingual
lumbar

malleolar
mammary
masseteric
mastoid
maxillary
median (hand, spinal cord)
mediastinal
meningeal
mental
mesenteric
metacarpal
metatarsal
musculophrenic

nasal
nasopalatine
neubauer's
nutrient (femur, fibula, tibia, humerus)

obturator
occipital
ophthalmic
ovarian

palatine
palmar
palpebral
pancreatica
pancreaticoduodenal
penis
perforating (of thigh)
pericardiacophrenic
perineal
peroneal
pharyngeal
phrenic
plantar
pontine
popliteal
preventricular
princeps cervicis
princeps hallucis
princeps pollicis
profunda brachia
profunda femoris
profunda linguae
pterygoid canal, artery of
pudendal
pulmonary
pyloric

radial
ranine
recurrent (tibial, ulnar, radial)
renal

sacral
saphenous
scapular circumflex
scapular transverse
sciatic

scrotal
septal, posterior (nose)
sigmoid
spermatic
sphenopalatine
spinal
spiral
splenic
stapedial
sternocleidomastoid
stylomastoid
subclavian
subcostal
sublingual
submental
subscapular
supraorbital
suprarenal
suprascapular
sural

tarsal
temporal
terminal
testicular
thoracic
thoracoacromial
thoracodorsal
thymic
thyrocervical trunk
thyroid
tibial
tonsilar
trabecular
transverse (facial, neck, perineal, scapular)
tympanic

ulnar
umbilical
urethral
uterine

vaginal
vasa brevia
vertebral
vesical
vidian
volar (digital, radial)

Wilkie's (supraduodenal)
Willis, circle of

Zinn's
zygomatico-orbital

Veins

accessory, cephalic
accessory, hemiazygos
accessory, saphenous
angular
anterior auricular
anterior bronchiole
anterior coronary
anterior facial
anterior jugular
anterior mediastinal
anterior parotid
anterior tibial
anterior vertebral
articular (knee, mandible)
ascending lumbar
axillary
axygos

basilic
basivertebral
branchial
bronchial

cephalic
cerebellar
cerebral
choroid
colic
comitans (lateralis, medialis)
coronary
costoaxillary
cystic

deep cervical
deep circumflex iliac
deep iliac circumflex
deferentiales
dental
digital
diploic
dorsal digital (hand, foot)
dorsal metacarpal
dorsal metatarsal
dorsal (of penis)
ductus venosus
duodenal

emissary
esophageal
external iliac
external jugular
external nasal
external pubic

femoral
femoropopliteal
frontal

galen
gastroepipoloic
gluteal
great saphenous

hemiazygos
hepatic
hypogastric

ileocolic
iliolumbar
inferior epigastric
inferior gluteal
inferior mesenteric
inferior ophthalmic
inferior palpebral
inferior petrosal sinus
inferior phrenic
inferior thyroid
inferior vena cava

innominate
intercapitular
intercostal
internal auditory
internal circumflex
internal iliac
internal jugular
internal mammary
internal maxillary
internal pudendal
internal pubic
internal vertebral
intervertebral

jugular

labial
lateral circumflex femoral
lateral plantar
lateral sacral
lienal (splenic)
lingual
lumbar

marginal right
median
median antebrachial
median temporal
meningeal
metacarpal
middle cardiac
middle colic
middle hemorrhoidal
middle sacral
musculophrenic

nasofrontal

obturator
occipital
ophthalmic
orbital
ovarian

palatine
palmar
pancreatic
pancreaticoduodenal
paraumbilical
pericardial
peroneal
pharyngeal
plantar
popliteal
portal
posterior auricular
posterior bronchiole
posterior facial
posterior mediastinal
posterior parotid
posterior scrotal
posterior tibial
prostatic
pubic
pudendal
pyloric

radial
renal

short gastric
short saphenous
sigmoid
spermatic
sphenoparietal
splenic
stylomastoid
subclavian
supraorbital
suprarenal

temporal, superficial

testicular
thoracic
thoracoepigastric
transverse cervical
transverse facial
transverse scapular

ulnar

urethral
uterine
uterovaginal

vaginal
vertebral
vesicular
volar

Muscles

abductor digiti minimi (foot, hand)
abductor hallucis
abductor pollicis (brevis, longus)
accelerator urinae
accessorius
adductor brevis
adductor hallucis
adductor hallucis transversus
adductor longus
adductor magnus
adductor minimus
adductor pollicis
agitator caudae
anconeus
antitragicus
arrectores pilorum
articularis genus
aryepiglottic
arytenoepiglotticus
arytenoid (oblique, transverse)
attollens aurem
attrahens aurem
auricularis anterior
auricularis superior
auricularis posterior
axygos uvulae

biceps brachii
biceps femoris
biventer cervicis
brachialis
brachioradialis
broncho-oesophageus
buccinator
buccopharyngeus
bulbocavernosus

caninus
cephalopharyngeus
ceratocricoideus
ceratopharyngeus
cervicalis ascendens
chondroglossus
chondropharyngeus
ciliary
coccygeus
complexus
compressor naris
compressor urethrae
compressor vaginae
constrictor of pharynx (inferior, middle, superior)
coracobrachialis
corrugator cutis ani
corrugator supercilii
costalis
costocervicalis
costocoracoideus
cremaster
cricoarytenoid (lateral, posterior)
cricopharyngeus
cricothyroid
crureus

dartos
deltoid
depressor alae nasi
depressor anguli oris
depressor epiglottidis
depressor labii inferioris
depressor septi
depressor urethrae
detrusor urinae
diaphragm
digastric

dilator naris
dilator pupillae

ejaculator seminis
epicranius
erector clitoridis
erector penis
erector pili
extensor brevis digitorum
extensor brevis pollicis
extensor carpi radialis brevis
extensor carpi radialis longus
extensor carpi ulnaris
extensor coccygis
extensor digiti quinti proprius
extensor digitorum brevis
extensor digitorum longus
extensor hallucis brevis
extensor hallucis longus
extensor indicis proprius
extensor ossis metacarpi pollicis
extensor pollicis brevis
extensor pollicis longus

flexor brevis hallucis
flexor carpi radialis
flexor carpi ulnaris
flexor digiti quinti brevis
flexor digitorum brevis
flexor digitorum longus
flexor digitorum profundus
flexor digitorum sublimis
flexor hallucis brevis
flexor hallucis longus
flexor sublimis digitorum
frontalis

gastrocnemius
gemellus (inferior, superior)
genioglossus
geniohyoid
glossopalatinus
glossopharyngeus
gluteus maximus
gluteus minimus
gracilis

helicis major
helicis minor
hyoglossus
hypopharyngeus

iliacus
iliococcygeus
iliocostalis cervicis
iliocostalis dorsi
iliocostalis lumborum
iliocostocervicalis
iliopsoas
infracostals
infraspinatus
intercostal (external, internal)
interossei, dorsal (of hand, foot)
interossei, plantar
interossei, volar
interspinalis
intertransversarii
ischiocavernosus
ischiofemoralis

latissimus dorsi
levator anguli oris
levator ani
levator costae
levator glandulae thyroideae
levator labii inferior
levator labii superior
levator labii superioris alaeque nasi
levator menti

levator palati
levator palpebrae superioris
levator prostatae
levator scapulae
levator veli palatini
levatores costarum
longissimus capitis
longissimus cervicalis
longissimus dorsi
longissimus thoracis
longitudinalis dorsi
longitudinalis inferior
longitudinalis superior
longus capitis
longus colli
lumbricals (toes, fingers)

masseter
mentalis
multifidus
mylohyoid
mylopharyngeal

nasalis

obliquus abdominis externus
obliquus abdominis internus
obliquus auriculae
obliquus capitis inferior
obliquus capitis superior
obliquus oculi inferior
obliquus oculi superior
obturator externus
obturator interus
occipitalis
occipitofrontalis
omohyoid
opponens digiti quinti (hand, foot)
opponens pollicis
orbicularis oculi
orbicularis oris
orbicularis palpebrarum
orbitalis

palatoglossus
palatopharyngeus
palatosalpingeus
palmaris brevis
palmaris longus
pectinatus
pectineus
pectoralis major
pectoralis minor
peroneus accessorius
peroneus brevis
peroneus tertius
pharyngopalatinus
piriformis
plantaris
platysma
popliteus
procerus
pronator pedis
pronator quadratus
pronator teres
psoas major
psoas minor
pterygoideus externus
pterygoideus internus
pterygopharyngeus
pubocavernosus
pubococcygeus
puboprostaticus
puborectalis
pubovesicalis
pyramidalis abdominis
pyramidalis auriculae
pyramidalis nasi
pyriformis

quadratus femoris

quadratus labii inferioris
quadratus labii superioris
quatratus lumborum
quadratus plantae
quadriceps femoris

rectococcygeus
rectus abdominis
rectus capitis anterior
rectus capitis anticus major
rectus capitis anticus minor
rectus capitis lateralis
rectus capitis posterior major
rectus capitis posterior minor
rectus femoris
rectus oculi inferior
rectus oculi internus
rectus oculi lateralis
rectus oculi medialis
rectus oculi superior
retrahens aurem
rhomboideus major
rhomboideus minor
risorius
rotatores

sacrococcygeus
sacrolumbalis
sacrospinalis
salpingopharyngeus
sartorius
scalenus anterior
scalenus medius
scalenus posterior
semimembranosus
semispinalis capitis
semispinalis cervicis
semispinalis dorsi
semitendinosus
serratus anterior
serratus posterior inferior
serratus posterior superior
soleus
sphincter ani externus
sphincter ani internus
sphincter oris
sphincter pupillae
sphincter urethrae membranaceae
sphincter vaginae
sphincter vesicae
spinalis capitis
spinalis cervicis
spinalis dorsi
spinalis thoracis
splenius cervicis
splenius colli
stapedius
sternalis
sternoclavicularis
sternocleidomastoid
sternocostalis
sternohyoid
sternothyroid
styloauricularis
styloglossus
stylohyoid
stylolaryngeus
stylopharyngeus
subanconeus
subclavius
subcostals
subcrureus
subscapularis
supinator
supinator longus
supinator radii brevis
supraspinalis
supraspinatus

tarsalis (inferior, superior)
temporal

tensor fasciae latae
tensor palati
tensor tarsi
tensor tympani
tensor vaginae femoris
tensor veli palatini
teres major
teres minor
thyroarytenoid
thyroepiglottic
thyrohyoid
thropharyngeus
tibialis (interior, posterior)
tibiofascialis anterior
trachelomastoid
tragicus
transversalis colli
transversospinalis
transversus abdominis
transversus auriculae
transversus linguae
transversus menti
transversus nuchae
transversus pedis
transversus perinei profundus
transversus perinei superficialis
transversus thoracis
trapezius
triangularis
triangularis labii (inferior, superior)
triangularis sterni
triceps brachii
triceps surae
trochlearis

uvulae

vastus externus
vastus intermedius
vastus internus
vastus lateralis
vastus medialis
ventricularis
verticalis linguae
vocalis

zygomatic

Diseases

ABC hemolytic
Acosta's
Adams-Stokes
adaptation
Addison's
Adenocystic
air sac
Akueyri
Albers-Schönberg
Albert's
Albright's
Aleutian
Alexander's
alkali
alligator skin
Alper's
Alzeimer's
amyloid
Ander's
Andersen's
Andes
anserine
Apert's
Aran-Duchenne
arc-welder's
Armstrong's
attic
Aujeszky's
Australian X
autoimmune
aviator's
Ayerza's

Babinski-Froehlich
bagasse
Balo's
Bamberger-Marie
Bamle's
Bang's
Bannister's
Banti's
Barcoo
Barlow's
Basedow's
Bateman's
Batten-Mayou's
Bazin's
Beau's
Behr's
Bekhterev's
Bell's
Bernhardt's
Besnier-Boeck-Schaumann
Best's
Biermer's
Billroth's
Binswanger's
Boeck's
Bornholm
Bostock's
Bouillaud's
Bourneville's
Bouveret's
Bowen's
Bright's
Brill's
Brill-Symmers
Brodie's
Buaki
Buerger's
Buhl's
Buschke's
Busquet's
Busse-Buschke's
Byler's

Caffey's
caisson
California
Calvé-Perthes

Carrión's
Castellani's
cat-scratch
celiac
Chargas'
Charcot-Marie-Tooth
Chauffard-Still's
Chiari's
Christian-Weber
Christmas
cobalt deficiency
collagen
communicable
Concato's
congenital
congenital polycystic
constitutional
contagious
Cooley's
Cooper's
Corrigan's
Cowden's
Coxsackie
Crohn's
Crouzon's
Cruveilhier's
Cushing's
cutaneous caisson
cystic d. of breast
cystine
cytomegalic inclusion

Da Costa's
Carier's
Darling's
David's
de Beurmann-Gougerot
deficiency
degenerative
degenerative joint
demyelinating
Dercum's
Devic's
DiGuglielmo's
Duchenne-Aran
Duchenne's
Duhring's
Duke's
Dupuytren's
Durand-Nicolas-Favre
Durand's
Durante's
Duroziez's

Eale's
Ebstein's
Economo's
Eddowe's
Eisenmenger
endemic
Engelmann's
Engel-Recklinghausen's
epidemic
epizootic
Erb-Charcot

Fallot's
Fanconi's
Favre
Fete-Riga's
fibrocystic
Fiedler's
Flajani's
Fleischner's
Forbes'
Fordyce's
Fox-Fordyce
Freiberg's
Friedländer's
Frei's
Friedman's
Friedreich's
functional

Gaisböck's
Gamna's
Garré's
Gaucher's
Gee-Herter
Gee's
Gee-Thayson
Gierke's
Gilchrist's
Glisson's
glycogen storage
Gougerot's
Graefe's
Grave's
Guillain-Barré
Gull and Sutton's

Habermann's
Hailey-Hailey
Hammond's
Hand-Schüller-Christian
Hanot's
Hansen's
Hashimoto's
Haxthausen's
Heberden's
Hebra's
Heine-Medin
hemorrhagic
hemorrhagic d. of the newborn
hepatolenticular
hereditary
Heubner-Herter
Hippel-Lindau
Hirschsprung's
His's
Hodgkin's
Hoffa's
Hunosh's
Hopf's
Huntington's
Hurler's

hyaline membrane
hydatid
hypertensive vascular

idiopathic
immune-complex
inclusion
intercurrent
Isambert's

Jaffé-Lichtenstein
Jaksch's
Johne's
Jüngling's

Kahler's
Kaiserstuhl
Kakke
Kaposi's
Kashin-Beck
Kempf's
Kienböck's
Kimmelstiel-Wilson
Kleb's
Köhler's
König's
Korsakoff's
Krabbe's
Kufs'
Kümmel's

Laennec's
Landry's
Lane's
Larsen-Johansson
Legg-Calvé-Perthes
Legionnaires'
Léiner's
Leriche's
Leri's
Letterer-Siwe
Lewandowsky's

Leyden's
Libman-Sacks
Lignac-fanconi
Looser-Milkman's
Lutembacher's
Lindau's
Lipoid storage
Little's
Lobstein's
loco
Lyme

Majocchi
malignant
maple syrup urine
Marie's
McArdle's
Mediterranean
Ménière's
Mikulicz's
milkman's
Milroy's
Mitchell's
Möbius
Moeller-Barlow
Monge's
Morquio-Brailsford
mosaic
Mya's

Newcastle
Niemann-Pick
Norrie's

Ollier's
Opitz's
organic
Osgood-Schlatter
Osler's
Osler-Rendu-Weber
Osler-Vaquez
Owren's

Paget's
pandemic
Panner's
pararheumatic
parasitic
Parkinson's
Parry's
Pel-Ebstein's
periodic
periodontal
Perthe's
Peyronie's
Pfeiffer's
Phoca's
Pick's
Picto
Pinkus'
Plummer's
pneumatic hammer
policeman's
Pollitzer's
polyhedral
Pompe's
Poncet's
porcupine
Posada-Wernicke's
Potain's
Pott's
Poulet's
Preiser's
Pringle's
Profichet's
Puente's
pullorum
Purtscher's
pyramidal

Quervain's
Quincke's
Quinquand's

Raugier's

Rayer's
Raynaud's
Recklinghausen's
Recklinghausen-Applebaum
Reclus'
Reed-Hodgkin
Refsum's
Reichmann's
Reiter's
Rendu-Oslo-Weber
Renikhet
rheumatic heart
rheumatoid
Ribas-Torres
Riedel's
Riga's
Riga-Fede
Riggs'
Ritter's
Rivolta's
Robinson's
Robles'
Roger's
Rokitansky's
Romberg's
Rose
Rosenbach's
Roth's
Roth-Bernhardt
Roussy-Lévy's
Rowland's
Rummo's
Runneberg's
Rust's
Ruysch's

Sachs'
sacroiliac
St. Agatha's
St. Aignon's
St. Aman's
St. Anthony's
St. Appolonia's
St. Avertin's
St. Blasius'
St. Clair's
St. Dymphna's
St. Erasmus'
St. Fiacre's
St. Francis'
St. Gervasius'
St. Gete's
St. Giles'
St. Gotthard's tunnel
St. Hubert's
St. Job's
St. Main's
St. Mathurin's
St. Modestus'
St. Roch's
St. Sement's
St. Valentine's
St. Zachary's
salivary gland
San Joaquin Valley
Sander's
sartian
Saunders'
Savill's
Schamberg's
Schanz's
Schaumann's
Scheuermann's
Schilder's
Schimmelbusch's
Schlatter's
Schmorl's
Scholz's
Schönlein's
Schönlein-Henoch
Schottmüller's
Schriddes'
Schroeder's
Schüller's

Schüller-Christian
Schultz's
Secretan's
Selter's
Senear-Usher
senecio
septic
serum
Sever's
Shishito
shuttlemaker's
sickle-cell anemia
silage
silo-filler's
Simmonds'
Simons'
Sjogren's
Skevas-Zerfus
Smith's
Spencer's
Spielmeyer-Stock
Spielmeyer-Vogt
sponge-divers'
sporadic
Stargardt's
Steinert's
Sterbe
sterility
Sternberg's
Stieda's
Still's
Stiller's
Stokes'
Stokes-Adams
Stokvis'
Strachan's
Strümpell's
Strümpel-Leichtenstern
Strümpell-Marie
Stuhmer's
Sturge's
Sturge-Weber-Dimitri
Stuttgart
subacute
subchronic
Sudeck's
Sutton's
Sutton and Gull's
Swediaur's
Swift's
Swift-Feer
Sylvest
Symmers'

Taenzer's
Talfan
Talma's
Tangier
tarabagan
tartaric
Tay's
Tay-Sachs
Taylor's
Teschen
Thaysen's
Theiler's
Thomsen's
Thomson's
Thornwaldt's
Tietze's
Tillaux's
Tomaselli's
Tourette's
Traum's
Trevor's
Trousseau's
tsetse fly
tsutsugamushi
Tyzzer's

Underwood's
Unna's

Unverricht's

Urbach-Oppenheim
Urbach-Wiethe's
Vagabonds'
vagrants'
Valee's
Valsuani's
van Buren's
Vaquez'
Vaquez-Osler
veldt
venereal
Verneuil's
Verse's
Vidal's
Vincent's
Virchow's
Vogt's
Vogt-Spielmeyer
Volkmann's
Voltolini's
von Economo's
von Gierke's
von Hippel's
von Jaksch's
von Recklinghausen's
von Willebrand's

Vrolik's

Wagner's
Waldenstrom's
Wardrop's
Wartenberg's
Wassilieff's

Weber's
Weber-Christian
Weber-Dimitri
Wegner's
Weil's
Weingartner's
Weir Mitchell's
Wenckebach's
Werdnig-Hoffman
Werlhof's
Werner-His
Werner-Schultz
Wernicke's
Westberg's
Westphal-Strümpell
Whipple's
White's
Whitmore's
Whytts'
Widal-Abrami
Wilks'
Willis'
Wilson's
Wilson-Brocq
Winckel's
Windscheid's
Winkelman's
winter vomiting
Winton
Woillez's

Zagari's
Zahorsky's
Ziehen-Oppenheim
zymotic

Syndromes

Aarskog's
Abercrombie's
Achard-Thiers
Adair-Dighton
Adams-Stokes
addisonian
Adie's
adiposogenital
adrenogenital
Albright's
Albright-McCune-Sternberg's
Aldrich's
Alper's
Alporet
amnestic
amyostatic
Andersen's
Angelucci's
anginal
anginose
anterior cornual
Apert's
Arnold's nerve reflex
Arnold-Chiari
Ascher's
Asherman's
asphyctic
auriculotemporal
Avellis's
Ayerza's

Babinski's
Babinski-Frolich
Babinski-Nageotte
Babinski-Vacquez
Banti's
Bárány
Bard-Pic
Bardet-Biedl
Barré-Guillain
Barrett's
Bassen-Kornzweig
Beau's
Behcet's
Benedikt
Bernard's
Bernard-Horner
Bernard-Sergent
Bernard-souliur
Bernhardt-Roth
Bernheim's
Bertolotti's
Bianchi's
Biedl's
Biemond's
Binney-Bow
Blatin's
Bloch-Sulzberger
Bloom's
Blum's
Bonnevie-Ullrich
Bonnier's
Booek
Bouillaud's
Bouveret's
Brenneman's
Briquet's
Brissaud-Marie
Brissaud-Sicard
Bristow's
Brock's
Brown-Sequard
Brugsch's
Brun's
Bud-Chiari
bundle of Kent
Burnett's
Bywater's

Caffey's

callosal
Capgras's
capsulothalamic
carotid sinus
carpal tunnel
Cauchois-Eppinger-Frugoni
cauda equina
cavernous sinus
centroposterior
cerebellar
cervical
cervical rib
cervicobrachial
Cestan's
Cestan-Chenais
Cestan-Raymond
Charcot-Weiss-Barber
Chargot's
Charlin's
Chauffards's
Chauffard-Still
Chiari's
Chiari-Arnold
Chiari-Frommel
chiasma
chiasmatic
chorea
Chotzen's
Christian's
Citelli's
Clarke-Hadfield
Claude's
Claude-Bernard-Horner
Clough and Richter's
Collet's
Collet-Sicard
Conradis
cor pulmonale
corpus striatum
Costen's
costoclavicular
Cotard's
Courvoisier-Terrier
Crigler-Najjar
Cruveilhier-Baumgarten
cubitan tunnel
Curtius
Cushing's
Cyriax's

Da Costa's
Dandy-Walker
Danlos'
defibrination
Dejerine's
Dejerine-Roussy
de Lange's
de Toni-Fanconi
diencephalic
DiGeorge
Dighton-Adair
Di Guglielmo
Doan and Wiesman's
Down's
Dresbach's
Duane's
Dubin-Johnson
Dubin-Sprinz
Dubreuil-Chambardel
Duchenne's
Duchenne-Erb
dumping
Duplay's
Dupre's
dysglandular
dystrophia-dystocia

ectopic ACTH
Eddowes'
Edwards
Ehlers-Danlos
Eisenmenger's
Ellis-van Creveld
EMG

encephalotrigeminal vascular
epiphysial
Epstein's
Erb's

Fisher
Fitz-Hugh Curpis
Forssman carotid
Foster Kennedy's
Foville's
Frey's
Friedmann's vasomotor
Frolich's
Froin's
Fuch's

Gailliard's
Gaisbock's
Ganser's
Gardner's
Gasserian
gastrocardiac
Gee-Herter-Heubner
Gelineau's
general adaptation
Gerhardt's
Gerlier's
Gerstmann's
Gilles de la Tourette
globus pallidus
Goodpasture's
Goplan's
Gougerot's
Gouley's
Gower's
Gradenigo's
Graham-Little
Gronblad-Strandberg
Guillian-Barré
Gunn's

Hadfield-Clark
Hakim's
Hallermann-Screiff
Hallervorden-Spatz
Hamman's
Hamman-Rich
Hand's
Hand-Schuller-Christian
hand-shoulder
Hanot's
Hanot-Chauffard
Harada's
Hare's
Harris'
Hartnup
Hassin's
Hayem-Widal
hemi
hemiparaplegic
hemohistioblastic
hemopleuropneumonic
hemorrhagic fever
Hench-Rosenberg
hepatorenal
Heyd's
Hines-Bannick
Hoffmann-Werdnig
Holmes-Adie
Homen's
Horner's
Horner-Bernard
Horton's
humoral
Hunter's
Hunt's
Hunt's striatal
Hunterian glossitis
Hurler's
Hutchinson's
Hutchinson-Gilford
hyaline membrane
hypercalcemia
hyperkinetic

hyperophthalmopathic
hypophyseal

inspissated bile
irritable bowel
Iuemark's

Jackson's
Jacquet's
Jahnke's
jejunal
job's
jugular foramen

Kanner's
Karroo
Kartagener's
Kast's
Kawasaki
Kennedy's
Kernohan
Kimmelstiel-Wilson
Kleine-Levin
Klinefelter's
Klippel-Feil
Klotz
Klumpke-Dejerine
Kocher's
Konig's
Korsakoff's

Ladd's
Landry's
Lasegue's
Laubry-Soule
Launois'
Laurence-Biedl
Laurence-Moon-Biefl
Lawen-Roth
Legg-Calvé-Perthe's
Lëitner
Lenz's
Leredde's
Leriche's
Lermoyez's
Leschke
Levi's
Levy-Roussy
Lhermitte and McAlpine
Libman-Sacks
Lichtheim's
Lightwood's
Lignac's
loculation
Loffler's
Lowe's
Lutembacher's
lymphoproliferative

McArdle
McCune-Albright
Mackenzie's
Maffucci's
malabsorption
Malin's
Maranon's
Marchiafava-Micheli
Marcus Gunn
Marfan's
Marie's
Marie-Robinson
Meigs'
Ménière's
Menkes'
mesodermal
metameric
middle radicular
Mikulicz's
Milian's
milkman's
Millard-Gubler
Minkowski-Chauffard
Mobius
Monakow's

Moore's
Morel's
Morgagni's
Morgagni-Steward-Morel
Morquio's
Morton's
Morvan's
Mosse's
Munchausen's
Murchison-Sanderson
myasthenia gravis
myeloproliferative

Naegeli's
Naffziger's
Nelson's
nephrotic
neurocutaneous
Nezelof's
nitritoids
Noack's
Nonne's
Nonne-Milroy-Meige
Noonan
Nothnagel's

oculocerebrorenal
Ogilvie's
orodigitofacial
orofacial-digital
Ostrum-Furst

paleostriatal
pallidal
pallidomesencephalic
Pancoast's
pancreaticohepatic
paralysis agitans
paratrigeminal
Parinaud's
Parke's
Parkinson's
parkinsonian
Pasqualini
Paterson's
Patton's
Paxson
Pellazzi's
Pepper
pericolic-membrane
Peutz
Peutz-Jeghers
Pfeiffer's
phrenogastric
physiopathic
Picchini's
Pick's
pickwickian
Pierre Robin
pineal
Pins'
pituitary
Plummer-Vinson
pluriglandular
polyglandular
pontine
postcommissurotomy
posterolateral
postgastrectomy
postirradiation
postpericardiotomy
Potain's
Pozzi's
Prader-Willi
premenstrual
premotor
Profichet's
Putnam Dana

radicular
Ramsay Hunt
Raymond-Cestan's
Refsum's
Reichmann's

Reifenstein
Reiter's
Renon-Delille
retroparotid space
Reye's
Rieder
Rieger's
Riley's
rolandic vein
Romberg-Paessler
Rosenbach's
Roth's
Rothman-Makai
Rothmund's
Roussy-Levy
Russel's
Rust's

salt-losing
Sawii
scalenus
scalenus anticus
scapulocostal
Schanz's
Schaumann's
Schmidt's
Schonlein-Henoch
Schroeder's
Schuller's
Schuller-Christian
Schultz
Schwachman
Seabright bantam
Seckel
segmentary
Selye
Senear-Usher
Sezary
Sezary reticulosis
Sheehan's
shoulder-hand
Sicard's
Siemens
Silverskiold's
Silverstrini-Corda
Simmonds'
Sipple's
Sjogren's
Sludder's
Sotos
Spens's
Spurway
Stein-Leventhal
Stevens-Johnson
Stewart-Morel
Still-Chauffard
Stokes's
Stokes-Adams
striatal
Stryker-Halbeisen
Sturge's
Sturge-Kalischer-Weber
Sturge-Weber
subclavian steal
Sudeck-Leriche
sudden infant death
superaspinatus
superior mensenteric artery

Tapia's
Taussig-Bing
Tay-Sachs
tegmental
temporomandibular joint
Terry's
testicular feminization
thalamic
Thibierge-Weissenbach
Thiele
thromboembolic
Tietze's
Timme's
Toland's
Tolosa-Hunt

Tomaselli's
Treacher-Collins
trisomy
Troisier's
Turcot's
Turner's

Ullrich-Feichtiger
Unverricht's

vago-accessory
Van Buchem
van der Hoeve's
van der Woude's
vascular
Vernet's
Villaret's
Vogt's
Vogt-Koyanagi
Volkmann's
von Welty's

Wallenberg's
Waterhouse-Friderichsen
Weber
Weber-Christian
Weber-Dubler
Weingarten's
Werdnig-Hoffman
Werner's
Wernicke's
Widal
Wilson's
Wilson-Mikity
Wolff-Parkinson-White
Wright's

Young's

Zeman-King
Zieve's
Zollinger-Ellison

Commonly Performed Tests

Abderhalden's
Abelin's
Abrams'
acetanilid
acetic acid
aceto-acetic acid (blood, urine)
acetone (blood, urine)
acetonitril
Achard and Castaigne's
acidity reduction
acidosis
Acree-Rosenheim
acrolein
Adamkiewicz's
Adam's
Addis'
Adler's
Admirality
adrenalin
adrenocorticotropic hormone
agglutination
Agostini's
Aiello's
Albarran's
albumin (blood, urine)
albumin globulin ratio
alcohol
aldehyde
Aldrich-McClure
Alfraise's
alizarin
alkali
alkaloid
alkaptone bodies
Allen's
Allen-Doisy
Allesandri-Guaceni
Almen's
aloin
Alper's
alpha
alphanaphthol
Althausen
Amann's
Ames
amidopyrine
amino-acid nitrogen
aminopyrine
ammonia
ammonium sulfate
amylase
amyl nitrite
amylopsin
Anderson-Collip
Andersch and Gibson
Anderson's
Anderson and Goldberger's
Andre's
Andreasch's
Andrewes
androsterone
Anstie's
antiformin
antimony
antipyrine
antiostreptolysin O
antithrombin
antitrypsin
Antonucci
anvil
Apgar
Apley's
apomorphine
aptitude
Arakawa's
Archetti's
Arloing-Courmont
Arnold's
Aron's
arsenic

arsphenamine
Aschheim-Zondek
Aschner-Danini
Ascoli's
Atkinson and Kendall's
atropine
Auricchio and Chieffi's
Australian antigen
autohemolysis
auto-urine
Axenfeld's
Ayer's
Ayer-Tobey
A-Z
azorubin

Babcock's
Babinski
Babinski-Weil
Bachman
Bachmeier's
bactericidal
bacteriolysin
bacteriolytic
Baeyer's
BAJ
Baldwin's
Balfour's
Bang
Barany's
Barberio's
Bardach's
Bareggi's
Barfoed's
Bargehr
Barral's
Basham's
basophil
Bass-Watkin
Bauer's
Baumann's
Baumann and Goldmann's
Bayer's
Bayrac's
B.C.G.
Bechterew's
Becker's
Bedson's
Behre and Benedict's
Bekhterev's
Bell's
Bellerby's
Bence Jones protein
Bendien's
Benedict's
Benedict and Denis'
Benedict and Murlin's
bentonite
benzidine
benzidine peroxidase
benzoin
Bercovitz
Berenreuther
Bergmann-Meyer
Berthelot's
Bertoni-Raymondi
Bertrand's
Berzelius's
beta
beta-oxybutyric acid
Bettendorff's
Bettmann's
Bial's
bicarbonate tolerance
bicolor guaiac
bile pigment
bilirubin
Binet's
Binet-Simon
Bing's entotic
Binz's
biological
Birkhaug
Bischoff's

bismuth
bitterlung
biuret
Black's
Blackberg and Wanger's
blanche
Blaxland's
Block-Steiger
blood cholesterol
blood-urea clearance
Bloor's
Bloxam's
Blum's
Blumenau's
Blyth's
Boas'
Bodal's
Boedeker's
Beorner-Luckens
Bohmansson's
Bolen
Boltz's
Bonanno's
Borchardt's
Borden's
Bordet-Gengou
Bordet's
Boston's
Botelho's
Bottger's
Bottu's
Bouchardt's
Bouin and Ancel
Bourdon's
Bourget's
Boveri's
Boyksen's
Bozicevich's
Brahmachari's
Bram's
Brande's
Braun's
Braun-Husler
Bremer's
Brieger's
bromine
bromsulphalein
Brouha
Brown's
brucellin
Brugsch's
Bryce's
Bufano
Burchard-Liebermann
Burger's
Burnam's
Busacca's
Buscaino's
butyric acid
Bychowski's

caffeine
Caillan's
Caillu's
calcium
Callaway's
Calmette's
caloric
Calvert's
Cammidge's
Campani's
Campbell's
camphor
Cantani
capillary resistance
capon comb growth
Cappagnoli's
Capranica's
carbohydrate
carbon dioxide content
carbon monoxide
Carnot's
carotine
Carr-Price

Carrez's
Casamajor's
casein
Casilli's
Casoni's intradermal
Castellani's
catecholamines
catoptric
cellulose
cephalin-cholesterol
flocculation
Chapman's
Chautard's
Chediak's
Chick-Martin
Chiene's
Chimani-Moos
chloride
chlorophyll
cholera red
cholesterol
choline
cholinesterase
Chopra's antimony
Chorine's
Chovstek
Chrobak
chromatin
chromic acid
Ciamician and Magnanini's
Cipollina's
citochol
Clark's
Clauberg
Clieve's
coagulation
cobra venom
coccidiodin
cockscomb
coffee
Cohen's
Cohn's
coin
colchicin
cold agglutinins
cold pressor
Cole's
colloidal benzoin
colloidal gold
Comessatti's
complement-fixation
concentration
Congo red
conjugate glycuronates
conjunctival
connective tissue
contact
Contejean
Cooke's
Coombs'
coproporphyrin
Cope's
Corner-Allen
cortisol
Costa
Cowie's guaiac
Craft's
Craig's
Cramer's
Crampton's
creatine
creatinine
Crismer's
Cronin Lowe
CT scan
Cuboni's
Cuignet's
Cunisset's
currant
Curschmann
Cutler-Power-Wilder
Cutola
Cutting's
cysteine

cystine
cytosin

Daclin
Dalldorf's
D'Amato's
Daranyi
dark-adaptation
Davy's
Day's
Dedichen's
Deen's
Degener's
Dehio's
dehydrocholate
Dejust's
Delff's
Deniges'
Dennis and Silverman's
Derrien's
desmoid
dextrose
diaçetic acid
diacetyl
Diagnex
dialysis
Diamond slide
diastase
diazo
Dick
Dicken's
Dienst
digestive function
digitalin
dilution
dimethylamino-azrobenzene
DNase
Doerfler's Stewart
Dold's
Dolman's
Donaldson's
Donath's
Donath-Landsteiner
Donders'
Donne's
Donogany's
Dorn-Sugarman
double-blind
Dowell
Dragendorff's
Draize
Drechsel's
Dreyer's
Duane's
Dugas'
Duke's
Dumontpallier's
Dungern's
Dupont's
Dwight-Frost

Eagle
Ebbighaus'
Eberson's
edestin
Edlefsen's
Ehrard's
Ehrlich's
Ehrmann's
Eijkman's
Einhorn's
Eiselt's
Eitelberg's
Ellermann and Erlandsen's
Elton's ring
Ely's
Emanuel-Cutting
epinephrine
epiphanin
Erdman's
Erichsen
erythrocyte sedimentation
Esbach's
Escatrich's

Escherrich's
Escudero's
ether
ethyl acetate
ethyl butyrate
euglobulin lysis
Eustis's
Ewald's
extinction
Exton's
Exton and Rose

Fabre's
Fahraeus'
Falk and Tedesco's
Falls'
Farber's
Faust's
Fearon's
Fehling's
fermentation
ferric chloride
Feulgen's
fibrinogen
Fieux's
Finckh's
Fischer's
Fishberg
Fishberg and Friedfeld
fistula
fixation
Flack
Fleig's
Fleischl's
Fleitmann's
flocculation
Florence
fluorescent treponemal
antibody-absorption
Flushmann's
Focker's
Folin's
Folin and Denis'
Folin and McElroy's
Folin and Wu's
formaldehyde
formalin
formol-gel
Fornet's ring
Foshay's
Foubert's
Fouchet's
Fournier
fragility
Francis'
Frank and Goldberger
Frank and Nothmann's
Fränkel's
Franken's
Frei
Fridweichsen's
Friedman's
Friedman-Hamburger
Fröhde's
Frohn's
Frommer's
fructose
Fuchs's
Fuld's
Fuld-Goss
Furbringer's
furfurol

Gairdner's coin
galactose
Gali Mainini
Gallois'
gamma globulin
Ganassim's
Gannther's
Gardiner-Brown
Garriga's
Garrod's
Gate and Papacostas'

Gault
Gauran
Gawalowski's
Gay-Force
Gayer
Geissler's
Gelle's
Gentele's
Geraghty's
Gerhardt's
Garrard's
Ghedini-Weinberg
Gibbon and Landis
Gies' biuret
Glenard's
globulin
glucose
glutoid
Gluzinski's
glycerol
glycerol-cholesterol
glycerophosphate
glycuronates
glycyltryptophan
glyoxylic acid
Gmelin's
Goetsch's
Goldscheider's
gold-sol
Gordon's
Gothlin's
Graefe's
Graham's
Grandeau's
Graupner's
Gregerson and Boas'
Greig
Greppi-Villa
Griess's
Grigg's
Grobly's
Grocco's
Gross'
Gruber's
Gruber-Widal
Grünbaum's
Grünbaum-Widal
Gruskin
guaiac
Gunning's
Gunning-Lieben
Gunzburg's
Guterman
Gutzeit's

Hager's
Haines'
Hallion's
Halstead-Reitan
Ham
Hamburger's
Hamel's
Hamilton-Swartz
Hamilton's
Hammarsten's
Hammer's
Hammerschlag's
Hanfmann-kasanin
Hanganatziu-Deicher
Hanger's
Hanke and Koessler's
Harding and Ruttan's
Harrington-Flocks
Harris and Ray
Harrison spot
Harrower's
Hart's
Hassall's
Hawk's
Hay's
Heaf
Hecht's
Hecht-Weinberg
Hecht-Weinberg-Gradwohl

Heichelheim's
Heller's
hematein
hematocrit
hematoporphyrin
hemin
hemoglobin
hemosiderin
Hench-Aldrich
Henderson's
Henie-Coenen
Hennebert's
Henry's
Henshaw
hepatic function
Hering's
Herman-Perutz
Herring's
Herring-Binet
Herter's
Herz's
Herzberg's
Hess capillary
heterophil antibody
Heynsius'
Hildebrandt's
Hindenlang's
Hines and Brown
Hinton
hippuric acid
Hirschfeldt's
Hirst
Hirst and Hare
histamine
histidine
Hitzig
Hoffmann's
Hofmeister's
Hogben
Holmgren's
Holten's
Hopkins' thiophene
Hopkins-Cole
Hoppe-Seyler
hormone
Horsley's
Hotis
Houghton's
Howell's
Huddleson's
Huggins
Huhner
Hunt's
Huppert's
Huppert-Cole
Hurtley's
hydrobilirubin
hydrochloric acid
hydrogen peroxide
hydrophilia skin
hydrostatic
hydroxylamine
hyperemia
hyperpnea
hypochlorite-orcinol
hypoxanthine

icterus index
Ide
Iefimov
Ilimow's
Iloxvay's
Imhof's
imidazole
immunologic pregnancy
indican
indigo carmine
indole
indophenol
inoculation
inosite
intelligence
intracutaneous tuberculin

intradermal salt solution
inulin clearance
iodine
iodipin
iodoform
Ishihara's
Israelson's
Ito-Reenstierna

Jacobsthal's
Jacoby's
Jacquemin's
Jadassohn's
Jadassohn-Bloch
Jaffe's
Jaksch's
Janet's
Jansen's
Javorski's
Jendrasic's
Jenner-Kay
Jenning's
Johnson's
Jolles'
Jones and
Cantarow
Jorissen's
Justus'

Kabatschnik's
Kafka's
Kahn
kairin
Kamnitzer's
Kantor and Gies'
Kapeller-Adler
Kaplan's
Kapsinow's
Kashiwado's
Kastle's
Kastle-Meyer
Katayama's
Kathrein
Katzenstein's
Kauffmann's
Keller's ultraviolet
Kelling's
Kelly's
Kendrick's
Kentmann's
Kerner's
Killian's
Kinberg's
Kitzmiller
Kiutsi-Malone
Kjeldahl's
Klausner's
Klein
Klemperer's
Klimow's
Kline
Kline-Young
Knapp's
Kober
Kobert's
Koch's
Koenecke's
Koh's
Kolmer's
Kondo's
Konew's
Knosuloff's
Korotkoff's
Kossel's
Kottmann's
Kowarsky's
Krauss'
Krokiewicz's
Kuhlmann
Kultz's
Kurzrok-Miller
Kustallow's
Kveim
Kveim-Silpzvach

Laborde's
lactose
Ladendorff's
Landau color
Lang's
Lange's
Laughlen
Lautier's
Leach's
Lebbin's
Lechini's
Lee's
Legal's
Leiner's
Le Nobel's
lentochol
Leo's
lepromin
Lesser's
Lesieur-Privey
leucine
Levinson
levulose
Lewis and Pickering
Lichtheim
Lieben's
Lieben-Ralfe
Liebermann's
Liebermann-Burchardt
Liebig's
Ligat's
Lignieres'
Lindemann's
Lindner's
Links'
Linzenmeier's
lipase
Lipps'
Lipschuetz's
lithium level
litmus mild
liver function
Livierato's
Loewe's
Loewi's
Lombard's
Lowenthal's
Lowy's
Lucke's
Luebert's
Luenbach-Koeppe
luetin
lupus induction
Luttge-Mertz
Luttke's
Lyle and Curtman's
lysis time

McClure-Aldrich
MacDonagh's
Macdonald's
Macht
McKendrick
McKinnin's
Maclagan's
MacLean
MacLean-de Wesselow
MacMunn's
MacQuarrie
MacWilliams
magnesionitric
Magpie's
Malerba's
Malmejde's
Malot's
maltose
Maly's
Mandel's
Manoiloff's
Manson evaluation
Mantoux
Manzullo's

Marechal's
Marechal-Rosin
Marie's three-paper
Markee
Marlow's
Marquardt's
Marquis's
Marris atropine
Marsh's
Marshall's
Maschke's
Masselon
Masset's
Master's
mastic
Matas'
Matefy
Mathews'
Maumene
Mauthner's
Mayer-Tanret
Mayer's
Mayerhofer's
Mazer-Hoffman
Mazzini
Mazzotti
Mehu's
Meigs's
Meinicke
melanin
melitin
Meltzer-Lyon
Mendel's
Mendeleeff's
Mendelsohn's
mercury
Mérieux-Baillion
Mester's
methemoglobin
methylene blue
methyl-phenyl-hydrazine
Mett's
Meyer's
Michaelides'
Michailow's
microprecipitation
Middlebrook-Dubos
Millard's
Miller-Kurzrok
Millon's
Mills's
miostagmin
Mitscherlich's
Mitsuda-Rost
Mittlemeyer's
Mohr's
Molisch's
Moloney
monosaccharide
Montigne's
Moore's
Morelli's
Moretti's
Moritz
Morner's
Moro's
morphine
Morton's
Moschowitz
Mosenthal's
Moynihan's
mucic acid
mucification
Muck's
Mulder's
Muller's
Muller-Jochmann
Murata
murexide
Murphy's
mucobiologic
mycologic
Myersand
Fine

Mylius'

Naffziger's
Nagle's
Nakayama's
Napier's serum
Nasso's
Nathan's
Neisser and Wechsberg's
Nencki's
neosalvarsan
Nessler's
Neubauer and Fischer's
Neufeld's
Neukomm's
neutralization
Newcomer's
Nickerson-Kveim
Nickles'
ninhydrin
Nippe's
nitrate reduction
nitric acid
nitric acid-magnesium sulfate
nitrites
nitrogen partition
nitropropiol
nitroprusside
nitroso-indole-nitrate
Nobel's
Noguchi's
Nonne's
Nonne-Apelt
nonverbal
Nothnagel's
nuclear
nucleus
nucleo-albumin
Nyiri's
Nylander's
nystagmus

Ober's
Obermeyer's
Obermuller's
obturator
occult blood
Oliver's
one-stage prothrombin time
orcinol
organoleptic
orientation
orthotoluidine
osazone
Osgood-Haskins'
osmotic resistance
Osterberg's
Otani's
Ott's
oxyphenylsulfonic acid

Pachon's
Page and van Slyke's
Paget's
palmin
palmitin
pancreatic function
Pandy's
Papanicolaou
para-dimethyl-amino
benzaldehyde
parallax
Parnum's
partial thromboplastin time
paternity
Patrick's
Patterson's
Paul's
Paul-Bunnell
Paunz's
Pavy's
Peck
Pelouse-Moore

Pels and Macht
pentose
Penzoldt's
Penzoldt-Fischer
peppermint
pepsin
peptone
perchloride
percutaneous tuberculin
Peret's
Peria's
Perls'
permanganate
peroxidase
Perthes'
Peterman's
Petri's
Pettenkofer's
Petzetaki's
phenacetin
phenol
phenolphthalein
phenolsulfonphthalein
phenoltetrachlorophthalein
phenylalanine
phenylhydrazine
phlorizin
phloroglucin
phosphatase
phosphoric acid
phrenic-pressure
phthalein
phytotoxin
Piazza's
picrotoxin
Pincus
Pintner-Patterson
Piorkowski's
Piria's
Pirquet's
plasmacrit
Plesch's
Plugge's
Poehl's
Pohl's
Politzer's
Pollacci's
Pollatschek-Porges
polyuria
Porges-Meier
Porges-Pollatschek
Porges-Salomon
porphobilinogen
Porter's
Porteus maze
Posner's
potassium iodide
Pratt's
precipitin
precipitation
Pregl's
pregnancy
Prendergast's
presumptive
Preyer's
Proetz
prostigmine
protein
protein-bound iodine
protein tyrosin
proteose
prothrombin
protozoan
psychometric
Purdy's
purine bodies
pyramidon
pyridine
pyrocatechin

quadriceps
Queckenstedt's

quelling
Quick's
quinine
Quinlan's

Raabe's
Rabuteau's
Ralfe's
Ramon
flocculation
Randolph's
Rantzman's
Raygat's
Rees'
Reh's
Rehberg's
Rehfuss'
Reichi's
Reid Hunt's
Reinsch's
Remont's
rennin
Renton's
resorcinol
resorcinol-hydrochloric acid
Reuss's
Reynold's
Rh
rhubarb
Rieckenberg's
Riegel's
Riegler's
Rimini's
Ringold
Rinne's
Rivalta's
Roberts'
Roffo's
Roger's
Roger-Josue
Romer's
Ronchese
Rorschach
Rose's
rose bengal
Rose-Waaler
Rosenbach's
Rosenbach-Gmelin
Rosenheim's
Rosenheim-Drummond
Rosenthal's
Rosenzweig
Rosett's
Rosin's
Ross's
Ross-Jones
Rossel's aloin
Rothera's
Rotter's
Rous's
Roussin's
Rowntree and Geraghty's
Rubin's
Rubner's
Ruge and Phillipp's
Ruhemann's
Rumpel-Leede
Russo's
Ruttan and Hardisty's
Ryan's skin
Rytz

Saathoff's
Sabrazes
saccarimeter
Sachs-Georgi
Sachs-Witebsky
Sachsse's
safranine
Sahli's
Sahli-Nencki
salicylaldehyde
salicylate
Salkowski's

Salkowski and Schipper's
salol
Salomon's
salvarsan
Sandrock
Sanford's
santonin
Saundby's
scarification
Schaffer's
Schalfijew's
Scherer's
Schick
Schiff's
Schiller's
Schilling
Schirmer's
Schlessinger's
Schmidt's
Schneider
Schneider's
Schonbein's
Schopfer's
Schroeder's
Schubert-Dannmeyer
Schulte's
Schultz-Charlton
Schultze's
Schultze's indophenol
  oxydase
Schumm's
Schurmann's
Schwabach
Schwartz's
Schwartz-McNeill
Schwarz's
scintiscan
Scivoletto's
secretin
Seidel's
Seidlitz powder
Selivanoff's
Sellards'
semen
Senn's
senna
sensitized sheep cell
Sereny
sero-enzyme
serologic
serum neutralization
Sgambati's
shadow
Shaw-Mackenzie
Shear's
sheep cell agglutination
Sicard-Canteloube
sickling
Siddall
Siebold and Bradbury's
sigma
Simonelli's
Sims'
Sivori and Rebaubi
skatole
Smith's
Snellen's
Snider match
sodium chloride balance
Soldaini's
Solera's
solubility
Sonnenschein's
specific gravity
sphenopalatine
Spiegler's
Spiro's
Staehlin's
Stanford-Binet
steapsin
Stein's
Steinle-Kahlenberg
Stenger
Stern's

Stern's fermentation
Stewart's
Stieglitz
Stock
Stokes's
Stokvis'
Storck's
Strange's
Strassburg's
Straus's biological
Strauss's
streptolysin
Struve's
strychnine
Stypven time
sulfonal
sulfosalicylic acid
sulfur
Sulkowitch's
Sullivan's
Suranyi's
syphilis
Szabo's

Takata-Ara
Taliqvist's
tannic acid
tannin
Tanret's
Tardieu's
Targowla's
taurine
Taylor's
Teichmann's
tellurite
Terman
thalleioquin
thermoprecipitin
thiocyanate
Thomas-Binetti
Thompson's
Thormahlen's
Thorn
thromboplastin generation
Thudichum's
thumb-nail thymol turbidity
thyroid
Tidy's
Tizzoni's
Tobey-Ayer
Tollens'
Tollens, Neuberg and Schwket's
Topfer's
Torquay's
tourniquet
Trambusti
trapeze
Trendelenburg's
Tretop's
Triboulet's
trichophytin
triketohydrindene
Trommer's
Trousseau's
trypsin
tryptophan
Tschernogowbou's
Tsuchiya's
tuberculin
Tuffier's
Twort
typhoidin
tyrosine
Tyson's
Tzanck

Ucko's
Udranszky's
Uffelmann's
Uhlenhuth's
Ulrich's

Ultzmann's
Umber's
Unterberger's
uracil
urea
urease
Urecholine
uric acid
urobilin
urochromogen
urorosein
Urriolla's

Valenta's
Valsalva's
van Deen's
van den Bergh's
van der Velden's
vanillin
Van Slyke
Van Slyke and Cullen's
Vaughn and Novy's
Venning Browne
ventilation
Vernes'
virulence
Visscher-Bowman
Vitali's
vocabulary
Voelcker and Joseph's
Voge's
Vogel and Lee's
Vogus-Proskauer
Volhard's
Vollmer's
von Aldor's
von Dungern's
von Frisch
von Jaksch's
von Maschke's
von Pall's
von Pirquet's
von Recklinghausen's
von Zeynek and Mencki's
Vulpain

Waaler-Rose
Wagner's
Walter's bromide
Wang's
Warren's
Wassermann
Waterhouse pus
Watson-Schwartz
Weber's
Webster's
Weichdrodt's
Weidel's
Weil-Felix
Weinberg's
Weinstein's
Weisman's
Weiss permanganate
Weiss's
Well-Felilx
Welland's
Weltmann's serum
Welty's
Wender's
Wenzell's
Weppen's
Wernicke's
Wetzel's
Weyl's
Wheeler and Johnson's
Whipple's
Widal's
Wideroe's
Widmark's
Wilbrand's prism
Wilbur and Addis'
Wildbolz's
Wilkinson and Peter's
Williamson's blood

Wilson's
Winckler
Winslow's
Winternitz's
Wishart
Witz's
Wohlgemuth's
Woldman's
Wolff-Eisner
Wolff-Junghans
Woodbury's
Woods's
Worm-Muller
Wormley's
worsted
Wreden's
Wurster's
Wys's

xanthemia
xanthine
xanthroproteic
Xenopus
xylidine
xylose concentration

Yakinoff's
Yefimov's
Yerkes-Bridges
Young
Yvon's

Zaleski's
Zambrini's
Zangemeister
Zappacosta's
Zeisel's
Zeller's
Zenoni's
Ziechen's
Ziffern's
Zitovitch's
Zondek-Aschheim
Zouchlos'
Zsigmondy's gold number
Zwenger's

Surgical Incisions

Auvray

Banks and Laufman
Bar
Battle
Bergmann
Bevan
buttonhole

celiotomy
Chernuy
circumscribing
confirmatory
crescent
crosshatch
crucial (cruciate)

Deaver
Dührssen

endaural
exploratory

Fergusson
Fowler

Gatellier
Gluck

Halsted
Halwarth's
Harmon
Hayes Martin
Heerman
hockey-stick

Kehr

Kocher
Kustner

Lamm
Langenbeck
lateral rectus
Lempert
Longuet

MacFee
Mackenrodt
Mason's
Maylard's
Mayo-Robson
McArthur
McBurney
median
Meyer

Ollier

paramedian
Parker
Perthe
Pfannenstiel
Phemister

relief
Ruddy's

saber cut
semilunar

Wilde

Visscher

Dental Surfaces

axial

basal
buccal

distal

glenoid

incisal

labial
lingual

masticating
masticatory
mesial

occlusal

subocclusal

Descriptive Positions, i.e., Anatomical

Albert's

Bonner's
Bonnet's
Bozeman's
Brickner's

Casselberry's
centric

dorsal
dorsoanterior
dorsoposterior
dorsosacral
Duncan's

eccentric
Edebohls

Fowler's
frontoanterior
frontoposterior
Fuch's

genucubital
Genupectoral

hinge candylar
hinge mandibular
hinge terminal

intercuspal

knee-chest
knee-elbow
Kraske's

lateral recumbent
leapfrog
lithotomy

Mayo Robson's
mentoanterior
mentoposterior
Mercurio's

Noble's
Nuchal-hitch

occipitoanterior
occipitoiliac
occipitolevoanterior
occipitolevoposterior
occipitoposterior
occlusal

prone
protrusive

Robsen's

sacroanterior
Scultetus'
semiprone
Simon's
Sim's
supine

Trendelenburg's

Valentine's

Walcher

Section VI

OFTEN USED ABBREVIATIONS

- Word Abbreviations
- Prescription Abbreviations

Word Abbreviations

ā	before
A.A.	achievement age
AAL	anterior axillary line
abbr.	abbreviation
a.c.	ante collation or before meals
ACTH	adrenocorticotrophic hormone
a.d.	right ear
ADH	antidiuretic hormone
ad lib	at pleasure
adm.	administration
AEq	age equivalent
A/G ration	albumin-globulin ration
AHD	arteriosclerotic heart disease
AID	Acute Infectious Disease; Alto Immune Disease; Artificial Insemination Donor
AMI	Acute Myocardial Infarction
anat.	anatomy
ant.	anterior
ante	before
anti.	antidote
AP; A.P.; A-P	anter-posterior or front to back; anterior pituitary gland
A.P.L.	anterior pituitary like
app.	appendix
A.Q.	achievement quotient
Aq.	water
aq. dest.	distilled water
ARD	acute respiratory disease
art.	artery
a.s.	left ear
AS	Anglo-Saxon
ASAP	as soon as possible
ASCVD	arteriosclerotic cardiovascular disease
ASHD	arteriosclerotic heart disease
assn.	association
Asso; Assoc.	associate
AT-10	dihydrotachysterol
at. no.	atomic number
at. wt.	atomic weight

a.u.	ears (both)
A.V.	arteriovenous; atrioventricular
A-Z	Ascheim-Zondek
bact.	bacteriology
BBB	Bundle Branch Block
BAL	British Anti-Lewisite
baso.	basophil
BBA	born before arrival
BBT	basal body temperature
BCG	Bacillus Calmette-Gúerin
bd.	board
B.E.	barium enema
bet.	between
b.i.d.	twice daily
biol.	biology
BM	bowel movement
B.M.R.	basal metabolic rate
BP	blood pressure
BPH	Benign Prostatic Hypertrophy
br	branch, branches
brp	bathroom privileges
B.S.	blood sugar
BSC	bedside commode
BSP	bromsulphalein
BTU; B.Th.U.	British thermal unit
BUN	blood urea nitrogen
BX	biopsy
c̄	with
C	carbon
C	centigrade, Celsius
c; cert; ct	certified
CBC	complete blood count
Ca	calcium
ca	carcinoma
Cal.	large calorie
cal.	small calorie
caps.	capsules
carbo.	carbohydrates
card; cardiog	cardiography
cardiol	cardiologist, cardiology

CAT	Computerized Axial Tomography
c.c.	chief complaint
cc.	cubic centimeter
CCU	Coronary Care Unit; Critical Care Unit
CDC	Center for Disease Control
cent.	centigrade
cf.	compare
cg.	centigram
CHD	congestive heart disease
chem.	chemistry
chm	chairman
CIPD	Chronic Intermittant Peritoneal Dialysis
Cl	chlorine
cm.	centimeter
C.M.A.	Certified Medical Assistant
C.N.M.	Certified Nurse Midwife
CNS	central nervous system
commun	communicable
comp.	composition
cons	consultant, consulting
contra.	contraindication
conv.	convalescent
C. P.	cerebral palsy
cran	cranial
CSF	cerebrospinal fluid
CT scan	computerized tomography scan
Cu	copper, cuprum
CVA	cerebrovascular accident
CVD	cardiovascular disease
CVRD	cardiovascular renal disease
d.	daily
DCA	Deoxycorticosterone Acetate
D.D.S.	dentist
DDT	dichloro-diphenyl-trichloroethane
def.	deficiency
der.	derivative
derm	dermatology
DES	Diethylstilbestrol
diag	diagnosis
dir	director
dis	disease

DJD	degenerative joint disease
DMSO	dimethyl sulfoxide
DNA	deoxyribonucleic acid
D.O.	Doctor of Osteopathy
DOA	dead on arrival
DOCAL	Deoxycorticosterone Acetate
DPH	Doctor of Public Health
DPT	Diphtheria, Pertussis, Tetanus
Dx.	diagnosis
E.	English
(e	alternate word ending
EENT	ear, eye, nose and throat
ECHO	entero-cytopathogenic human orphan virus
EDC	expected date of confinement
EDTA	ethylenediaminetetraacetate
EE	eye and ear
EEE	Encephalitis, Eastern Equine
EEG	electroencephalogram
e.g.	for example
EKG; ECG	electrocardiogram
EKY	Electrokymogram
elect.	electricity
elix	elixir
E.M.F.	Electromotive Force
EMG	electromyography
encephalog	encephalography
endocrin	endocrinology
EOM	extraocular movements
eos.	eosinophils
ESP	extrasensory perception
esp.	especially
ESR	erythrocyte sedimentation rate
EST	electroshock therapy
etiol.	etiology
ETOH	alcohol
ex.	example
ext.	exterior, external
F	Fahrenheit
F.A.	first aid
FAD	flavine-adenine dinucleotide

FDA	Food and Drug Administration
Fe	iron, ferrum
fem.	female, feminine
ff. ind.	fact-finding index
FH	family history
fl	fluid
Fr.	French
frict.	friction
FSH	follicle stimulating hormone
funct.	function
FUO	fever of undetermined origin
FX	fracture
G.	Greek
g; gm	gram
gas-int; G.I.	gastro-intestinal
gastroent; ge	gastroenterology
GB	gall bladder
Ger.	German
ger	geriatrics
GH	Growth Hormone
GH-RF	Growth-Hormone-Releasing Factor
GI	gastrointestinal
GP	general practice
gr.	grain
grad.	graduate
Grav.I, Grav.II, etc.	primagravida, secundigravida, etc. indicating a woman of so many pregnancies
GTH	gonadotropic hormone
GTT	glucose tolerance test
gtt	one drop
gtts	drops
G-U	genito-urinary
gyn; gyec	gynecology
H	hydrogen
h.	hour
H & E	hematoxylin and eosin
HAV	Hepatitus A Virus
Hb	hemoglobin
HBP	high blood pressure
HBV	Hepatitus B Virus

hematol	hematology
HEW	Health, Education and Welfare
HMD	Hyaline Membrane Disease
HMO	Health Maintenance Organization
H_2O	water
hosp	hospital
HS	at bedtime
HSV	Herpes Simplex Virus
ht.	height
HTLV	Human T-Lymphotropic Retro Virus
I	iodine
I & O	intake and output
ICM	intercostal margin
ICP	Intracranial Pressure
ICS	intercostal space
ICU	Intensive Care Unit
ICSH	interstitial cell-stimulating hormone
i.e.	that is
IgA	Immunoglobulin A (Gamma A globulin)
IM	infectious mononucleosis
I.M.	intramuscular injection
immun	immunology
ind.	indication
Ind Med	industrial medicine
ind sur	industrial surgery
inf.	inferior
Infec. dis.	infectious disease
INH	isoniazid
inst.	institute
int.	intern; internal; interior
int med	internal medicine
IOP	intraocular pressure
IPPB	intermittent positive pressure breathing
I.Q.	intelligence quotient
I.U.	international unit
IUD	intrauterine device
IV	intravenous
IVP	intravenous pyelogram
JRA	Juvenile Rheumatoid Arthritis
jt.	joint
K	potassium, kalium

kg	kilogram
KUB	kidney, ureter and bladder
KV	kilovolt
KW	kilowatt
L.	Latin
L & A	light and accommodation
LBW	Low Birth Weight
LDH	Lactic Acid Dehydrogenase; Lactatie Dehydrogenase
L & W	living and well
lab	laboratory
LAO	left anterior oblique
lar; laryng	laryngology
lat.	lateral
lb.	pound
LCM	lymphocytic chorio-meningitis
LD	Lethal Dose; Learning Disability
LE	lupus erythematosus
LH	luteinizing hormone
LL.	late Latin
LLQ	left lower quadrant
L.M.D.	local medical doctor
L.M.P.	last menstrual period
L.O.A.	left occiput anterior
L.O.P.	left occiput posterior
LP	Lumbar Puncture
L.P.N.	licensed practical nurse
LPO	left posterior oblique
LSD	lysergic acid diethylamide
L.S.P.	left sacroposterior
LTH	luteotropic hormone
LVN	licensed vocational nurse
LUQ	left upper quadrant
m.	male, minum
M.Sc.	Master of Science
MA	mental age
malig	malignant
mat	maternity
MBD	Minimal Brain Dysfunction
mCi	millicuries

MC	Medical Corps
MCH	mean corpuscular hemoglobin
MCHC	mean corpuscular hemoglobin concentration
mcg	microgram
MCV	mean corpuscular volume
med	medicine, medical
metab.	metabolism
mEq	milliequivalent
MetHB	Methemoglobin
Mg	magnesium
mg.	milligram
mgh.	milligram-hour
MHMR	Mental Health/Mental Retardation
MI	mycardial infarction
min	one drop of water
min.	minim
ml.	milliliter
MLD	minimal lethal dose
MM	mucous membrane
mM	millimole
mm.	millimeter
MOM	Milk of Magnesia
mos.	months
MS	Multiple Sclerosis
M.S.L.	midsternal line
Mt	membrane tympana
mu; u	micron
MW	Molecular Weight
N	nitrogen
N and V	nausea and vomiting
Na	sodium
neur	neurologist, neurology
neuropath	neuropathology
N.F.	National Formulary
NFIP	National Foundation for Infantile Paralysis
NIH	National Institutes of Health
NND	new and nonofficial drugs
N.N.R.	new and nonofficial remedies
NP	nursing procedure
NPH insulin	neutral protamine hegedorn insulin
N.P.N.	nonprotein nitrogen

NREM	Non-Rapid Eye Movement
NS soln.	normal saline solution
nut.	nutrients
NVD	nausea, vomiting and diarrhea; Newcastle virus disease
NYD	not yet diagnosed
O	oxygen
ob; obst	obstetrician, obstetrics
OBS	Organic Brain Syndrome
o.d.	right eye
O. Fr.	Old French
o.l.; o.s.	left eye
O.M.	otitis media
OMPA	otitis media, purulent, acute
ONP	operating nursing procedure
OPD	outpatient department
oph; ophth	ophthalmology
opp.	opposite
O.R.	operating room
or; orth	orthopedics, orthopedist
orig.	origin
os	mouth
O.T.	old tuberculin; Occupational Therapy
OTC	Over the Counter
ot; oto; otol	orolaryngology
O.U.	both eyes
o.v.	both eyes
oz.	ounce
P	phosphorus
p.	page
P.A.	pernicious anemia, professional association, Physician Assistant
P & A	percussion and auscultation
P.A.	pernicious anemia, professional association
PAL	posterior axillary line
PAS	para-amino salicylic acid
PAT	Paroxysmal Atrial Tachycardia
path	pathological, pathologist, pathology
PBI	protein bound iodine
p.c.	after meals

pcu	packed cell volume
PDR	Physician's Desk Reference
ped; pd	pediatrics, pediatrician
periph vas dis	peripheral vascular disease
pert.	pertaining
P-G	post-graduate
PH	Public Health, past history
phar	pharmacology, pharmacy
Ph.G.	graduate pharmacist
phy. phys	physician
phy med	physical medicine
phys	physiology
physiol	physiological, physiologist, physiology
physiother	physiotherapy
PI	present illness
PICU	psychiatric intensive care unit
PID	pelvic inflammatory disease
PKU	phenylketonuria
pl.	plural
plast sur	plastic surgery
PM & Rehab	physical medicine and rehabilitation
PMI	point of maximum impulse
p.o.	by mouth
post.	posterior
p.p.	post prandial
PPLO	pleuropneumonia-like organism
pre.	prefix
prenat	prenatal
pro.	protein
proct	proctology, proctologist
prog.	prognosis
prof	professor
PSRO	Professional Standards Regulatory Organization
psy	psychiatrist, psychiatry
psych	psychologist, psychology
PT	physical therapy
pt.	pint
PTA	plasma thromboplastin component
q:	each, every
q.d.	every day
q.h.	every hour

q.i.d.	four times daily
q.o.d.	every other day
q.s.	as much as suffices
qt.	quart
q.v.	which see
r	roentgen
RAO	right anterior oblique
RBC	red blood cell
RBDB	Right Bundle-Branch Block
RCM	right costal margin
rel.	relating
REM	rapid eye movement
RES	reticuloendothelial system
RHD	rheumatic heart disease
rheum	rheumatic, rheumatism
RLF	retrolental fibroplasia
Rh	Rhesus blood factor
RLQ	right lower quadrant
R.N.	registered nurse
RNA	ribonucleic acid
R.O.A.	right occiput anterior
roent	roentgenologist, roentgenology
ROM	Range of Motion
R.O.P.	right occiput posterior
R.Q.	respiratory quotient
RS	related subjects
R.T.	x-ray technician
R.U.	roentgen unit
RUQ	right upper quadrant
RVH	right ventricular hypertrophy
Rx	prescription, take
s̄	without
s.	left
SBE	sub-acute bacterial endocarditis
SCUBA	self-contained underwater breathing apparatus
S.G.O.	Surgeon General's Office
SGOT	serum glutamic oxalopyruvic transaminase
SH	social history
SIDS	Sudden Infant Death Syndrome
sig.	let it be labeled

sing.	singular
SOB	shortness of breath
soc.	society
sp. gr.	specific gravity
SPCA	serum prothrombin conversion accelerator
ss, $\overline{ss}$	half - ½
STD	Sexually Transmitted Disease
STS	serologic test for syphilis
sup.	superior
supt.	superintendent
sur; surg	surgeon, surgery
sym	symptoms
symb	symbol
syn	synonym
syph	syphilologist, syphilology
T.	temperature
T & A	tonsillectomy and adenoidectomy
TAT	tetanus antitoxin
TAO	triacetyloleandomycin
THC	Tetrahydrocannabinol
Tb; Tbc	tuberculosis
Thor sur	thoracic surgery
tid	thrice daily
TLC	tender loving care
TMJ	Temporomandibular joints
TPR	temperature, pulse and respiration
tr.	tincture
TSH	thyroid stimulating hormone
UCHD	usual childhood diseases
UHF	Ultrahigh Frequency
USA	United States Army
USN	United States Navy
U.S.P.	United States Pharmacopeia
U.S.P.H.S.	United States Public Health Service
URI	upper respiratory infection
UV	Ultraviolet
v.	volt
VA	Veteran's Administration
Vas Dis	vascular disease

VC	Vital Capacity
VCG	Vetrocardiogram
VD	venereal disease
V.D.R.L.	venereal disease research laboratory test
viz.	namely
VOD	vision right eye
VOS	vision left eye
VSD	Ventricular Septal Defect
WBC	white blood cell
WEE	Western Equine Encephalitis
WHO	World Health Organization
WN, WD	well nourished, well developed

Prescription Abbreviations

āā (ana)	of each (equal parts)
a.c. (ante cibum)	before meals
aq. (aqua)	water
b.i.d. (bis in die)	twice a day
caps. (capsula)	capsule
chart. (chartulae)	papers (powders)
ft. (fiat)	make
h.s. (hora somni)	at bedtime
M. (misce)	mix
m. dict. (modo dictu)	as directed
non rep. (non repetatur)	do not repeat (do not refill)
o.d. (oculus dexter)	right eye
o.s. (oculus sinister)	left eye
p.c. (post cibum)	after meals
p.r.n. (pro re nata)	as needed
q.h. (quaque hora)	every hour
q.i.d. (quater in die)	four times a day
q.s. (quantum sufficit)	a sufficient quantity
R (recipe)	take (thou) a recipe
sig. (signa)	write on label
stat. (statim)	immediately
t.i.d. (ter in die)	three times a day
ut dict. (ut dictum)	as directed
gr.	grain or grains
gtt. (gutta(e))	drop(s)
m.	minim
3 iss	one and one-half drams
3 i	one ounce
3 s̄s̄	one-half ounce
cc.	cubic centimeter
gm.	gram
mg.	milligram
mcg.	microgram
ml.	milliliter

Section VII

COMMONLY PRESCRIBED PHARMACEUTICALS

- Proprietary and Corresponding Generic Names
- Generic and Corresponding Proprietary Names
- Schedule II Drugs—Proprietary and Corresponding Generic Names

PROPRIETARY	*GENERIC*
Achromycin-V	tetracycline HCl
Aldactazide, Aldactone	spironolactone
Aldomet	methyldopate hydrochloride
Amoxil	amoxicillin
Antivert	meclizine HCl
Apresoline, Apresazide	hydralazine hydrochloride
Atarax	hydroxyzine hydrochloride
Ativan	lorazepam
Atromid-S	clofibrate
Benadryl	diphenhydramine hydrochloride
Bentyl	dicyclomine hydrochloride
Brethine	terbutaline sulphate
Butazoladin Alka	phenylbutazone
Butisol Sodium	sodium butabarbital
Catapres	clonidine hydrochloride
Ceclor	cefaclor
Chlor-Trimeton Tabs.	chlorpheniramine maleate
Choledyl	oxtriphylline
Clinoril	sulindax
Cogentin	benztroprine mesylatalate
Compazine	prochlorperazine
Cortisporin Otic	polymyxin B-neomycin-hydrocortisone
Coumadin	warfarin sodium
Dalmane	flurazepam hydrochloride
Darvocet-N-100	propoxyphene napsylate
Darvon	propoxyphene HCl
Diabinase	chlorpropamide
Dilantin Sodium	phenytoin sodium
Diuril	chlorothiazide sodium
Dyazide	triamterine & hydrochlorothiazide
Elavil	amitriptyline HCl
Elixophyllin	theophylline
Enduron	methclothiazide
Equanil	meprobamate
Esidrix	hydrochlorothiazide
Fastin	phentermine hydrochloride
Feldene	piroxicam
Flagyl	metronidazole
Flexeril	cyclobenzaprine HCl
Gantrisin systemic	sulfisoxazole

PROPRIETARY	*GENERIC*
Garamycin	gentamicin sulfate
Gyne-Lotrimin	clotrimazole
Halcion	triazolam
Haldol	haloperidol
HydroDiuril	hydrochlorothiazide
Hygroton	chlorthalidone
Inderal	propranolol HCl
Indocin	indomethacin
Ionamin	phentermine resin
Isordil	isosorbide dinitrate
Keflex	cephalexin
Kenalog Derm.	triamcinolone acetonide
Lanoxin	digoxin
Larotid	amoxicillin
Lasix	furosemide
Librium	chlordiazepoxide
Lidex	fluocinonide
Lopressor	metroprolol tartrate
Lotrimin	chlotrimazole
Medrol	methylprednisolone acetate
Mellaril	thioridazine HCl
Minipress	prazosin HCl
Minocin	minocycline HCl
Monistat-7	miconazole nitrate
Motrin	ibuprofen
Nalfon	fenoprofen calcium
Naprosyn	naproxen
Neosporin Ophth.	polymixin B-bacitracin-neomycin
Nitrobid, Nitrostat	nitroglycerin
Norinyl	norethindrone
Norpace	disopyramide phosphate
Omnipen	ampicillin
Orinase	tolbutamide
Pavabid	papaperine HCl
Pen-Vee-K	penicillin V potassium
Periactin	cyproheptadine HCl
Persantine	dipyridamole
Phenergan	promethazine HCl
Polaramine Tabs.	dexchlorpheniramine maleate
Polymox	amoxicillin
Premarin	conjugated estrogens

PROPRIETARY	GENERIC
Procardia	nifodipine
Proloid	thyroglobulin
Provera	medroxyprogesterone acetate
Quibron	theophylline-guaifenesin
Restoril	teazepam
Robaxin	methocarbamol
Rufen	ibuprofen
Salutensin	hydroflumethiazide, reserpine
Septra DS	sulfamethoxazole
Serax	oxazepam
Sinequan	doxepin HCl
Slo-Phyllin Gyrocaps	theophylline, anhydrous
Slow-K	potassium chloride
Sorbitrate	isosorbide dinitrate
Stelazine	trifluoperazine hydrochloride
Sumycin	tetracycline
Synalar	fluocinoclone acetonide
Synthroid	levothyroxine sodium
Tagamet	cimetidine
Tenormin	atenolol
Tenuate	diethylopropion hydrochloride
Theo-Dur	theophylline (anhydrous)
Thorazine	chlorpromazine
Tigan	trimethobenzamide HCl
Timoptic	timolol maleate
Tofranil	imipramine hydrochloride
Tolectin	tolmetin sodium
Tolinase	tolazamide
Tranxene	clorazepate dipotassium
Valisone	betamuthasone valerate
Valium	diazepam
Vanceril	declomethasone dipropionate
Vasodilan	isoxsuprine HCl
V-Cillin K	penicillin V potassium
Ventolin	albuterol
Vibramycin	doxycycline hyclate
Vistaril	hydroxyzine panoate
Xanax	alprazolam
Zaroxolyn	metolazone
Zyloprim	allopurinol

GENERIC	*PROPRIETARY*
albuterol	Ventolin
allopurinol	Zyloprim
alprazolam	Xanax
amitriptyline HCl	Elavil
amoxicillin	Amoxil,Polymox
ampicillin	Omnipen
atenolol	Tenormin
benztroprine mesylatalate	Cogentin
betamuthasone valerate	Valisone
cefaclor	Ceclor
cephalexin	Keflex
chlordiazepoxide	Librium
chlorothiazide sodium	Diuril
chlorpheniramine maleate	Chlor-Trimeton Tabs.
chlorpromazine	Thorazine
chlorpropamide	Diabinase
chlorthalidone	Hygroton
chlotrimazoe	Lotrimin
cimetidine	Tagamet
clofibrate	Atromid-S
clonidine	Catepres
clonidine hydrochloride	Catapres
clorazepate dipotassium	Tranxene
clotrimazole	Gyne-Lotrimin
conjugated estrogens	Premarin
cyclobenzaprine HCl	Flexetril
cypropheptadine HCl	Periactin
declomethasone dipropionate	Vanceril
dexchlorpheniramine maleate	Polaramine Tabs.
diazepam	Valium
dicyclomine hydrochloride	Bentyl
diethylopropion hydrochloride	Tenuate
digoxin	Lanoxin
diphenhydramine hydrochloride	Benadryl
dipyridamole	Persantine
disopyramide phosphate	Norpace
doxepin HCl	Sinequan
doxycycline hyclate	Vibramycin
fenoprofen calcium	Nalfon
fluocinoclone acetonide	Synalar
fluocinonide	Lidex
flurazepan hydrochloride	Dalmane

GENERIC	*PROPRIETARY*
furosemide	Lasix
gentamicin sulfate	Garamycin
haloperidol	Haldol
hydralazine hydrochloride	Apresoline, Apresazide
hydrochlorothiazide	HydroDiuril
hydrochlorothiazide	Esidrix
hydroflumethiazide, reserpine	Salutensin
hydroxyzine hydrochloride	Atarax
hydroxyzine panoate	Vistaril
ibuprofen	Motril
ibuprofen	Rufen
imipramine hydrochloride	Tofranil
indomethacin	Indocin
isosorbide dinitrate	Isodril
isosorbide dinitrate	Sorbitrate
isoxsuprine HCl	Vasodilan
levothyroxine sodium	Synthroid
lorazepam	Ativan
meclizine HCl	Antivert
medroxyprogesterone acetate	Provera
meprobamate	Equanil
methclothiazide	Enduron
methocarbamol	Robaxin
methyldopate hydrochloride	Aldomet
methylprednisolone acetate	Medrol
metolazone	Zaroxolyn
metronidazole	Flagyl Oral
metroprolol tartrate	Lopressor
miconazole nitrate	Monistat-7
minocycline HCl	Minocin
naproxen	Naprosyn
nifodipine	Procardia
nitroglycerin	Nitrobid, Nitrostat
norethindrone	Norinyl
oxazepam	Serax
oxtriphylline	Choledyl
paperine HCl	Pavabid
penicillin V potassium	Pen-Vee-K
penicillin V potassium	V-Cillin K
phentermine hydrochloride	Fastin
phentermine resin	Ionamin
phenylbutazone	Butazoladin Alka

GENERIC	*PROPRIETARY*
phenytoin sodium	Dilantin Sodium
piroxicam	Feldene
polymixin B-bacitracin-neomycin	Neosporin Ophth.
polymyxin B-neomycin-hydrocortisone	Cortisporin Otic
potassium chloride	Slow-K
prazosin HCl	Minipress
prochlorperazine	Compazine
promethazine HCl	Phenergan
propoxyphene HCl	Darvon
propoxyphene napsylate	Darvocet-N-100
propranolol HCl	Inderal
sodium butabarbital	Butisol Sodium
spironolactone	Aldactazide, Aldactone
sulfamethoxazole	Septra DS
sulfisoxazole	Gantrisin systemic
sulindac	Clinoril
teazepam	Restoril
terbutaline sulphate	Brethine
tetracycline	Sumycin
tetracycline HCl	Achromycin-V
theophylline	Elixophyllin
theophylline, anhydrous	Slo-Phyllin Gyrocaps
theophylline (anhydrous)	Theo-Dur
theophylline-guaifenesin	Quibron
thioridazine HCl	Mellaril
thyroglobulin	Proloid
timolol maleate	Timoptic
tolazamide	Tolinase
tolbutamide	Orinase
tolmetin sodium	Tolectin
triamcinolone acetonide	Kenalog Derm
triamterene & hydrochlorothiazide	Dyazide
triazolam	Halcion
trifluoperazine hydrochloride	Stelazine
trimethobenzamide HCl	Tigan
warfarin sodium	Coumadin

Commonly Prescribed Schedule II Drugs

Brand Name	Dosage Form	Generic Name	Manufacturer
Amytal	tablet/elixir/injection	(amobarbital)	Lilly
B & O	suppository	(belladonna and opium)	Webcon
Benzedrine	tablet/Spansule	(amphetamine)	SKF
Biphetamine	capsule	(amphetamine)	Pennwalt
Delcobese	tablet/capsule/time-release capsule	(amphetamine)	Delco
Demerol	tablet/elixir/injection	(meperidine)	Winthrop
Demerol APAP	tablet	(meperidine/acetaminophen)	Breon
Demerol, APC with	tablet	(meperidine/a.p.c.)	Winthrop
Desoxyn	tablet/Gradumet	(methamphetamine)	Abbott
Dexamyl	tablet/Spansule	(dextroamphetamine and amobarbital)	SKF
Dexedrine	tablet/Spansule	(dextroamphetamine)	SKF
Dilaudid	tablet/syrup/injection/suppository	(hydromorphone)	Knoll
Dolophine	tablet/injection	(methadone)	Lilly
Eskatrol	Spansule	(dextroamphetamine/prochlorperazine)	SKF
Hycodan	powder (*not* tablet/syrup)	(hydrocodone)	Endo
Innovar	injection	(fentanyl)	Critikon (McNeil)
Leritene	tablet/injection	(anileridine)	MSD
Levo-Dromoran	tablet/injection	(levorphanol)	Roche
Mepergan	injection	(meperidine/promethazine)	Wyeth
Mepergan Fortis	capsule	(meperidine/promethazine)	Wyeth
Nembutal	capsule/elixir/injection (*not* suppository)	(pentobarbital)	Abbott
Numorphan	injection/suppository	(oxymorphone)	Endo
Obetrol	tablet	(amphetamine)	Obetrol

Section VIII

LIST OF RECOGNIZED MEDICAL AND DENTAL SPECIALTIES

Allergist—A physician who treats diseases caused by sensitivity to substances found in food, water, air, etc.

Anesthesiologist—A physician specializing in the administration of drugs for the relief of pain and discomfort, usually during operative procedures.

Cardiologist—A physician who diagnoses and treats diseases of the heart and blood vessels.

Dermatologist—A physician who diagnoses and treats disease of the skin and integument.

Endocrinologist—A physician, usually a specialist in internal medicine, who manages problems associated with the endocrine (glandular) system.

Endodontist—A dentist who specializes in the diagnosis and treatment of diseases and injuries of the dental pulp and periapecal tissues of the teeth.

Exodontist—A dentist who extracts teeth.

Gastroenterologist—A physician, usually an internist, who treats disease of the stomach, intestine and associated organs.

General Practitioner—A physician who diagnoses and treats general disease of the entire body, usually of all ages.

Geriatrician—A physician who handles medical problems of the elderly.

Gynecologist—A physician specializing in medical and surgical disorders of the female reproductive system.

Industrialist—A physician who specializes in medical problems of industry.

Internist—A physician who specializes in diagnosis and treatment of non-surgical medical diseases.

Neurologist—A physician who diagnoses and treats nonpsychiatric disease of the nervous system.

Obstetrician—A physician who cares for a woman before, during and after childbirth.

Oncologist—A physician who specializes in the diagnosis and treatment of tumors.

Ophthalmologist—A physician who specializes in caring for diseases of the eye.

Oral Surgeon—A dentist who surgically treats natural or traumatic diseases of the mouth and adjacent tissue.

Orthodontist—A dentist trained to treat malformed teeth and oral problems.

Orthopedist—A physician who specializes in disease of the bones, joints, muscles, etc.

Osteopath—One who has been awarded a degree of Doctor of Osteopathy (D.O.). This field encompasses all of medicine with particular emphasis on the manipulation of the skeletal system to treat illness.

Otolaryngologist—A physician specializing in the disorders of the ear, nose and throat.

Pathologist—A physician who specializes in the disorders of diseased tissue or body fluids, usually under laboratory conditions.

Pediatrician—A physician who specializes in the treatment and care of infants, children and adolescents.

Pedodontist—A dentist who specializes in the treatment and prevention of disease of the gums.

Physiatrist—A physician specializing in the rehabilitation of patients following disease, trauma or surgery.

Plastic Surgeon—A physician who specializes in the reconstruction and repair of diseased, damaged or poorly functioning tissue.

Preventive Medicine—A medical specialty practiced by a physician who is mainly interested in preventing diseases and halting their spread.

Proctologist—A physician who treats diseases of the rectum, anus and large intestine.

Psychiatrist—A physician who treats and prevents mental health disorders.

Oncologist—A physician who specializes in the diagnosis and treatment of tumors.

Ophthalmologist—A physician who specializes in caring for diseases of the eye.

Oral Surgeon—A dentist who surgically treats natural or traumatic diseases of the mouth and adjacent tissue.

Orthodontist—A dentist trained to treat malformed teeth and oral problems.

Orthopedist—A physician who specializes in disease of the bones, joints, muscles, etc.

Osteopath—One who has been awarded a degree of Doctor of Osteopathy (D.O.). This field encompasses all of medicine with particular emphasis on the manipulation of the skeletal system to treat illness.

Otolaryngologist—A physician specializing in the disorders of the ear, nose and throat.

Pathologist—A physician who specializes in the disorders of diseased tissue or body fluids, usually under laboratory conditions.

Pediatrician—A physician who specializes in the treatment and care of infants, children and adolescents.

Pedodontist—A dentist who specializes in the treatment and prevention of disease of the gums.

Physiatrist—A physician specializing in the rehabilitation of patients following disease, trauma or surgery.

Plastic Surgeon—A physician who specializes in the reconstruction and repair of diseased, damaged or poorly functioning tissue.

Preventive Medicine—A medical specialty practiced by a physician who is mainly interested in preventing diseases and halting their spread.

Proctologist—A physician who treats diseases of the rectum, anus and large intestine.

Psychiatrist—A physician who treats and prevents mental health disorders.

Radiologist—A physician who specializes in the use of radiation to diagnose and/or treat disease.

Surgeon—A physician who operates to cure or prevent disease.

Urologist—A physician who specializes in the treatment of disease of the urogenital system (bladder, kidneys, penis, etc.).

METRIC—APOTHECARIES' LIQUID MEASURE

Milliliters	*Minims*	*Milliliters*	*Fluidrams*	*Milliliters*	*Fluid ounces*
1	16.231	5	1.35	30	1.01
2	32.5	10	2.71	40	1.35
3	48.7	15	4.06	50	1.69
4	64.9	20	5.4	500	16.91
5	81.1	25	6.76	1000 (1 L.)	33.815
		30	7.1		

METRIC—APOTHECARIES' LIQUID MEASURE

Milliliters	*Minims*	*Milliliters*	*Fluidrams*	*Milliliters*	*Fluid ounces*
1	16.231	5	1.35	30	1.01
2	32.5	10	2.71	40	1.35
3	48.7	15	4.06	50	1.69
4	64.9	20	5.4	500	16.91
5	81.1	25	6.76	1000 (1 L.)	33.815
		30	7.1		

APOTHECARIES - METRIC WEIGHT

Grains	Grams
1/150	0.0004
1/120	0.0005
1/100	0.0006
1/80	0.0008
1/64	0.001
1/50	0.0013
1/40	0.0014
1/30	0.0022
1/25	0.0026
1/16	0.004
1/12	0.005
1/10	0.006
1/9	0.007
1/8	0.008
1/7	0.009
1/6	0.01
1/5	0.013
1/4	0.016
1/3	0.02
1/2	0.032
1	0.065
1½	0.097 (0.1)
2	0.12
3	0.20
4	0.24
5	0.30
6	0.40
7	0.45
8	0.50
9	0.60
10	0.65
15	1.00
20	1.30
30	2.00

METRIC-APOTHECARIES' WEIGHT

Scruples	*Grams*
1	1.296 (1.3)
2	2.592 (2.6)
3	3.888 (3.9)
Drams	
1	3.888
2	7.776
3	11.664
4	15.552
5	19.440
6	23.328
7	27.216
8	31.103
Ounces	
1	31.013
2	62.207
3	93.310
4	124.414
5	155.517
6	186.621
7	217.724
8	248.828
9	279.931
10	311.035
11	342.138
12 (1lb.)	373.242
Milligrams	*Grains*
1	0.015432
2	0.030864
3	0.046296
4	0.061728
5	0.077160
6	0.092592

Obstetrical Table to Determine Date of Confinement

Numbers shown on the top lines in each section represent the first day of the last menstrual period. Those appearing directly below indicate the probable date of the parturition.

Jan.	1	2	3	4	5	6	7	8	9	10	11	12	13	14	15	16	17	18	19	20	21	22	23	24	25	26	27	28	29	30	31	
Oct.	8	9	10	11	12	13	14	15	16	17	18	19	20	21	22	23	24	25	26	27	28	29	30	31	1	2	3	4	5	6	7	Nov.
Feb.	1	2	3	4	5	6	7	8	9	10	11	12	13	14	15	16	17	18	19	20	21	22	23	24	25	26	27	28				
Nov.	8	9	10	11	12	13	14	15	16	17	18	19	20	21	22	23	24	25	26	27	28	29	30	1	2	3	4	5				Dec.
Mar.	1	2	3	4	5	6	7	8	9	10	11	12	13	14	15	16	17	18	19	20	21	22	23	24	25	26	27	28	29	30	31	
Dec.	6	7	8	9	10	11	12	13	14	15	16	17	18	19	20	21	22	23	24	25	26	27	28	29	30	31	1	2	3	4	5	Jan.
April	1	2	3	4	5	6	7	8	9	10	11	12	13	14	15	16	17	18	19	20	21	22	23	24	25	26	27	28	29	30		
Jan.	6	7	8	9	10	11	12	13	14	15	16	17	18	19	20	21	22	23	24	25	26	27	28	29	30	31	1	2	3	4		Feb.
May	1	2	3	4	5	6	7	8	9	10	11	12	13	14	15	16	17	18	19	20	21	22	23	24	25	26	27	28	29	30	31	
Feb.	5	6	7	8	9	10	11	12	13	14	15	16	17	18	19	20	21	22	23	24	25	26	27	28	1	2	3	4	5	6	7	Mar.
June	1	2	3	4	5	6	7	8	9	10	11	12	13	14	15	16	17	18	19	20	21	22	23	24	25	26	27	28	29	30		
Mar.	8	9	10	11	12	13	14	15	16	17	18	19	20	21	22	23	24	25	26	27	28	29	30	30	31	1	2	3	4	5	6	April

July	1	2	3	4	5	6	7	8	9	10	11	12	13	14	15	16	17	18	19	20	21	22	23	24	25	26	27	28	29	30	31	
April	7	8	9	10	11	12	13	14	15	16	17	18	19	20	21	22	23	24	25	26	27	28	29	30	1	2	3	4	5	6	7	May
Aug.	1	2	3	4	5	6	7	8	9	10	11	12	13	14	15	16	17	18	19	20	21	22	23	24	25	26	27	28	29	30	31	
May	8	9	10	11	12	13	14	15	16	17	18	19	20	21	22	23	24	25	26	27	28	29	30	31	1	2	3	4	5	6	7	June
Sept.	1	2	3	4	5	6	7	8	9	10	11	12	13	14	15	16	17	18	19	20	21	22	23	24	25	26	27	28	29	30		
June	8	9	10	11	12	13	14	15	16	17	18	19	20	21	22	23	24	25	26	27	28	29	30	1	2	3	4	5	6	7		July
Oct.	1	2	3	4	5	6	7	8	9	10	11	12	13	14	15	16	17	18	19	20	21	22	23	24	25	26	27	28	29	30	31	
July	8	9	10	11	12	13	14	15	16	17	18	19	20	21	22	23	24	25	26	27	28	29	30	31	1	2	3	4	5	6	7	Aug.
Nov.	1	2	3	4	5	6	7	8	9	10	11	12	13	14	15	16	17	18	19	20	21	22	23	24	25	26	27	28	29	30		
Aug.	8	9	10	11	12	13	14	15	16	17	18	19	20	21	22	23	24	25	26	27	28	29	30	31	1	2	3	4	5	6		Sept.
Dec.	1	2	3	4	5	6	7	8	9	10	11	12	13	14	15	16	17	18	19	20	21	22	23	24	25	26	27	28	29	30	31	
Sept.	7	8	9	10	11	12	13	14	15	16	17	18	19	20	21	22	23	24	25	26	27	28	29	30	1	2	3	4	5	6	7	Oct.

Reprinted from *Medifacts*, page 32, with permission of the Lilly Research Laboratories.

Section X

179 TROUBLESOME MEDICAL WORDS AND HOW TO SPELL THEM

ab′scess
ac″e tab′u lum
ach″a la′si a
al″o pe′ci a
am″y loi do′sis
an″a phy lax′ia
an′eu rysm
ar″rhe no blas to′ma
ath″er o scle ro′sis
ba cil′li form
bac te′ri o phage
bar″bi′tu rate
bleph′a ron
bron″chi ec′ta sis
bron′chi ole
buc′ca
ca chex′i a
cal ca′ne us
cal′lus
ca′lyx
cap″i tel′lum
car′ci no gen
ca′se ous
cau′dad
cha la′zion
cho re′i form
chyle
cir rho′sis
coc′cyx
con″tre coup′
co ry′za
cul-de-sac
cy a no′sis
de cid′u a
de his′cence
di″a pho re′sis
di u re′sis
dys cra′si a
dys″men or rhe′a
dys to′ci a
ec″chy mo′sis
ec′ze ma
em″phy se′ma
en ceph″a li′tis
en″do me″tri o′sis
e piph′y sis
er″y sip′e las
ex san′gui nate
fa′ci es
fen″es tra′tion
fim′bri a
fis′tu la
flat′u lence
fol′li cle
fu′run cle
gan′gli on
gas″tro en″ter i′tis
gas″tro en″ter os′to my
gin′gi vae
glo mer′u lus
glu te′al
gyn″e co mas′ti a
hal′lux
he man″gi o′ma
he″ma tem′e sis
he ma tu′vi a
hem″i an op′si a
he mop′ty sis
her ni or′rhaphy
ho″me os′ta sis
hor de o′lum
hy′dro cele
hy per em′e sis
hys″ter ec′to my
i at″ro gen′ic
id″i o syn′cra sy
il″e i′tis
il′e us
in cip′i ent
in ner va′tion
in sid′i ous
in si′tu

ab′scess
ac″e tab′u lum
ach″a la′si a
al″o pe′ci a
am″y loi do′sis
an″a phy lax′ia
an′eu rysm
ar″rhe no blas to′ma
ath″er o scle ro′sis
ba cil′li form
bac te′ri o phage
bar″bi′tu rate
bleph′a ron
bron″chi ec′ta sis
bron′chi ole
buc′ca
ca chex′i a
cal ca′ne us
cal′lus
ca′lyx
cap″i tel′lum
car′ci no gen
ca′se ous
cau′dad
cha la′zion
cho re′i form
chyle
cir rho′sis
coc′cyx
con″tre coup′
co ry′za
cul-de-sac
cy a no′sis
de cid′u a
de his′cence
di″a pho re′sis
di u re′sis
dys cra′si a
dys″men or rhe′a
dys to′ci a
ec″chy mo′sis
ec′ze ma
em″phy se′ma
en ceph″a li′tis
en″do me″tri o′sis
e piph′y sis
er″y sip′e las
ex san′gui nate
fa′ci es
fen″es tra′tion
fim′bri a
fis′tu la
flat′u lence
fol′li cle
fu′run cle
gan′gli on
gas″tro en″ter i′tis
gas″tro en″ter os′to my
gin′gi vae
glo mer′u lus
glu te′al
gyn″e co mas′ti a
hal′lux
he man″gi o′ma
he″ma tem′e sis
he ma tu′vi a
hem″i an op′si a
he mop′ty sis
her ni or′rhaphy
ho″me os′ta sis
hor de o′lum
hy′dro cele
hy per em′e sis
hys″ter ec′to my
i at″ro gen′ic
id″i o syn′cra sy
il″e i′tis
il′e us
in cip′i ent
in ner va′tion
in sid′i ous
in si′tu

in″tus sus cep′tion
is che′mi a
is′chi um
jaun′dice
je ju′num
ker nic′ter us
ke″to gen′e sis
ke″to nu′ri a
ky pho′sis
la′bile
lab″y rin thi′tis
lam″i nec′to my
lar′ynx
leu″ko pe′ni a
lin′gual
li thi′a sis
lym phad″e ni′tis
lym phad″e nop′a thy
mal le′o lus
mas″toid ec′to my
me a′tus
me″di as ti′num
meg″a kar′y o cyte
me nin′ge al
me nin″go en ceph″a li′tis
men″or rha′gi a
me″tror rha′gi a
my″as the′ni a
nar cis′sism
ne phri′tis
neph″ro li thi′a sis
neph″ro scle ro′sis
neu ri′tis
nys tag′mus
ol″i ge′mia
ol″i gu′ri a
om phal′ic
o″o pho rec′to my
oph″thal mol′o gist
or″chi ec′to my
os″te o my″e li′tis
pach″y men″in gi′tis
pal′pe bra
pan″cre a ti′tis
pa pil″le de′ma
par″a cen te′sis
par″a ple′gi a
par″o nych′i a
per″i or″te ri′tis
per″i stal′sis
pe te′chi a
phe″o chro″mo cy to′ma
phle bi′tis
pit″y ri′a sis
pneu″mo en ceph″a log′ra phy
pneu″mo tho′rax
pol″y cy the′mi a
pop″li te′al
pres″by o′pi a
proc″i den′ti a
pro″te in u′ri a
pseu″do cy e′sis
pto′sis
pu″er pe′ri um
py″e lo ne phri′tis
quad″ri ple′gi a
ra chi′tic
ra″di o paque′
re″cru des′cence
re sus″ci ta′tion
rheu′ma tism
rhi ni′tis
ron″geur′
scir′rhous
scle′ro sis
se″ro san guin′e ous
si″al ad″e ni′tis
sphe′noid
spon″dy li′tis
ster″e og no′sis
stra bis′mus
syn′cope

syn o′vi a
tach″y car′di a
tel an″gi ec′ta sis
tho″ra cen te′sis
throm bo phle bi′tis
tin ni′tus
ty′pa num
ur″ti ca′ri a
u′vu la
var′i co cele″
ver ru′ca
xan″tho chro′mi a
xiph′oid
zy′go ma